ENDURING QUESTIONS
IN GERONTOLOGY

Debra Sheets, PhD, RN, is assistant professor in the Department of Health Sciences and Coordinator of the Interdisciplinary Gerontology Program at California State University–Northridge. Her research interests include aging and disability, intergenerational service learning, and aging, health, and disability policy. She is a fellow of the Gerontological Society of America and the Association for Gerontology in Higher Education.

Dana Burr Bradley, PhD, is the director of the Center for Gerontology and the Cliff Todd Distinguished Professor of Gerontology at Western Kentucky University. Her research interests include cohort effects in volunteerism, history of retirement policy, and intergenerational service learning. She is a fellow of the Gerontological Society of America and the Association of Gerontology in Higher Education.

Jon (Joe) Hendricks, PhD, is dean of the University Honors College, Oregon State University. He served as president of the Association for Gerontology in Higher Education (AGHE), as chair of the sections on Sociology of Aging and Life Course, American Sociological Association, and Behavioral and Social Sciences, Gerontological Society of America. He received the 2004 AGHE Clark Tibbitts Award, the 1994 Distinguished Career Contribution Award, and the 1998 Kalish Innovative Publication Award from the Gerontological Society of America. Dr. Hendricks has authored numerous articles, chapters, and books and edits the *Society and Aging* series. He is also the coeditor-in-chief of *Hallym International Journal of Aging*.

Enduring Questions in Gerontology

edited by

DEBRA J. SHEETS, PhD, RN

DANA BURR BRADLEY, PhD

JON HENDRICKS, PhD

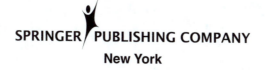

SPRINGER PUBLISHING COMPANY

New York

Springer Publishing Company, Inc.
11 West 42nd Street, 15th Floor
New York, NY 10036-8002

Acquisition Editor: Helvi Gold
Production Editor: Print Matters, Inc.
Cover Design: Mimi Flow
Composition: Compset, Inc.

Library of Congress Cataloging-in-Publication Data

Enduring questions and in gerontology / Debra J. Sheets, Dana Burr
   Bradley, Jon Hendricks [editors].
      p. cm.
   Includes bibliographical references and index.
   ISBN 0-8261-6415-3
      1. Gerontology. I. Sheets, Debra J. II. Bradley, Dana Burr. III. Hendricks, Jon, 1943-
   HQ1061.E543 2005
   305.26—dc22

                                                                      2005054063

06 07 08 09 10 5 4 3 2 1

Printed in the United States by Bang Printing

Dedication

With gratitude to those dear to our hearts who enrich our lives with love, joy and steadfast support:

> *Bill Tomlinson*
> *Krist, Saralinda and Daniel*
> *Hazel Reeves*

Contents

About the Contributors

W. Andrew Achenbaum, PhD, teaches history and social work at the University of Houston, where he heads the Gerson David Consortium for Vital Aging. He has written broadly on the history of aging, the history of gerontology, and the evolution of age-related policies, as well as spirituality and aging. A past chair of the board of the National Council on the Aging, he is the author most recently of *Life's Uncertain Voyage*, an overview of societal aging.

Steven N. Austad, PhD, is professor of cellular and structural biology and affiliated with the Barshop Center for Longevity and Aging Studies at the University of Texas. His research focuses on the biology of aging in humans, mammals, and birds. In 2003, he received the Robert W. Kleemeier Award, given annually for outstanding research by the Gerontological Society of America. Dr. Austad has written widely on the social, political, and ethical obstacles to human life extension.

James E. Birren, PhD, DSc, is the associate director of the UCLA Center on Aging and professor emeritus of gerontology and psychology at the University of Southern California. Dr. Birren has published extensively and is series editor of the internationally recognized *Handbooks on Aging*. He has more than 250 publications in academic journals and books. Dr. Birren's awards include the Brookdale Foundation Award for Gerontological Research, the Gerontological Society of America Award for Meritorious Research, the 1989 Sandoz Prize for Gerontological Research, and the 1990 Award for Outstanding Contribution to Gerontology by the Canadian Association of Gerontology.

Kenneth Brummel-Smith, MD, is professor of geriatrics and founding chair of the Department of Geriatrics at Florida State University College of Medicine. He is a past president of the American Geriatric Society. He is board certified in family medicine and has a certificate of added qualifications in geriatrics. He is a fellow of the American Geriatric Society. Dr. Brummel-Smith has published four geriatric medicine textbooks and hundreds of articles and chapters on geriatric medicine, dementia, and rehabilitation.

Alissa Dark-Freudeman, MS, is a graduate student in developmental psychology at the University of Florida. Her research focuses on the development of possible selves across the adult life span. She recently published "Memory and Goal Setting: The Response of Older and Younger Adults to Positive and Objective Feedback" (coauthored with R. L. West and D. K. Bagwell) in *Psychology and Aging.*

Manfred Diehl, PhD. is associate professor in developmental psychology at the University of Florida. His research focuses on the development of self and personality across the adult life span, as well as everyday problem solving, competence, and functional health in late life. His recent publications include "Self-Concept Differentiation across the Adult Life Span" (coauthored with C. T. Hastings and J. M. Stanton), published in *Psychology and Aging,* and "Agency and Communion Attributes in Adults' Spontaneous Self-Representations" (coauthored with S. Owen and L. Youngblade), published in the *International Journal of Behavioral Development.*

Christine L. Fry, PhD, is professor of anthropology, emerita at Loyola University of Chicago. She has written extensively on culture and aging, cultural aspects of the life course, the meaning of a good old age, and the meaning of age. She is co-author of *The Aging Experience* (Sage Publications): *Diversity and Commonality across Cultures* and winner of the Kalish Award from the Gerontological Society of America, 1995. She was also a codirector of Project AGE, a major cross-cultural study of aging in seven communities around the world. She currently lives and writes in Bisbee, Arizona.

Martha Holstein, PhD, teaches bioethics at DePaul University and ethics for human service providers at the Spertus Institute for Jewish Studies. Her research interests include ethics, policy, and community-based long-term care. Her most recent coedited book (with P. Mitzer), *Ethics in Community-based Elder Care* (Springer Publishing Company), is a theoretical and practical guide for practitioners. Dr. Holstein serves as an ethics consultant to the Office of the Inspector General, Illinois Department of Child and Family Services, and to the Selfhelp Home (Chicago) and is a nationally recognized trainer and expert on ethics.

Phoebe S. Liebig, PhD, is associate professor of gerontology and public administration at the Andrus Gerontology Center, University of Southern California. Her research interests include supportive housing policies, federalism, aging and disability, and aging in India. She is a fellow of the Gerontological Society of America and the Association for Gerontology in Higher Education and the recipient of the 2003 Clark Tibbits award from AGHE. Liebig has numerous publications, and her most recent book is *An Aging India* (2003).

George L. Maddox, PhD, is professor emeritus of medical sociology at Duke University. He joined Duke in 1959 as an investigator in the Longitudinal Studies of Normal Aging, later becoming director. He has served as president of the Gerontological Society of America and received the society's Kleemeier Award for Research. A founding director of the National Council of the National Institutes of Health, he was editor-in-chief of the first three editions of *The Encyclopedia of Aging* and currently edits *Contemporary Gerontology.*

Chris Phillipson, PhD, is professor of applied social studies and social gerontology at Keele University, where he is a pro vice-chancellor for the university. He is president of the British Society of Gerontology. His research interests include problems relating to poverty and social exclusion in old age, the impact of urban change on older people, and developing social theory in gerontology. Recent publications include *Social Theory, Social Policy and Old Age* (Open University Press, 2003, coauthored) and *Social Networks and Social Exclusion* (Ashgate, 2004, coedited).

Mark Waymack, PhD, is codirector of Graduate Programs in Health Care Ethics in the Department of Philosophy, Loyola University–Chicago. He has been interested and active in the area of health care ethics since 1987, and has a particular interest in questions concerning ethics and aging.

Preface

During the past half century the abiding questions in gerontology have become even more compelling as contexts changed in the light of breakthroughs and emerging knowledge. Pressing issues are unlikely to go away; instead, they will continue to influence the emerging policy formulations, research agenda, and practice priorities. To illuminate the shadows and to cast attention on what is coming from just over the horizon, we invited some of the most creative thinkers currently contributing to the gerontological literature to reflect on their disciplines, to consider how key questions have emerged, how they have changed in the decades since gerontology entered the fray, and what may lie ahead. The resulting collection of essays provides a comprehensive perspective on the enduring questions in gerontology and how they have shaped our understanding of differences in the experience of old age.

Clearly, no single disciplinary approach has an exclusive claim on insight, nor can any particular point of view chart a course for the next few decades without being cognizant of advances in related disciplines and areas of research. The authors represented here consider which questions within each discipline comprising the field of gerontology will persist and elucidate the ways in which disciplinary approaches advance the field over time. As new initiatives are undertaken, new vistas have opened, raising more questions and prompting innovative approaches and solutions that reflect the disciplinary lens brought to the task at hand. By suggesting ways in which a discipline has influenced other disciplines, or benefited from the influence of other foci, the authors show how, in tandem, progress emerges when boundaries are pushed between what we know and what remains elusive. Lessons are both imported and exported, and progress in one area often leverages progress in another, creating the momentum that propels science and scholarship ahead. By juxtaposing broad disciplinary perspectives through the lenses of a cadre of innovative and forward-thinking gerontologists, *Enduring Questions* prepares readers to sift the details as well as to make their own contributions to the knowledge base necessary to affect the lives of the elderly. The impact of the contributions is to move beyond a "history of ideas" to incorporate events and developments unfolding outside the realm of narrowly focused scholarly research. An overarching framework was sought by asking authors to address cross-cutting themes that included technology, global aging, and the influence of changing contexts and to provide the basis for readers to stand higher and see farther in their own efforts to provide meaningful contributions.

Scholars new to the field will be particularly interested to see how leaders in the field arrived at their current suppositions and where they are likely to go next. Emerging and seasoned scholars alike should find insight in the ways in which each disciplinary focus grapples with societal transitions, identifies emerging issues, and lays out strategies and salient perspectives for what should come next. None of the contributors represented in this volume will consider their efforts a success if they do not prompt others to step forward and offer a change for the better.

Debra J. Sheets
Dana Burr Bradley
Jon Hendricks

PROLOGUE

Finding New Beacons

Searching for Timeless and Interdisciplinary Perspectives

George L. Maddox

My four decades in the young discipline of gerontology have been characterized by continual exposure to changing perspectives and some questions that seem to endure. Changing perspectives in scientific inquiry are natural and expected. Enduring questions result from our discovery, sooner or later, that not all the questions worth answering have neat, definitive answers. My gerontology career began with a chance encounter with Ewald "Bud" Busse in 1959. Dr. Busse, recently arrived at Duke Medical Center as chair of the Department of Psychiatry, had convinced the university administration that an all-university, multidisciplinary center for the study of aging was a good idea. The National Institutes of Health funded five such university centers. The Duke Longitudinal Studies of Aging was just under way at the new center, with psychologist Carl Eisdorfer as research director. A sociologist was needed. I had recently arrived at Duke Medical Center as a Russell Sage Foundation postdoctoral fellow with the mandate to study how medical students are trained. Because my earlier research was on adolescent development, the idea of inquiring about the life at the other edge of adulthood seemed reasonable, even interesting. I decided to take a look at gerontology. This was an early invitation to broaden my perspective on life course development.

   The research of a large group of multidisciplinary scholars proved to be intellectually stimulating, and the weekly Monday night meeting of investigators was an extraordinary exposure to the evolving theoretical perspectives and paradigms of medicine, psychiatry, psychology, and sociology as well as

1

specialists in research methodology and computer technology. A firm rule was that current research involving the longitudinal studies being prepared for publication had to be presented to all the other investigators for critique. Any myopic disciplinary perspective was assured of a challenge and discussion of alternative perspectives. Most research on aging had focused on older adults in hospitals or served by social welfare agencies; the inevitable outcome was that the dominant images of older adults was primarily negative, portraying them as sick, poor, and depressed.

In contrast, the Duke studies focused on the majority of adults who live most of their lives in a community. In part, because all the principal investigators were a self-taught cohort of gerontologists, the intellectual atmosphere at Duke emphasized changing perspectives rather than enduring questions. Over the next 4 decades, I became research director of the Duke Longitudinal Studies and eventually director of the Duke Aging Center. The exhilaration of the developments and the changing perspectives on human aging only intensified. In retrospect, four broad generalizations about aging derived initially from the Duke Studies of Aging and tested subsequently against other evidence are prominent in my thinking. These generalizations were summarized in my Kleemeier Research Award Lecture, *Aging Differently* (Maddox, 1987). These generalizations leave a wide latitude for incorporating new evidence and changing perspectives, but they appear to be central to the prospect of understanding aging and aging well.

FOUR USEFUL GENERALIZATIONS

Evidence from the Duke Longitudinal Studies of Normal Aging carried out between 1955 and 1980 (Busse & Maddox, 1987) suggested the changing perspectives of human aging summarized briefly here. Evidence from a wide range of other sources has helped my evolving understanding of their implications.

Differentiation and Variety

The focus of the Duke studies on community-dwelling older adults and on sampling with attention to gender, ethnicity, and social status recognized the importance of place and social location in understanding later life. Place calls attention to variations in living accommodation, neighborhood, community, and culture. Social location calls attention to cultural preferences regarding allocation of essential social resources (e.g., education, income, status) to individuals based on gender, ethnicity, and presumed merit. In the extreme case, medical demographers have noted the extraordinary differences in life expectancy at birth that distinguish less and more developed societies. The most common explanations of these observed differences are the availability of clean water and a stable food supply, and more recently the availability of health care. Confirmation of these explanations lies in the observed improvement in life expectancy in less developed societies when life-supporting conditions change. Research has broadened our perspective on why social status and educational exposure were found to be important variables in understanding differences in the experience of aging among community-dwelling older adults.

The effects of social location (e.g., education, occupation, income, status) in differentiating individuals within a society are dramatic but often quite subtle. In the United States, for example, the relationship between social status and health observed among individuals of all ages is one of the most consistently documented conclusions in epidemiology and medical sociology. Gender and ethnicity add dimensions to understanding this relationship. Sociologists who have documented the consequences of a lifetime of growing up poor and uneducated describe them as "cumulative disadvantage." Being Black as well as poor is insightfully viewed as double jeopardy. Being female in a culture historically characterized as male dominated can constitute double jeopardy. My own longitudinal research illustrates that when one controls for educational attainment and income, the observed differences in functional status and perceived health status between men and women and between Whites and Blacks tend to diminish. The persistent differentiation of older adults has some obvious practical implications for research and public policy. Sampling procedures must ensure that subpopulations are adequately represented and, if necessary, oversampled. Political and policy analysts are challenged to abandon the notion of "the elderly" who vote alike and have the same needs and preferences for social services.

Continuities

Societies typically promote some sense of orderly development that differentiates childhood, adolescence, adulthood, and old age. Our society's organization of the educational system fine-tunes such distinctions and adds suggestions of the preferred time for completing one's education, getting a job, marrying, and retiring. Considerable flexibility about age expectations persist, and recently age markers for development have become attenuated; however, our society is a long way from accepting the irrelevance of age.

The notion of continuities over the life course, that the past is inevitably prologue, is likely to get our attention when epidemiologists discuss risk factors as predictors of disease and disability. Risk factors are typically events and behaviors earlier in life that predict unwanted outcomes later in life. For decades now health advocates, magazines, and public health announcements have documented why, in the interest of health and well-being, we should eat right, exercise, avoid smoking and using noxious drugs, get adequate sleep, and learn to manage stress. These are more than good advice that mothers give their children. They are advice based on evidence about the predictors of health and illness. They are risk factors. They are the epidemiological analog of cumulative disadvantage.

Longitudinal research in aging regularly provides other confirmation of continuities. In longitudinal research, take any observation of a variable at time 1 and compare it with the same variable at time 2. The time 1 value is likely to be the best available predictor of that variable at time 2. More broadly, in a conversation with my colleagues of many years at Duke, economist Juanita Kreps noted that observed differences in adaptation to retirement were predictable from observed adaptations to work. Individuals who flourish at work tend to adapt well in retirement. Also, as clinicians observe about intergenerational relationships in families, 50-year-olds who exhibit hostility toward their aging parents are typically continuing tensions developed over a family lifetime. One cannot rule out the possible resilience of individuals and the capacity for change and resilience, as will be noted below. But continuity, not change, is the rule, in human development.

In passing, I note the importance of observed continuities over the life course that provide a compelling reason why gerontologists are often attracted to a life course perspective and why they understand and support advocacy for the resources necessary for development of children. Avoiding the cumulative deprivation initiated in childhood, or, restated positively, promoting the cumulative advantage of education, meaningful work, adequate income, and healthy lifestyles, has a demonstrable effect on the experience of later life.

Modifiability

At the turn of this century, Americans preferred a very optimistic view of the almost unlimited good that science and technology could offer individuals and society. Biomedicine promised major advances in health care and functional health, the extension of life expectancy, and even a longer life span. Science promised a better old age. This optimistic view of the modifiability of the biological life course is among the most significant changes in gerontology during my career. But this optimism has limits and a downside. The biogerontology of the last quarter of a century tended initially to be reductionistic.

Biology too easily became destiny. The focus was on what our biology made necessary rather than what it made possible. The importance of contextual factors that are the consequential ingredients of cumulative deprivation and advantage tended to be undervalued or, worse, ignored. I remember vividly a conversation on one occasion with Nathan Shock, a great scientist and one of the grand old men of American gerontology. As a physiologist, he documented evidence of declining function in the human biological system that was expressed as regression lines. These lines were often parodied as those damnable negative regression lines that show that, in the long run, we are all dead. Being especially aware of human variation, I called to his attention that his regression lines did not recognize variance. His response was simply, "Yes, regression lines should be reported."

Recognition of variance is important because one might inquire about an explanation of variance and follow with an inquiry about whether the poorer functional performances might be improved. Even more optimistically, one might ask not only about the change in performance at any point along the regression line but also, more audaciously, about the modifiability of the slope of the regression line. Others were also thinking about the modifiability of aging processes and, more broadly, about changes in the quality of later life.

In its early decades, the Duke Center for Aging hosted a lecture series that brought to our university a broad range of scholars and scientists exploring the course and experience of aging. Andrew Wallace, a cardiologist, was one of the young scientists invited as a lecturer. He began his presentation by pointing out that middle-aged men in the United States at that time had the worst record of cardiovascular disease and death in the world. He believed that this problem could be modified significantly by lifestyle change, particularly changes in diet and exercise. Andrew Wallace acted on his hypothesis and health promotion and disease clinical demonstrations proved he was right. Managing one's lifestyle is now a regular component of management, particularly for chronic conditions. His early observation now is taken for granted, and, significantly, the cardiovascular health of middle-aged men has improved.

But there is more. James Fries fired the shot heard round the world of gerontology in a paper he published in the *New England Journal of Medicine* that argued the onset of morbidity and related disability can be, in fact were being, delayed in the American population. The result was what he called a "compression of morbidity," so that older adults would experience more disability-free years of life. Some scoffed initially at his optimistic forecast. But increasingly evidence supports his optimism about improved functioning, though argument persists on whether reducing disability lies in individuals or in technological or environmental supports.

Although arguments persist about the extent of improvement in average functional status, there is no question that the economic and health status quality of life and well-being of older Americans has improved in recent decades, though certainly not as much as possible or desirable. The explanation lies in a broad range of social interventions. Social Security is one obvious explanation, accounting for the reduction of the poverty rate among older adults. Medicare and Medicaid have increased access of older adults to health care. Housing and home ownership have grown. Legislation for Americans with disabilities of all ages has improved access to public places. The dramatic increase in social resources available to older adults in the past half-century has enhanced the capacity for resilience in later life. The experience of resilience, in turn, potentially forecasts the development of a sense of self-efficacy in responding to subsequent life challenges.

There is no need to pit the contributions of gerobiology and geriatrics against social gerontology. Both have important contributions to make, and the challenge of the future is to ensure that gerontologists of all persuasions see the advantages of multidisciplinarity in improving the quality of life for older adults. Periodic focus on antiaging medicine and the prospect of grand extensions of life span, as well as average life expectancy, have seduced some but not most gerontologists, who continue to emphasize the enhancement of quality years of life within currently expectable life expectancy. This more moderate objective is clearly a multidisciplinary, not just a biomedical, task.

We do not know the limits of modifiability of the human life span or enhancement of quality years of life. The mood of contemporary gerontology, however, is to explore the limits. The eminent scientist Niels Bohr described the current mood: "If you want to understand something, try to change it." However, boundless optimism about unlimited improvement in the quality of life at the upper levels of longevity is not yet warranted. Paul Baltes and Jacqui Smith, in a paper prepared for a recent Second World Assembly on Aging (2003), used data from the Berlin Studies of Aging to argue that sizable losses in cognitive and subjective potential plus increased prevalence of dementia occur in "the Fourth Age" (those 90 year of age and older). The particular importance of contextual factors in modifying aging outcomes will be noted below.

Context

Historians are among the first to remind us that place, time, and culture are variables that matter in understanding the variability of the human life course and aging. Gerontological research has not been the same since Warner Schaie in the 1960s spoke persuasively about the importance of considering age, period, and cohort (APC) as key factors in understanding human development. (For a brief overview of the problems as well as the promise posed by APC analysis, see Maddox & Campbell, 1985.) Longitudinal research and cohort-sequential sampling are now recognized as the demanding essentials of life course research. Never mind that age and period are difficult to sort out. Never mind that historical factors implicit in period effects are complex and difficult to summarize as variables. We will never understand age as a factor in life course development without attention to the time of birth that places individuals in historically different and changing sociocultural contexts. Furthermore, to describe the outcomes for different cohorts is not possible with the longitudinal experiences of different cohorts.

I still remember my initial discomfort in imagining how any investigator could specify the complex variables implicit in a historical "period" and hope to trace the stochastic process that would evolve in the lives of the exposed individuals. The sorting out did seem to be a multidisciplinary task. On this point I remember a conversation with Paul Baltes, specifically at the Gerontological Society of America meeting in Puerto Rico in 1972. He presented a paper in which he referred to the relevance of social context. My observation was that the measurement of social context as a variable was poorly developed, and I asked what psychology was doing to address that. Baltes quipped, "I thought the measurement of social context is the responsibility of sociologists."

The longitudinal measurement of environmental, and particularly social, contextual effects still leaves a great deal to be desired. This is especially the case in social survey research using large probability samples. In the interest of generalizability and large samples, survey research has typically given up, in part from practical reasons, explicit measurement of contexts. One might add that such research has typically substituted a synthetic, composite view of individuals. Perhaps these are the more practical reasons for recognizing the value of what we euphemistically call qualitative research capable of focusing explicitly on identified selves and their perceived and actual contexts. In any case, work remains to be done on realizing the potential of APC analysis.

The importance of context has also been increasingly reinforced in biological research that at times in the recent past has been reductionistic in its interpretation of human as well as animal development. Caleb Finch, for example, early in his career as a gerobiologist, became so convinced that the environment in which experimental animals are housed affects their behavior and outcomes in experiments, that he promoted a mandatory declaration to accompany published research articles specifying the contextual factors of animal maintenance and handling. Finch (2005) discusses in a recent paper how developmental variations in experimental animals, despite identical genomes, arise and influence individual outcomes in aging. There is not, he argues, recognition that life spans of genetically similar animals are hugely plastic. He suggests that, contrary to former assumptions, there is no clear intrinsic life span maximum in a species that cannot be modified environmentally. He concludes that the future triumphs of genetics of the human lifespan will come through research documenting multigenerational environmental effects on the outcomes in aging. Such analysis will involve the collaboration of geneticists, demographers, and epidemiologists.

EXPLORING THE SIGNIFICANCE OF CHANGING PERSPECTIVES AND ENDURING QUESTIONS

The essays in this volume consistently document the changing perspectives observed in the recent history of gerontology. My brief overview has identified four major foci in the field—differentiation and variation, continuities, modifiability, and context. Each focus illustrates a currently enduring topic whose underlying theory and evidence continue to evolve and scholars continue to debate. The questions we continue to raise in each topical area are not expected to yield a final answer. The process of variation and differentiation will remain even as the basis and outcomes of these processes change. The balance of continuities and resilient change in human development will vary among and within populations by historical circumstance. Understanding the limits of aging and aging well remains to be established. The changing sociocultural contexts of societies with different values, expectations, and distributions of resources will continue to make a difference in aging and the experience of aging.

For some, I expect, the search for enduring rather than merely persistently unresolved questions in gerontology is of a different order. An enduring question would be one that has no definitive answer, at least not an answer that scientific inquiry might resolve. Among gerontologists, those who think of themselves as critical gerontologists correctly point out that societies construct socially binding and limiting characterizations of the life course and persons as they age. Scientists can and do superimpose their own characterizations of persons in whom they are interested and, in the case of late life, can describe older adults largely as composites of medical problems, not as people with problems. What would be a more tolerable, if not ultimately preferable, social construction of later life can and will be debated from various value perspectives. No harm in that. But this exercise has the quality of being enduring with little prospect of ultimate resolution, although one can imagine in the culture-building process that social groups will develop consensual definitions of aging well and justify distribution of social resources to implement a society that ages well according to a shared definition. Every society tends to arrive at some degree of consensus about what later life is, might be, or ought to be. Nothing unusual about that. The difficulty is likely to arrive when the prevailing consensus has no mechanism to critique the merit of evolving perspectives. Traditions of scholarship and science do tend to have at their center a commitment to challenging received wisdom. These traditions were a vital part of my early education and continue to guide my current thinking about later life.

EPOCHS, SYSTEMS, AND SCIENTIFIC REVOLUTIONS

I was an undergraduate philosophy major who received large doses of the Greek classics with an emphasis on epistemology, logic, and ethics. Less attention was given then to contemporary American philosophy. Although there was interest in the enduring questions Who am I?, What is justice?, and What is truth?, these questions had answers, not an answer. One book very distinctly remembered from undergraduate days about the apparent inevitable evolution of our thought and values is Suzanne Langer's *Philosophy in a New Key* (1942). Every historical epoch is characterized by its own questions, the generation of ideas that rise and decline, and notions of the limitations of our ideas. So it is that the quest for knowledge, not the certainty of our ideas, that forms the heart of inquiry. Finding a truth that endures is a leap of faith.

In my transition into a graduate student, I quite incidentally encountered a biologist turned general system theorist, Ludwig von Bertalanffy. His *Problems of Life* (1952) and later his *General System Theory* (1968) laid out the rationale for a theory of interaction between organism and context that had multiple alternative outcomes. Many of these possible options had an "equipotential of outcomes." The multiple potential, he argued, was grounded in the differential resources in various contexts and an organism's/person's differential initiative (for organization's differential leadership). Hence a variety of organismic/organizational responses can work in the same setting. Leadership and initiative are key factors in the choices made and implemented. This seemed to me a compelling reason in human development to consider the possible viability, if not preferability, of alternative responses and to expect to observe sustainable variety in aging processes.

Another seminal work was Thomas Kuhn's *The Structure of Scientific Revolutions* (1962). Here was a plausible rationale for challenging received wisdom and recognizing the vested intellectual interest in transmitting received wisdom in scholarship and science. All the alternative options for achieving well-being in later life lead one to anticipate changing perspectives and understandings of later life. Changing perspectives would be a normal and expected condition in science, and perhaps to a lesser degree in scholarship generally. So expecting consensual final answers to enduring questions would seem improbable.

MULTIDISCIPLINARITY

With a few exceptions, the essays in this volume refer to and illustrate the significance of multidisciplinary exposure in gerontological training for research and scholarship. But there is not much evidence of interdisciplinary action or how interdisciplinary training occurs or should occur. As I noted in my account of my career at the Duke Aging Center in the early days, exposure to and working with colleagues in a variety of disciplines were usual and expected. Even there, multidisciplinary exposure only occasionally led to conversations about, or actually pursuing, the potential for integrating disciplinary theory and thought styles of various disciplines. Such integration is intellectually challenging, but something more than that is involved.

A recent article in *Science* (Rhoten & Parker, 2004) reviewed evidence indicating that in programs around the nation designed to promote interdisciplinary research on complex issues in science, more than exposure to interdisciplinary opportunities is required. The younger scientists being studied perceived interdisciplinary research to be risky for their careers and foresaw negative effects on their careers. Realistically, gerontology in the near term may have to live with "interdisciplinary exposure" rather than interdisciplinary research training, in spite of the research challenges that appear to require multidisciplinary cooperation at a minimum.

One of the most obvious opportunities for multidisciplinary collaboration is posed by Warner Schaie's seminal conception of age, period, and cohort (APC) analysis in longitudinal research on aging. Creative attack on APC analysis requires investigators with theoretical and research skills from human development, psychology, sociology, history, demography, epidemiology, and the methodology of research design and analysis. Although the stimulus for interdisciplinary research in gerontology is not absent, it has certainly not been a feature of the field. Read the chapters in this book with this challenge in mind. Where does a more integrative interdisciplinary perspective potentially have useful applications? How might understanding of the unsolved, hence enduring, questions be advanced if not resolved?

REFERENCES

Baltes, P., & Smith, J. (2003). New frontiers in the future of aging: From successful aging of the young old to the dilemmas of the fourth age. *Journals of Gerontology, 49,* 123–135.

Bertalanffy, Ludwig von. (1952). *Problems of life.* London: Watts.

Bertalanffy, Ludwig von. (1968). *General system theory.* New York: Braziller.

Busse, E. W., & Maddox, G. L. (1987). *The Duke longitudinal studies of normal aging, 1955–1980.* New York: Springer.

Finch, C. (2005). Dialogues in biogerontology between molecular reduction and ecological integration. *Contemporary Gerontology, 11*(3) in press.

Fries, J. F. (1980). Aging, natural death and the compression of morbidity. *New England Journal of Medicine, 303,* 130–135.

Kuhn, T. (1962). *The structure of scientific revolutions.* Chicago: University of Chicago Press.

Langer, S. K. (1942). *Philosophy in a new key.* Cambridge, MA: Harvard University Press.

Maddox, G. L. (1987). Aging differently. *The Gerontologist, 27*(5), 557–564.

Maddox, G. L., & Campbell R. T. (1985). Scope, concepts and methods in the study of aging. In R. Binstock & E. Shanas (Eds.), *Handbook of aging and the social sciences* (2nd ed., pp. 3–31). New York: Van Nostrand Reinhold.

Rhoten, D., & Parker, A. (2004). Risks and rewards of an interdisciplinary research path. *Science, 306,* 2046.

CHAPTER 1

Identifying Enduring Questions in Gerontology

Jon Hendricks, Debra Sheets, and Dana Burr Bradley

IDENTIFYING KNOWLEDGE AND MAKING SENSE

As knowledge of aging has expanded over the past half-century, pioneering questions were posed, new perspectives emerged, and innovative method-ologies came to the fore. With each advance in our knowledge, new horizons have come into view, raising further questions and promoting groundbreak-ing approaches and solutions. Nevertheless, ongoing issues continue to in-form gerontological research and theorizing even as new issues emerge. To make sense of the way gerontology advances, it is important to be aware of the "enduring" questions within disciplines comprising the field and to ap-preciate the ways in which these disciplinary approaches change as advances occur and interdisciplinary propagation takes root. The intent of this vol-ume, *Enduring Questions and Changing Perspectives in Gerontology*, is to speak to exactly these issues as a means of pointing the way toward tomorrow's gerontology.

As George Maddox so convincingly acknowledges in the Prologue, the complexity of aging requires interdisciplinary approaches necessitating ger-ontologists to remain current in their knowledge of neighboring disciplines. By suggesting ways in which a discipline has influenced other disciplines or benefited from the influence of other foci, the authors in this volume show how, in tandem, progress emerges when boundaries are pushed between what we know and what remains ambiguous. The perspicacious and vision-ary gerontologists in this volume bring broad perspective to address ongoing questions, cross-cutting influences, and likely developments just visible on the horizon. The authors elucidate which parameters are stable and which change in the context of emergent concerns and contextual transformation. As James Birren contends in the epilogue, and the other contributors make clear, the diverse nature of aging issues has resulted in a greater need to integrate knowledge from each disciplinary focus. Collectively, the authors identify emerging issues and provide a context for current foci within the field of aging that will prepare readers to make their own contributions to the knowledge base necessary to make a difference.

What are the enduring questions of gerontology? As noted above, and by Maddox in the Prologue, to a certain extent these questions reflect disciplinary viewpoints. To further our knowledge of gerontology, we turn to received wisdom, established methodologies, and familiar procedures. Our scholarly traditions determine the routes taken, establish the boundaries for exploration, and validate what counts as discovery. It is small wonder that some questions recur as the mere practice of a way of doing things provides corroboration of the logic of a particular way of knowing and facilitates the creation of communities of knowledge (Turner, 1994). The philosopher-mathematician Alfred North Whitehead was prescient as he pointed out that knowledge is a matter of perspective, of points of view, and any chosen vantage point will obscure alternative itineraries. As we explore the further reaches of what is known, certain nagging questions remain unresolved, and we often simply elect to move on. As Lewis-Williams (2001) pithily points out, "We do not have to explain everything in order to explain something." Jigsaw puzzles can be assembled in a reasonable way, even if some of the pieces are missing.

To acquire knowledge, we must also be able to discern whether or not something is that same question, regardless of appearances. When, in light of new information, does a question ask a different question even while appearing the same? For example, when Newtonian physics was shunted aside in favor of the Einsteinian framework, were physicists asking the same questions about velocity? Einstein's answer is different and is figured differently, so is it the same question with a different answer, or has the definition of velocity in the new context changed meaning and morphed into a different question that only appears the same? In gerontology, questions that appear the same may have different answers because of the changing meanings and contexts in which they are asked. As the authors illustrate, consider how definitions of who is old are influenced by politics. Similarly, our notions of what is normal with age have changed as we separate out aging per se from age-related conditions. As a result, dementia is now recognized as a disease, and so the possibilities for a solution have changed.

As gerontologists, our training necessarily involves an implicit bridge to disciplinary traditions and ways of knowing. Accordingly, when progress occurs, it is not surprising that it does so in fits and starts; subject to strictures imposed by professional knowledge communities (Hendricks, 1995; Katz, 1996). Coming under the sway of an influential éminence grise, as W. Andrew Achenbaum phrases it in chapter 8, molds the next generation of scholars whose undertakings reflect the intellectual nimbus of luminaries in their field. Achenbaum artfully highlights a dozen themes near and dear to the heart of gerontologists that have been sifted through by successive generations of gerontologists and that serve as the polestar for charting the course of scholarly agendas for a significant portion of the gerontological community. Despite the inspiration and guidance thus provided, the remaining to-do list is daunting indeed.

GERONTOLOGY: ENDURING QUESTIONS

The task at hand requires moving past relativism and realizing that enduring questions are those that occur on a more general level and that are universally applicable. Enduring questions involve concerns that are invariant over time, places, and worlds. However, they are not questions that are, in fact, a focus of all cultures, but rather those questions about aging that should be the focus of all cultures. For this we will need a general sense of what is fundamentally the same, even though details and definitions may differ. Complicating things further is the self-referential nature of our field in which knowledge is adopted and influences the phenomenon (i.e., aging) being investigated. Therefore, as we have learned about the importance of context, or in the case of human beings, lifestyle, in relation to aging, that information has influenced behaviors among older adults in ways that affect later research. Of course, as soon as we think we have a handle on universally applicable principles of aging processes, someone discovers that everyday life choices are more important than even genetics in explaining what happens later in life (Rowe & Kahn, 1998).

What are the enduring questions in gerontology across cultures or across time? We propose that among the disciplines comprising gerontology there is a shared common focus on the processes of change over time and in context. For example, in biology an enduring question is "What is the nature of senescence?" In psychology a lasting issue is "How do developmental processes affect the mind?" Some might argue that the most fundamental enduring question in gerontology is "What is the nature of aging?" Steven Austad in chapter 2, Maddox, and others might add "How do contexts influence basic aging processes?" But these questions do not seem to capture the entirety of what gerontology is concerned about. To a significant extent, gerontology focuses on pragmatic concerns associated with the processes of aging (Bengtson & Schaie, 1999). In this latter sense, Chris Phillipson in chapter 5 notes that gerontology is an applied science, and the focus and scope of scholarship selected for inclusion here reflect sectors that include human services professions and administrative and policy sciences. At the same time, gerontology is bifurcated between those who see it as a life science and those who see it as a cultural science. Gerontology is concerned with how to do things, how to change things, and it has a profound interest in knowing what should be changed when grappling with the process of aging.

To illustrate this pragmatic concern, we propose that a key enduring question in social gerontology is "How should we treat people by virtue of their age to maximize the quality of their life?" By "treat," we mean not only physical behaviors but also how we should think about people by virtue of their age. Maddox reiterates a familiar point as he notes that every society arrives at reasonable consensus about the nature of later life. Christine Fry in chapter 6 adds emphasis to Maddox's point as she ponders how utile ideological perspectives contour the configuration of aging, implying that age is even more of a relativizing cultural construct than a chronological categorization. Achenbaum addresses this issue when he notes that an abiding concern in historical gerontology has focused on understanding how civic-minded people constructed the conclusions they did and how the service industry has developed the way it has to address the needs of an aging society. In other words, neither science nor practice arises ex nihilo; each reflects implicit normative judgments. Although the issue of how to treat the old is not the main focus of contemporary gerontology, it may just be a matter of emphasis at this time.

Whereas gerontology purports to be about the processes of aging, in fact, the field has largely focused on the problems of the aged by framing issues as a dichotomy between the elderly and nonelderly. As Phoebe Liebig makes clear, this paradigm has fueled much of the policy sciences research agenda, leading to a pragmatic narrowing of the question to "How should the nonelderly treat the elderly?" We suggest that concerns reflected in the questions "How should the elderly treat themselves?" and "How should the elderly treat the nonelderly?" are also fundamental in gerontology, though they presently receive little emphasis.

As successive cohorts experience longer life expectancies, the nature of the issues surrounding the aging of the population has itself changed. It is one thing to hold a positive attitude about a phenomenon that is relatively rare, but quite another thing to hold those same values when it becomes an everyday fact of life. Until the 20th century, only a small percentage of any birth cohort survived to reach what we might consider an advanced age. As Austad avers, it has become commonplace for most people to reach an advanced age, and the most rapid growth is occurring among those age 85 and older. Simultaneously, the pace of societal change foreshadowed other changes, smaller families, geographic mobility, the advent of industrialization and its displacement by technological production, and ultimately the proliferation of broad-based service industries. The spread of technology and the changing economy have both shifted and expanded boundaries, resulting in the general trend toward globalization. Meanwhile, medical breakthroughs and biotechnologies hold the portent of equally dramatic changes; but what has been made even more probable is increasingly described as a drain on national resources, and the specter of rationing and shifting of responsibilities is very much in the air. In the epilogue Birren refers to the "agequake" that has taken place and comments on the increasing impersonality and economic criteria used to determine the good and the worthwhile. How does a gerontologist go about trying to decide on an appropriate course of action or research agenda, formulate policy recommendations, or determine what would be fair and appropriate? No easy questions are these, and, as will be seen, no easy answers, either.

SEARCHING FOR ANSWERS INSIDE AND OUT

One obvious and necessary circumstance of old people is that for each day they live and grow older, they are one day further from birth and one day closer to death. Indeed, mortality can be graphed as an exponential equation in what has been termed a Gompertz plot. In modern societies the science has become ever more exact, and actuaries are able to predict mortality rates under a multitude of conditions with remarkable accuracy. Even so, explaining biological causes of aging is not self-evident. Proximate and ultimate explanations are routinely offered, but as Austad makes clear, evolutionary theories of aging have generated scant consensus. Scientists who delve into how organisms age point to a variety of cellular processes, including replication limits, mutation, free radical accumulation, and so on, to more systemic but still proximate circumstances revolving around immunological, neuroendocrine, and reproductive change, but they do not offer particularly satisfactory explanations (Phelan, 2001). Even evolutionary theory provides partial understanding because deleterious effects as far as longevity are concerned would have to occur prior to the cessation of reproduction. If they occurred earlier, it would lead to the demise of the species, and advantageous late-onset mutations cannot be transmitted across generations. Evolutional biologists continue to grapple with the ultimate causes of aging but have recognized the causes may not operate independently of one another and may not operate in the same fashion for different individuals. Then, too, as Austad points out, the presence of extrinsic risks and hazards exerts yet another effect, serving to compound explanation even further.

In the evolutionary scheme of reproduction, menopause is a relatively recent phenomenon. There is no obvious point for iteroparous species, such as our own, to expend energy on somatic repairs necessary for prolonging longevity in the postreproduction period; there simply is no phylogenetic reason for doing so. Those in the know are quick to admit that even in terms of fundamental ontogenetic processes, any number of questions persist despite the remarkable breakthroughs of the past 2 decades. As will be seen, Austad is struck by the way antiaging goods and services have attracted as much hucksterism as effective intercession. Even so, the priorities of aging research are being affected by trends in antiaging medicine. As the bright light of scientific inquiry is shone on the prospect of life extension, a new set of questions has surely come to the fore.

If all other things were equal, perhaps biologists and geneticists might explain aging, but the fact is that few things are equal. Austad's contribution highlights how differential hazards and risks serve as crucial intervening factors, and it certainly can be claimed that what is true for animals is no less true for humans; it is just that the nature of the hazards is different. Indeed, as Austad points out, environmental hazards and lifestyle risks are crucial intervening factors, and a well-informed interdisciplinary approach in our field is essential in the development of knowledge. Maddox makes much the same point as he notes that a systems model demands that all inputs be taken into consideration. Interestingly, in the groundbreaking MacArthur Study on Successful Aging, Rowe and Kahn (1998), found that aging patterns are neither predetermined nor inflexible; heredity and genetic background matter less than do personal lifestyle practices and socioenvironmental contexts that increase risk for disease and disability. All societies, no matter their state of development, can expect to confront the issue of age-related chronic illness. This and other problems will be permanent and worsen over time, and we would expect this difference for the elderly, as a social class, to be universal and to occur across cultures. In chapter 3, Kenneth Brummel-Smith is unequivocal: The costs of medical care, new technologies, and the desire of the baby boom generation for holistic health care are on a collision course that will only deepen the divisions between the haves and the have-nots. One group will be better positioned to grapple with off-setting environmental factors, whether natural or social, whereas the other group experiences the full force of those factors in the ways they experience aging.

One telling facet of the above is the chasm between social class categories. Along with shaping retirement experiences or the pacing and structure of the life course, social class gives rise to diverse outcomes, ranging from ability to buffer stress to health outcomes. Included among the social causes of disease identified by epidemiologists is the power to control commonplace challenges of daily life, stress, personal relationships, diet, and health-risk behaviors (Hayward, Crimmins, Miles, & Yang, 2000; Link & Phelan, 1995). Once again the implications are that there is an indelible connection between environmental circumstances and fundamental experiences that accrue with age.

It is likely that the impact of age-related disease and disability will be lessened by scientific discoveries and geriatric cures, but it is highly probable that social class cleavages will deepen. For instance, Alzheimer's disease and related dementias may at some point in the future be mitigated for a significant portion of the population. However, there will likely always be age-related illnesses and disabling conditions that show up in differential patterns among that same population due to disparities in access to effective mitigation. Thus we expect gerontology will forever be concerned with those issues, and the relative impact of created or organizational risks will remain.

Brummel-Smith draws attention to recent organizational changes within the health care system, and in hospitals specifically, which are ostensibly designed to ensure appropriate care for geriatric patients. The goal of these changes is to provide cost-effective care at recoverable rates by shifting medical attention away from the most costly providers to parallel professionals who can service the needs of the patient base less expensively through a four-step system of care. Not surprisingly, there is considerable controversy surrounding these steps, ranging from the American College of Physicians Internal Medicine group, to the American Academy of Family Physicians, and by consumers themselves who are concerned about quality issues.

The costs of health care are likely to fuel continuing controversies about resource allocation and efficacy of care in the years ahead. The development of new drugs that are genetically targeted is costly, and absent adequate assurances, pharmaceutical companies are not likely to undertake the costly process necessary to bring products to market. Medical technology is increasingly expensive and is already being rationed on the basis of effective treatment, resumption of economic contributions, and costs for intervention. Consider anticholinesterase inhibitors. Even if they are shown to reduce Alzheimer's symptoms, the question of their cost effectiveness is prominent on the national policy agenda. Brummel-Smith raises a compelling question as he points out that despite its efficacy in treating rheumatoid arthritis, in 2005 Etanercept cost $2,000 a week and was not covered by Medicare. One way or another health care rationing looms large on the horizon, and as Liebig reminds us, the question remains how the policy systems will effectively deal with the trend.

BEYOND THE MIND OF NEANDERTHALS

Among the enigmas of human evolution is one that receives attention from a very narrow segment of the scholarly community: How people think about themselves and how that view has changed over time. Whether the focus is on the evolution of the species or the evolution of individual consciousness, there are more questions than answers. Lewis-Williams (2001) is representative of those who offer a convincing case that the way we humans think about ourselves is no more static than anything else in our histories. Aries (1962) wrote convincingly that conceptions of childhood revealed a dramatic shift with the advent of industrialization and what might be considered the modern age, but that is hardly where it all started. Whether we look to Altamira or any of the caves near and dear to UNESCO and anthropologists, part of their significance is that they reveal a marked shift in how the artisans conceived of themselves, their fellow cave dwellers, other animals, even their relative place in the world. The polychromatic images and engravings suggest a step change in the evolution of consciousness, and the creation of meaning from what had gone before and the way we think of ourselves today is different still. According to Lewis-Williams (2001), the Upper Paleolithic evidence suggests synthetic linkages between self-conscious mental processes, social activities, and context. Modern-day psychologists have rediscovered this same relationship; they use a comparable model in their analysis of the life course, consciousness, subjectivity, and the creation of meaning. They certainly emphasize ongoing interactions between circumstances, worldview, the accretion of experience, and the self-conscious traveler.

Whether discussing intelligence, cognitive change, psychomotor performance, memory, the development of meaning, self-consciousness, or personality, psychology has moved from a straight-forward mimicking of biologically based models of growth, development, and decline to one in which what was once regarded as noise has turned out to be the signal. The scientific community has come to realize we humans do not live life one variable at a time. Over the past several decades a new paradigm emerged, one emphasizing in-terpersonal and milieu synergies that once were seen as perturbations but in fact result in disparate, discrete patterns of aging. In chapter 4, Manfred Diehl and Alissa Dark-Freudeman maintain that most psychological processes turn out to be highly differentiated, yet reveal marked continuity, and go on evolving over the life course in a harmonic that resonates with situational factors.

When older adults experience decrements that affect performance, what constitutes a sufficient difference that might be construed as a disability? A significant change in reaction times or intellect compared to the nonelderly (as a class) could be addressed by adjusting standard, or by adapting an environment to accommodate a functional deficit. When are such age decrements realistically significant in their impact on ability? Psychological gerontologists are also left with thorny questions about whether such claims should be established in the laboratory or by real-world operations.

Interestingly, Diehl and Dark-Freudeman also underscore a kind of bio-social interconnection not unrelated to what Austad and others are trying to thrash out that affects psychological functioning. Depending on a combination of available resources filtered through contextual circumstances, person-environmental transactions, and cohort memberships, psychological functioning appears to be distinctly altered. Perhaps it is the seemingly limitless adaptability of the human condition that gives rise to enduring questions, and it is not a matter of whether change or influence occurs, but of establishing parameters of flexibility.

DEVELOPING CRITICAL AWARENESS

Across policy context, culture, and historical time is a similar enduring question in gerontology: "What are our obligations to those who have worked and now need help?" This question is really about larger issues that shape our obligations towards others. One way to examine this question is to ask, "How should the nonelderly treat the elderly?" The answer to this question occurs at a level just below the most general, because on the most general level we should treat everyone the same. One obvious answer is, "We should treat them as they deserve to be treated or as we would want to be treated when it is our turn." How might the circumstances or situations that the elderly find themselves in, or the differences in their nature in light of being elderly, require us to treat them differently? Is it possible that whatever characteristics are imputed to the elderly are given meaning by the ways societies are organized and by virtue of values espoused? People do not age without reference to the situations in which they have lived, nor do they grow old in isolation.

Culture and Social Justice

Notions of what is appropriate, acceptable, and in keeping with societal ideas of distributive justice are themselves subject to change and evolution. Both historical and now global reconfigurations are commonplace. As will be seen, Fry asks what has become of culture as a macro-level construct in gerontological analysis as both perspectives and methodologies have zoomed in on individuals as micro-level units of analysis. She points out that the most immediate application of culture is in the creation of age grading, accompanying age-appropriate prescriptions or social hierarchies, a contention she illustrates with her ethnographic sketch of aging among the Nacirema. The ramifications are obviously more momentous than as a fairly straightforward social organizing scheme. As Fry points out, they have fueled considerable research both here and abroad but fewer answers. By means of her "gentle fiction," Fry explores how the general concept of aging has been useful in shaping the meaning of age, its interaction with gender, social class, and the shape of the life course.

Though ideas about what is due the elderly pass under a variety of labels, they all fall within the larger rubric of culture. Ethical considerations are part of the picture, and determination of ethical standards is no more static than anything else in life. With the pace of biomedical technology running full tilt, the implications of prolongation of life for our societal obligations immediately become subject to calculations of cost–benefit analyses in determining the value of individual lives and whether the prospect should be extended to all citizens or a select subset (Moody & Kapp, 2001).

Embedded Ageism

One aspect of how we construct old age is found in negative stereotypes and prejudicial behavior toward old people. These ageist tendencies cannot be dismissed as simply the purview of uninformed individuals or those who have developed an age bias. Ageism is more than actions or attitudes of individuals; it is a propensity woven into the very fabric of our morality that is then internalized by individual actors. Gerontology has always had to work to dispel such mythology, and it may always have to do so. Accordingly, another of the enduring questions of gerontology is discovering the embedded ways of thinking about aging that need to be challenged if the elderly (and eventually each of us) are to achieve a better quality of life. If these preconceptions about aging are key barriers to a good old age, they merit concerted scrutiny.

Indeed, it might be argued that gerontologists have an obligation to change culture so that the elderly are perceived more positively. No one deserves to feel attenuated, useless, or unattractive, and feeling so is hardly conducive to subjective comfort or a good life. There are important quality of life reasons that extend all the way to health and sense of well-being to want to change this situation. Yet there are those who say that ageist predilections occur in the world of work, family life, access to one or another opportunity, and the distribution of social resources. Ageism exists in the social institutions and taken-for-granted assumptions that are the stuff of contemporary attitudes about aging. If the promulgation of instrumental reasoning, cost–benefit analysis, and bottom-line mindsets continues to carry the day, the relationship between ageism and the experience of old age will remain an important concern for gerontologists for the foreseeable future.

Meaning of Old Age

Those who are retired or are simply old and have need for help and assistance are likely to wonder about the meaning of life, at least the meaning of their life. This is consistent with the view that the meaning of one's life is determined by one's roles in society, obligations toward others, and ways of connecting to others. It seems likely that in every society, as we age our roles change, and a corresponding reevaluation of the meaning of our lives would be natural. Consequently, questions concerning the meaning of one's life are likely to endure. Yet, as Martha Holstein and Mark Waymack suggest in chapter 7, many people do not think about questions of meaning when their life is going well and they are preoccupied with myriad mundane tasks. It is more a question that concerns those with more time to think because the demands and pace of earning a living have lessened. It is then that thoughts often shift to "needing more" and searching for purpose or greater reason to live. So we would expect that gerontology might respond to concerns about meaning in old age by finding ways to help enrich the life of the elderly.

Holstein and Waymack raise a number of pointed questions about the applied ethical implications of gerontology as it is being plied. As they note so compellingly in their discussion of normative questions within the discipline, the way questions are asked frame the solutions proffered. They also say that the underlying and often implicit value orientations in those questions create biases of one kind or another. As they point out, assertions of autonomy and self-determination result in an implicit prejudicial attitude about those incapable of either. For example, the underlying voluntaristic model of in-terpersonal relationships results in gender, racial, and social class biases that label those not able to exercise their wills to the extent stipulated as some form of less successful being. As will become apparent, they urge caution and critical awareness before drawing conclusions about the marketplace of misfortune that has grown up around the issues of aging and other people's progress (Titmuss, 1968; Townsend, 1981).

PUBLIC POLICY: QUESTIONS OR ANSWERS

What are the persistent differences in situation between the elderly and non-elderly that might occur in modern societies and raise concerns? One possibility is situations that the elderly are more likely to hold or possess as a class, simply because of old age. Another possibility has to do with qualities that the elderly possess necessarily by virtue of being old. What are those situations that make the elderly generally different from the nonelderly?

To a great extent, policy rulings operate in a fashion akin to an invisible hand arraying assets, opportunities, entitlements, and responsibilities. In many respects, public policies establish parameters of meaning for age-based definitions more than any other single aspect of life. From definitions of dependency, to entitlement and eligibility, age-based and age-related policies generate what Fraser (1997) refers to as a "deep grammar" definitive of not only legal rights, standing, and the apportionment of opportunities, but the very notion of personhood. Once implemented, the parameters for participation in one or another publicly mandated provision assume a taken-for-granted status with social relations correspondingly ordered. No period of life is free of the penumbra of pronouncements of the polity, but the old and the young are seemingly more subject than other age categories. The canons of public policy are central to orchestrating movement across the life course, status passages, and entry to and exit from successive social statuses (Estes, 2001; Mayer & Muller, 1986). Given this context, gerontologists must necessarily address the issue of societal organization, prescriptions, or proscriptions as they relate to framing the meaning of old age. Policy decrees shape customary ways of looking at the world, standing as powerful social constructions delimiting one situation from another, frequently classified in terms of problems or needs. As both Liebig and Phillipson assert in their chapters, the dominance of public policy concerns about aging cannot be overestimated whether considering the United States, Europe, Great Britain, or any other country. Liebig acknowledges the impact of policy in her recounting of both the history of policy pronouncements and the specific public provisions on the lives of those they touch. As there is no gainsaying that policies pigeonhole people through the structures and order they create in our worlds, it may be that one of the enduring questions facing gerontologists is the degree to which public policy shapes the way we perceive old age.

Within the policy arena, especially in discussions of Social Security and other retirement sinecures, not to mention in ethical arenas, a familiar question is What do we owe individuals in later life for their work contributions to the larger society when they were younger? The answer likely varies from culture to culture. As Liebig makes clear, for much of the past century it seemed as though we had a sense of obligation to care for those who have worked hard and who need help in later life. These values were so strongly endorsed that the Social Security program was deemed the "third rail" of American politics; touching it would lead to untoward outcomes for anyone who tried. However, fundamental disagreements about the role of government in individuals' lives has led to forceful evaluations of the efficacy of the program.

THE WORLD AT THE DOORSTEP

Is the world becoming smaller, or are there cross-cutting international currents affecting aging? It used to be that policies were formulated in terms of proximate circumstances and in light of local forces. That is no longer the case; in fact, globalization is affecting economic, social, cultural, and familial realms in ways that reach well beyond the borders of nation-states. As Phillipson observes, the landscape of gerontology now includes economic and market considerations operating half a world away. What has been called the "globalization of capital" means markets are no longer local, and neither is production or determination of benefits. The world is now the forum in which production takes place; inordinate labor costs, retirement benefits, or health insurance demands in one locale mean production is likely to be relocated someplace else, and multinational corporations have the wherewithal to look hither and yon for the most advantageous arrangements.

Throughout most of the 20th century, there was a great deal of certainty about what was coming in the years ahead. In contrast, one of the hallmarks of the early years of the 21st century has been a future rife with uncertainty, as even the contours of working life cannot be forecast with any great clarity. A number of pundits are convinced that globalization will profoundly alter how age unfolds, reaching in to effect so fundamental a phenomenon as our perception of what is fair and appropriate (Estes & Phillipson, 2002; Hendricks, 2006). Despite its resolution being years away, if ever, it is a question sure to provoke persistent discussion.

WHAT DOES IT ALL MEAN?

If one were to ponder the most pressing issues facing gerontology, identifying key enduring questions would be listed among the top priorities, but they might not be the only priorities. Although a focus on a specific area or issue in gerontology may prevent it from being general enough to count as an enduring question, that does not mean that it is not important to answer it so that people can have better lives. So let us not assume that enduring questions are the only important questions.

As the contributors to this volume make clear, an enduring question is not a question so ambiguous as to be understood differently at different times, but a question general enough to always be of concern. Consequently, generality is a necessary condition for an enduring question in any science or scholarly endeavor. The question How should we treat the elderly? is not context specific, so when local conditions are added to the equation, fresh answers may emerge. How the elderly should be treated in 2005 will require a different focus than answering how they were treated in 1955 or might be treated in 2055. The general question is the same, but concern for what might be likely problems for the elderly in 2055 will be quite different if not stated in general terms. One could use the precedents to begin to formulate an answer, or one might muse about the significance of one or another trial balloon on what the future answers might be, but the context of the present will be different from the context of the future. In an era in which trial balloons literally dot the horizon, an important question to ponder is the extent to which they began to pinion possibilities for the future.

The chapters also make clear that because a question is deemphasized at some points in time and regarded as more compelling at other times does not count against it as being an enduring question. For example, Einstein regarded the quest for a unified field theory to be compelling, yet such concerns were not appreciated at the time or for quite a time thereafter. Recently, the concern has morphed into what is now being called finding the "theory of everything," which is seen as a necessary step for significant progress in the field. In the Prologue Maddox allowed as how gerontology has a number of cross-cutting themes and dilemmas, some of which might be considered primary, associated with the process of aging itself. Others might be called secondary, growing out of context, environmental, or policy impositions; still others might be classified as tertiary, arising out of unique circumstances not related to broadly based patterns. The enduring questions of gerontology require an examination of the characteristics or situations on each level, as some will likely always be associated with aging (barring completed science and perfect societies). Such issues may go across cultures, across species, across times, and across worlds; others are surely local and perhaps even individual. As we close in upon resolutions, we may have to think in general concepts to get an important universality to the question. This approach will identify what gerontology will need to know as long as something needs to be known about aging. These will be the enduring and eternal questions facing practitioners and researchers alike.

Clearly, no single disciplinary approach has an exclusive claim on insight, nor can any particular point of view chart a course for the next few decades without being cognizant of breakthroughs in sister disciplines and areas of research. Few of us are able to benefit from discourse at an interdisciplinary "Monday night meeting" of the ilk that Maddox describes. But in its stead, we offer the chapters of this volume. Taken as a whole, they provide an overview and identify a number of cross-cutting themes that, when viewed from a single disciplinary focus, may lose some of their salience when viewed across the constitutive elements of gerontology. One thing becomes abundantly apparent: Malleability and flexibility are watchwords of aging without the limits yet being clearly identified. As should be apparent, lessons are both imported and exported, and as progress in one area often leverages progress in another, science and scholarship move ahead. We may have overlooked some obvious or not so obvious processes that accompany aging, but as we discover new processes associated with aging, we will have "new" enduring questions, which may seem like a contradiction—an interesting problem, but one for consideration at another time perhaps.

REFERENCES

Aries, P. (1962). *Centuries of childhood: A social history of family life.* Trans. R. Baldick. New York: Alfred Knopf.

Bengtson, V. L., & Schaie, K. W. (1999). *Handbook of theories of aging.* New York: Springer.

Estes, C. L. (2001). *Social policy and aging.* Thousand Oaks, CA: Sage.

Estes, C. L., & Phillipson, C. (2002). The globalization of capital, the welfare state and old age policy. *International Journal of Heath Services, 32,* 279–297.

Fraser, N. (1997). The force of law: Metaphysical or political? In N. J. Holland (Ed.), *Feminist interpretations of Jacques Derrida* (pp. 157–163). University Park: The Pennsylvania State University Press.

Hayward, M. D., Crimmins, E. M., Miles, T. P., & Yang, Y. (2000). The significance of socioeconomic status in explaining the racial gap in chronic health conditions. *American Sociological Review, 65,* 910–930.

Hendricks, J. (2006). Moral economy: Cross cultural dialogue about values and ageing. In M. Johnson (Ed), *Cambridge handbook of age and ageing.* Cambridge: Cambridge University Press.

Hendricks, J. (1995). The social power of professional knowledge in aging. *Generations, 19,* 51–53.

Katz, S. (1996). *Disciplining old age: The formation of gerontological knowledge.* Charlottesville: University Press of Virginia.

Lewis-Williams, D. (2001). *The mind in the cave: Consciousness and the origins of art.* New York: Thames & Hudson.

Link, B., & Phelan, J. (1995). Social conditions as fundamental causes of disease. *Journal of Health and Social Behavior* (Suppl.), 80–94.

Mayer, K., & Muller, W. (1986). The state and the structure of the life course. In A. Sorensen, F. Weinert, & L. Sherrod (Eds.), *Human development and the life course: Multidisciplinary perspectives* (pp. 217–246). Hillsdale, NJ: Lawrence Erlbaum.

Moody, H. R., & Kapp, M. B. (2001). Ethics. In G. L. Maddox (Ed.), *The encyclopedia of aging* (3rd ed., pp. 352–355(1). New York: Springer.

Phelan, J. P. (2001). Evolutionary theory. In G. L. Maddox (Ed.), *The encyclopedia of aging* (3rd ed., pp.365–367). New York: Springer.

Rowe, J., & Kahn, R. (1998). *Successful aging.* New York: Pantheon Books.

Titmuss, R. M. (1968). *Commitment to welfare.* London: George Allen & Unwin.

Townsend, P. (1981). The structured dependency of the elderly: A creation of social policy in the twentieth century. *Ageing and Society, 1,* 5–28.

Turner, S. (1994). *The social theory of practices: Tradition, tacit knowledge, and presuppositions.* Chicago: University of Chicago Press.

CHAPTER 2

A Biologist's Perspective

Whence Come We, Where Are We, Whither Go We?

Steven N. Austad

At the beginning of the 20th century, life expectancy in the United States was about 48 years (47 for men, 49 for women) (Faber, 1982). Biologist Raymond Pearl, an early demographer and gerontologist, wrote semiseriously in the 1930s that there probably should be an upper age limit of 50 years or so on voting rights, because after that people became too foolish to be entrusted with such a vital social responsibility. One hundred years later—by the year 2000—much had changed. In particular, life expectancy had increased by nearly 30 years (Fig. 3.1). In Japan, the longest-lived country in the world, women in the year 2000 lived on average more than 84 years (U.S. Census Bureau, 2004). Now no one talked, seriously or otherwise, about 50 as an age of incipient senility. As a *New Yorker* cartoon aptly put it, "Good news, honey—70 is the new 50."

This dramatic increase in life expectancy was not simply the continuation of a long-term trend. It was unprecedented. Data from modern hunter-gatherers, as well as analysis of ancient skeletal remains, agreed that life expectancy for most of human history was likely around 20 years (Gage, 1988; Lovejoy et al., 1977). Therefore, there seems to have been as much increase in life expectancy during the last 100 years as since the dawn of civilization, when the development of agriculture first allowed humans to clump and cluster into villages and towns, freeing them from the daily hunting-gathering grind and allowing some to become inventors or engineers, artists, entrepreneurs, or biologists (Diamond, 1997). Even just prior to the

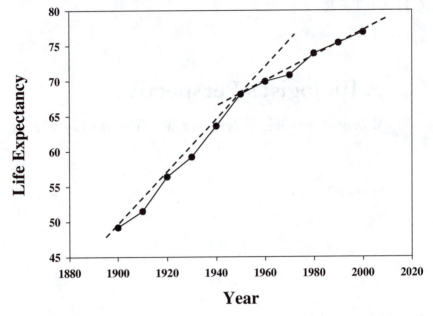

FIGURE 3.1 Changes in life expectancy in the United States over the course of the 20th century. The dotted lines emphasize that the rate of increase since 1950 was somewhat slower than in the first half of the century. (Data from Faber, 1982; U.S. Census Bureau, 2004.).

beginning of the 20th century changes were slower. The last three decades of the 19th century found British life expectancy increasing by 4 years, but during the next 3 decades life expectancy increased at 4 times that rate (Fogel & Costa, 1997).

Of course, life expectancy—the average age at death for all individuals—is a crude summary measure of how long people actually live. Deaths, particularly in high-mortality populations, do not follow a bell-shaped distribution where an average falls in the middle and therefore represents the most common case. No, in such populations, deaths are typically distributed in two clear peaks, one in infancy, the other in old age (see, for instance, Fig. 3.2). Such an enormous number of very early deaths has a huge impact on the overall average, that is, life expectancy. Consequently, just because life expectancy was only 20 years in Paleolithic times does not mean that 30-year-olds in those times had the physical capabilities of today's 80- or 90-year-olds. Those 30-year-olds that had been lucky enough to survive childhood and adolescence were physically probably pretty much like 30-year-olds today. There is no evidence, in other words, that the fundamental biology of human aging has changed during historical

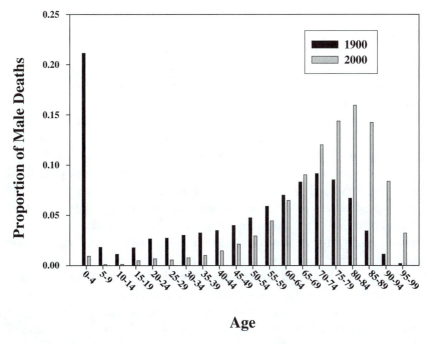

FIGURE 3.2 Distribution of male ages at death in the United States in 1900 compared with 100 years later.

time. That 20-year life expectancy meant that many more people, particularly young people, died compared with today from causes that had nothing to do with aging. Life was inherently more dangerous at all ages. Violence, famine, drought, and particularly pestilence have been much more significant hazards throughout history compared with the past century. As an illustrative example, the 17th-century English diarist Samuel Pepys lived to be 70 years old, and a number of his friends, including Isaac Newton (84 years), Robert Hooke (68 years), and the architect Christopher Wren (90 years), lived about as long or longer at a time when life expectancy was only about 30 years. However, three of Pepys's 10 siblings died before their first birthday, three more were gone before the age of 10, and his sister Mary succumbed at 13. Infectious diseases commonly carried off even those such as Pepys's brother John (age 36) and wife, Elizabeth (age 29) in their prime years (Tomalin, 2003). As late as 1900, the 5-year period of life during which most deaths occurred was between birth and 5 years (Fig. 3.2).

Although the ghastly infant mortality rate throughout most of human history inflates recent changes in life expectancy, there has also been a dramatic reduction in death rate at later ages over the past century (Figs. 3.3, 3.4). Life expectancy even at age 50 increased by more than 7 years during the 20th century. The most common age at death among adults was 72 years in 1900 compared with 81 years at the turn of the next century (Faber, 1982; University of California, Berkeley & Max Planck Institute for Demographic Research, 2004).

To what can we attribute this unparalleled lengthening of life? In all likelihood, what we think of today as modern medicine—high-tech clinical tests and procedures—played a relatively minor role. I say this because the biggest mortality rate changes (20- to 40-fold) during the 20th century occurred during the childhood years (Fig. 3.3), and decreases in mortality later in life become progressively smaller. If high-tech medicine played a significant role, it would probably be most obvious among the elderly. Thus the changes were probably mostly due to some combination of improved nutrition, increasing attention to public health measures, such as the provision of clean water and uncontaminated food, and the widespread availability of childhood vaccinations. For instance, smallpox was at one time a common, and commonly fatal, childhood disease. Although the smallpox vaccination had been available in the United States since about 1800, its use did not become widespread until

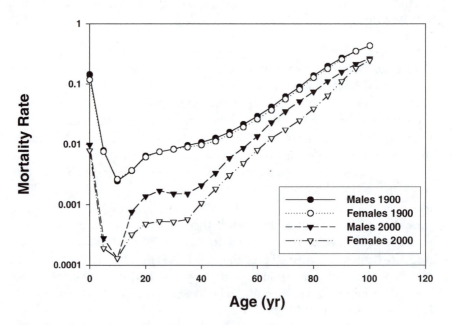

FIGURE 3.3 Age-specific mortality, the probability of dying at a given age, in the United States in the year 1900 compared with 2000.

the early 20th century, after the U.S. Supreme Court in *Jacobson v. Massachusetts* (1905) upheld a Massachusetts law making vaccination of all residents compulsory. As a consequence, the reported number of smallpox cases in the United States dropped from more than 100,000 in 1921 to between 5,000 and 15,000 by the 1930s to one in 1949, the last year any cases were reported ·(Bazin, 2000). In the 1940s and 1950s many additional childhood vaccinations were developed, and their large-scale administration became routine.

Another evident 20th-century trend was a dramatic decline in women's death rates during the childbearing years, again largely due to better hygiene surrounding birthing procedures. In the United States, maternal mortality fell from about 5,000 deaths per 100,000 live births in the late 1800s, to 670 deaths in 1930, to about seven deaths today—more than a 700-fold decrease over the course of less than 2 centuries (De Costa, 2002; Hayden, 1970; "Maternal mortality," 1998). For less obvious reasons, men's lives also grew substantially less dangerous in the young adult years over the past century, with death rates declining 4- to 5-fold. After age 50, in both sexes, there was a smaller but still very substantial change in death rate (Fig. 3.4). One

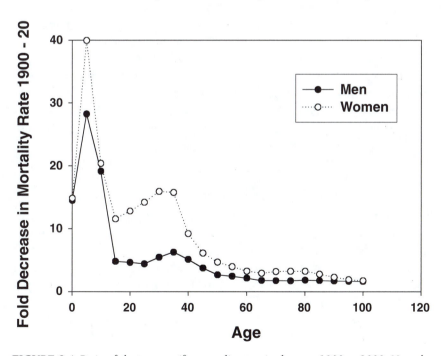

FIGURE 3.4 Ratio of the age-specific mortality rate in the year 1900 to 2000. Note the largest changes are in the infant and childhood death rates. There was also a dramatic change in female death rates during the childbearing years.

possible reason for this could be that the reduction in childhood infections in midcentury meant fewer long-term sequelae due to chronic inflammation (Finch & Crimmins, 2004).

Dramatically declining death rates are only part of the success story, however. Health of the elderly, at least as measured by a decline in chronic morbidity and disability, also improved rapidly (Fogel & Costa, 1997; Manton & Gu, 2001). For instance, a comparison of Civil War veterans who were 65 or older in 1910 and World War II veterans who were similar in age during 1985–1988 revealed that heart disease among old soldiers was about 3 times as prevalent, musculoskeletal and respiratory disease about 1.6 times as prevalent, and digestive diseases almost 5 times as prevalent in the early part of the century relative to the latter part (Fogel & Costa, 1997). Nor does this trend seem to be abating. The decline in disability among the elderly in the United States was even more rapid during the early 1990s than during the 1980s (Manton & Gu, 2001). Perhaps less tangibly but no less important, aspects of life such as amount of chronic pain and degree of sensory acuity have been improved by the development of better analgesics, joint replacement surgery, and widespread availability of effective treatment for cataracts and glaucoma, as well as continuously improving hearing aid technology.

So where do we go from here? If all of this improvement in the length and quality of life has come without any apparent alteration in the underlying human biological aging rate, then it has essentially come from better management of our environment with a dollop of help from modern medicine. But how long can such increases be sustained? Moreover, should we even wish that they be sustained? Increasing life expectancy has been a blessing thus far, but could it become a curse as it continues into the future?

THE FUTURE: GANYMEDE OR TITHONUS?

Even the most grimly pessimistic demographers expect life expectancy to continue increasing (Olshansky, Carnes, & Désesquelles, 2001). However, opinions differ sharply on the rate of future increase as well as when (and if) it will ultimately slow, stop, or reverse. Conservative projections have been made by the U.S. Social Security Administration as well as some demographers (Cheng, Miller, & Morris, 2004; Olshansky & Carnes, 1990; Olshansky et al., 2001). The Social Security Administration estimates that by the latter part of the current century, life expectancy in the United States will be about 83 years (81 for males, 85 for females) (Cheng et al., 2004) or about 5 to 7 years longer than at present. Though not making explicit time-specific predictions, Olshansky and colleagues have generally argued that the rate of life expectancy increase must necessarily slow dramatically and that, for both sexes combined, it is unlikely to rise much above 85 years, even in the very distant future, unless scientists discover how to retard the fundamental rate of aging. They base this claim on several lines of argument. First, they note that as mortality rates decline, proportionally greater and greater decreases are required to achieve a given amount of life expectancy increase. For instance, if the proportional mortality rate reductions that produced the roughly 30-year increase in longevity in the United States over the 20th century were repeated in the future, the further gain in life expectancy would only be about 10 years. If it were repeated again, only about 6 years would be gained (Olshansky et al., 2001). Framed slightly differently, to achieve a life expectancy of 90 years in the United States would require that 1985 mortality rates (life expectancy 74.7 years) be reduced by 70% at every age. Second, they note that mortality rates early in life are now so low in the United States that if all deaths before age 50 were eliminated, life expectancy would only rise by a little more than 3 years (Olshansky & Carnes, 1990). Furthermore, they calculate the surprisingly small longevity increase associated with the elimination of major causes of death. Thus eliminating all cancer deaths (using the 1985 census data) would increase life expectancy at birth by only about 3 years. Eliminating all cardiovascular diseases, diabetes, and cancer (more than 70% of all 1985 deaths) would produce a life expectancy increase of only about 15 years (Olshansky & Carnes, 1990).

Other demographers, more convinced of the ineluctability of biomedical progress, disagree. They forecast life expectancies from the mid-80s to as high as 100 years within this century (Lee & Carter, 1992; Manton, Stallard, & Tolley, 1991; Oeppen & Vaupel, 2002). Two approaches have been used to arrive at these forecasts. Most commonly, researchers have extrapolated from past mortality or longevity trends into the future. For instance, Oeppen and Vaupel (2002) noted that female life expectancy in the world's longest-lived country (which specific country is longest lived has changed several times over that period) has increased at a steady rate of about 2.5 years per decade since 1840. If that trend continues, they calculated that females in some country will have a life expectancy of 100 years by about 2060. Less dramatically, Tuljapurkar, Li, and Boe (2000) used observations that mortality rate at every age has declined exponentially at a roughly constant rate in the G7 industrialized countries since 1950 to make stochastic projections that some of these countries would have life expectancies in the high 80s or low 90s by the year 2050. A second approach has modeled chronic disease risk factors as extracted from populations with particularly healthy lifestyles to project that humans with optimized health habits could achieve life expectancies of

nearly 100 years (Manton et al., 1991). This latter study loses some credibil-
ity in that it projects slightly greater life expectancy for men than for women,
a phenomenon that is currently unknown among industrialized countries.
Among G7 countries (Canada, France, Germany, Italy, Japan, Great Britain,
United States), for instance, female life expectancy at birth now outpaces male
life expectancy by more than 6 years on average (U.S. Census Bureau, 2004).
The anomalous result from Manton and colleagues may be a consequence of
the fact that several of the population studies used for their analysis consisted
exclusively of males.

Regardless of which group of prognosticators turns out to be more accurate, the population of what are now considered elderly people will increase
dramatically over the ensuing decades. The key question for understanding
the social, political, and economic consequences of this increase will depend
to a large extent on the health and vitality of the growing elderly population.

In Greek mythology, two Trojan youths renowned for their beauty were
kidnapped by Eos, the randy dawn goddess, to be her lovers. They met very
different fates. Ganymede was soon stolen away from Eos by an equally en-
thralled Zeus, who made the lad like a god, forever young and beautiful. Eos
managed to keep Tithonus for herself and asked Zeus that he be granted eternal life, but in a now famous oversight she neglected to point out that what
she really meant was eternal youth. In one of those malicious pranks to which
Greek gods were prone, Zeus did give Tithonus eternal life but allowed him
to continue aging. Eventually he became feeble, withered, and demented,
until Eos could no longer stand it and turned him into a grasshopper.

The fates of Ganymede, long-lived yet still youthful, versus Tithonus,
long-lived but increasingly decrepit, illustrate two extreme scenarios about
how increased longevity during the next century could play out. In the night-
mare Tithonus scenario, we become better and better at keeping people alive
solely by better management of life-threatening diseases. Yet pain, isolation,
disability, and dementia characterize these extra years, because we have
not been able to address chronic problems like arthritis, weakened bones
and muscles, sensory loss, and the development of Alzheimer's disease.
The potential seriousness of this scenario can be appreciated by noting that
the prevalence of chronic pain increases with each decade of life (Davis &
Srivastava, 2003). Perhaps more frightening, by age 85 as many as 50% of
people become demented with Alzheimer's disease (Hy & Keller, 2000). One
third of the population lives to age 85 or beyond today, and a much larger
fraction will live than long in the future. As the over-85 population grows at
an increasing rate, the emotional, social, and economic costs of neurological
aging would become staggering.

By contrast, under the Ganymede scenario, the continuing extension of life will be accompanied by a medical reduction in rate of aging itself or by the development of multiple new therapies to combat much of the spectrum of debilitating late-life diseases. In either case, this scenario promises not only more life but a more pleasant life.

Of course, these scenarios represent diametric ends of a continuum. Although the lengthening of life over the past few hundred years has not been due to slowing the rate of aging itself, still there have been developed a wide range of interventions that mitigate the ailments of the elderly. These interventions are now so common that their impact on life's quality is often overlooked. For instance, high-quality eyeglasses and cataract surgery allow most people to continue reading or watching television until the very end of life. Compare this with the previously mentioned 17th-century English diarist Samuel Pepys, who gave up writing his diary at the age of 39, because what we now know to be typical middle-age farsightedness led him to fear total loss of his eyesight if he continued nighttime reading and writing in candle-lit rooms (Tomalin, 2003).

Where along the Tithonus–Ganymede continuum will people living in the late 21st century and beyond fall? Clearly, the social, political, and economic consequences will differ dramatically depending on the answer to this question. Although no one can predict for certain, some clues are now available from animal research where we already know multiple ways to extend life and health.

WHAT ANIMAL RESEARCH TELLS US

In retrospect, potentially the most exciting and surprising discovery about the biology of aging made during the 20th century may turn out to be a short note published in the scientific journal *Nature* in 1996. That note revealed that a particular dwarf mouse—the so-called Ames dwarf, which is about one third the normal mouse size—lives 50% to 65% longer than its standard-issue brothers and sisters (Brown-Borg, Borg, Meliska, & Bartke, 1996). Putting this in human perspective, it was as if we had discovered a hitherto unknown group of human pygmies with a life expectancy of 120 to 130 years. To appreciate the significance of this finding even in the animal world, it might be worth a brief historical summary of what we knew about making animals live longer up to the time this unexpected paper was published.

Prior to 1996, the only tried-and-true way to lengthen life and health in any species of mammal was by restricting the amount of food they ate (Weindruch & Walford, 1988). Over the years, there had been isolated reports that mammals lived longer if you castrated them (Hamilton, Hamilton, & Mestler, 1969; Hamilton & Mestler, 1969) or removed part of their pituitary gland and replaced some of the hormones thus lost (Everitt, 1973), but these findings proved difficult to repeat by other investigators and therefore were not widely believed (although it is worth noting that the Ames dwarf mouse validates Everitt's conclusions about the pituitary's role in aging). Caloric restriction as a way to increase longevity in laboratory rodents had been repeated scores of times.

Examining the caloric restriction effect in a little detail, if only to contrast it with the Ames dwarf discovery, is fruitful. Its essence is that if you cut back by 30% to 40% the number of calories eaten by laboratory rats and mice relative to what they would eat if given unlimited access to food, they live longer healthier lives. The longevity effect is not quite as dramatic as seen in the Ames dwarf, somewhere between 20% and 40% if started early in life. However, it is not bad, either. Note that I stress calories, because it does not appear to matter whether you reduce the intake of protein, fat, or carbohydrates. As long as the animals are not malnourished, they live longer. They clearly live healthier lives, too. Some rodent diseases, particularly a variety of cancers, are delayed until later in life in calorie-restricted animals; others disappear completely (Masoro, 2002). Restricted animals are also more resistant to toxins of many sorts, including carcinogenic ones, and they recover from surgery more quickly. In addition, they lose muscle mass more slowly as they grow older (although they have smaller muscles to begin with), and if given a running wheel to use if they wish will stay more active throughout life (McCarter et al., 1997; Weindruch & Walford, 1988). Mental function is also better preserved in most (Ingram, Weindruch, Spangler, Freeman, & Walford, 1987; Magnusson, 2001) but not all (Yanai, Okaichi, & Okaichi, 2004) studies, and some but not all parts of the immune system are enhanced as well (Effros, Walford, Weindruch, & Mitcheltree, 1991; Sun, Muthukumar, Lawrence, & Fernandes, 2001). For the most part, then, caloric restriction may be said to slow aging, rather than simply extend life—the Ganymede rather than the Tithonus effect.

The scientific difficulty raised by caloric restriction is that it has proven very difficult to figure out how it works. The best we can say after 70 years of fairly intense research is that we know a number of reasons why it *does not* work. For instance, it does not work because it slows metabolism. A general human intuition seems to be that metabolism, the slow-controlled fire by which we get our energy, must play a key role in aging, not least because using energy creates oxygen-free radicals as an unwanted but inevitable by-product. For some animals, in some circumstances, this is true. Put a house fly in the refrigerator, its metabolism slows, and it lives much longer. Put it in a hothouse, its metabolism increases, and it becomes short-lived. But mammal metabolism is more complex. Put you or me in a refrigerator, unlike the fly our metabolism increases, and we certainly will not live longer. By definition and design, calorie-restricted animals eat less and therefore must use less energy, but they are also smaller. If one calculates how much energy a restricted mouse uses per cell (or as the physiologists prefer, per lean body mass), it uses if anything slightly more energy than fully fed animals (McCarter & Palmer, 1992). The rate of energy consumption, at least as measured per cell of the entire animal's body, does not seem to be involved in the caloric-restriction effect.

What about exercise? We also know that calorie-restricted animals run around in their cages considerably more than fully fed animals and have much less body fat. Could the exercise or the lack of body fat, or both, play critical roles in the effect? The short answer is no. We know this because researchers have forced gluttonous, fully fed animals to exercise until they were as lean as restricted animals. It turns out that they live a bit longer as a consequence, mainly because deaths in middle age are rarer. Yet they did not live as long as restricted animals who simply lounged around their cages for their entire lives (Holloszy, 1997). We also know that if you restrict the diet of mice rendered grotesquely obese by a genetic mutation, they will still live a bit longer than normal mice, despite the fact that even calorie restriction has left these mice much fatter than normal mice (Harrison, Archer, & Astle, 1984). Parenthetically, it is worth noting that the long-lived Ames dwarf mice are decidedly portly, particularly early in life. Fat and exercise, alas, do not explain why calorie-restricted mice and rats age more slowly. Scientifically, the bottom line is that 70 years after the caloric-restriction effect was first discovered, after hundreds of studies from dozens of laboratories, we still do not have a clue how it works, mainly because restricting rodents' diets changes dozens to hundreds of physiological functions simultaneously. Hormone levels change (most go down, but a few go up), reproduction slows or stops, the fuel mix used to produce energy changes, body temperature decreases, cell turnover slows, and hundreds of genes alter their activity. Emerging technology such as deoxyribonucleic acid (DNA) microarrays, which can simultaneously monitor the activity of thousands of genes, could potentially give us novel insights into how the caloric-restriction effect works (e.g., Lee, Klopp, Windruch, & Prolla, 1999), but so far we are at a loss. Science works best when we can change only one or a few things at a time during our experiments. It should not be surprising, then, that we still do not know how caloric restriction works to slow aging.

This gets us back to a second key factor about the Ames dwarf mouse. It differs from its normal-size relatives only in bearing a mutation that disables just one of its approximately 25,000 genes. In other respects, it is a typical laboratory mouse. It is easy to imagine how a change in a single gene could shorten life. In fact, there are many (too many) human examples where a specific genetic mutation causes a horrific life-shortening disease, such as progeria or Tay-Sachs disease. Mutations generally make things worse. A life-extending mutation, on the other hand, has made something better. That is surprising, unusual, but scientifically quite a boon. In principle, with only a single genetic alteration, it should be much easier than for some complex alteration such as caloric restriction to follow the causal chain of events from the defective gene through the protein its normal variant makes through the other molecules with which the protein interacts to ultimately understand how the gene affects longevity.

There is a precedent for this. Before the Ames dwarf discovery, single gene modifications had been known to extend life dramatically in nearly microscopic worms. However, few people, including myself, thought that modifying a single gene in a larger, more complex animal such as a mouse could possibly have much effect on extending life. To provide some genetic context and meaning to the Ames dwarf mouse discovery, it is helpful to consider how dramatically worm research has altered thinking about the malleability of the rate of aging.

During the late 1980s and early 1990s a tiny roundworm about the size of a comma on this page had been admitted to the bestiary of animals used in the study of aging. Called by the rather inelegant name *C. elegans* (the *C.* standing for its tongue-twisting official name, *Caenorhabditis*), this worm species had been brought into the laboratory in the 1960s because of its unrivaled utility for the study of development (the process by which fertilized eggs eventually turn into adult animals) and neuroscience. You can make a persuasive case that we now know more about this worm than any other animal on the face of the earth, including humans. For instance, it was the first animal to have its genome completely sequenced (*C. elegans* Sequencing Consortium, 1998). Besides knowing its genome, we know that each adult has exactly 959 somatic cells. Of these, 302 are nerve cells, and 95 are striated muscle cells. We know the precursor cells from which each of the adult cells arose back as far as when it was a two-celled embryo. We even know that 131 cells die during the course of the worm's development. Moreover, the worm is transparent, so we can observe each of these cells when the worm is still alive and swimming around in its petri dish home. Adopting the worm as a laboratory animal turned out to be such a good idea that hundreds of laboratories throughout the world now dedicate themselves to the study of its biology, and the scientist responsible for its adoption, Sydney Brenner, received the Nobel Prize for Physiology and Medicine in 2002.

Thomas E. Johnson, of the University of Colorado, recognized in the 1980s that these worms had all the traits to make them extremely useful for aging studies, not least of which is that they only live about 2 weeks and can be kept in the laboratory by the millions. In 1988, he published the first paper describing a gene he called *age-1*, which when mutated extended worm life by about 60% (Friedman & Johnson, 1988). By the early 1990s a host of other *C. elegans* laboratories joined the field to search for other genes that when mutated extended life. They had no trouble finding them. In 1993, Cynthia Kenyon of the University of California–San Francisco discovered that mutations in another gene called *daf-2* could as much as double worm life span (Kenyon, Chang, Gensch, Rudner, & Tabtiang, 1993). Actually, this gene has an even greater effect than that. It doubles life span in the more common of the two worm sexes (hermaphrodites), but in the other sex (males), the same mutation increases longevity more than 6-fold (Partridge & Gems, 2002). In human terms, this is equivalent to changing one gene in men, and suddenly their life expectancy jumps to nearly 500 years.

What is the meaning of these startling findings even in worm terms? Biologically, at least three aspects of this discovery stand out. Foremost is the fact that if you alter only one DNA "letter" in the 100,000,000-letter DNA genome of the worm, it can live as much as 6 times longer than an unaltered worm. That such a seemingly miniscule change should have such a mind-bogglingly large effect, particularly on a trait—longevity—that many scientists assumed was fairly immutable, is pretty astonishing in itself. Equally astonishing, though, the gene alteration that leads to such a dramatically longer life does not enhance the activity of a gene that is already doing something pretty useful for the worm. It actually partially disables the gene, that is, reduces its activity. Whatever the normal form of the gene was doing shortened life. Also somewhat surprising is why, if such a dramatic increase in longevity can be accomplished by altering just this one DNA letter, has not nature already favored having this long-life letter in place? Worms captured in nature never have the long-life form of the gene. We will consider these issues in detail a bit later.

Moving ahead to 2004, we learn that alterations in more than 100 different worm genes had been found to be capable of extending life (Johnson et al., 2005) when mutated. Again, almost all of these alterations make the genes in question less active, not more active. Nature seems to abhor long life for worms. But making worms live longer by laboratory manipulations, it turns out, is easy. Gene alterations are not the only way to do it, either.

Worms also live substantially longer if you feed them less or shock them with a brief burst of heat, or if you destroy the cells they use to sense food in the environment, or if you remove their gonads (Apfeld & Kenyon, 1999; Butov et al., 2001; Hsin & Kenyon, 1999). Is this something unique to these worms or can the life of any animal be so easily extended?

Most likely worms are particularly easy creatures in which to extend life. In no other species have we come anywhere close to the 6-fold life extension that can be produced by genetic changes in worms. Worms have a specialized juvenile phase of their development that they enter in response to food short-age, and that may be part of the reason we can make them live so long. They can survive in this dauer (i.e., enduring) life phase for much longer than a normal adult worm can live. It is probable that many of the genetic and en-vironmental factors that extend worm life do so by stimulating biochemical pathways that have evolved to help maintain the dauer phase itself. On the other hand, some of the genes and environmental alterations that extend life in the worms clearly do so in other animals as well. For instance, laboratory fruit flies, which live several months compared with worms' several weeks, live longer if they are sterilized, if they are isolated from the other sex, if they are fed less, or if they are given a brief heat shock, just like worms (Chapman, Hutchings, & Partridge, 1993; Khazaeli, Tatar, Pletcher, & Curtsinger, 1997; Rose, 1991). Moreover, there is an equivalent of the worm *daf-2* gene, which, if partially inactivated, also extends fly life.

There are some differences in the effects of these genes between flies and worms, though. Although almost any mutation that reduces activity of this gene extends life in worms, only a few do in fruit flies. Most shorten life. Also, whereas there is a large effect in both sexes in worms, only females seem to live substantially longer in flies. Also, flies with this life-extending mutation are also dwarfs and infertile (Tatar et al., 2001). Worm mutants may be larger, smaller, or the same size. They have a reduced reproductive rate, but they are not sterile.

Ah, but what is the quality of life in a mutant worm that lives 6 times lon-ger than its more normal brethren? Is it experiencing a Tithonus-like period of extended decrepitude or a Ganymede-like extended youth? One problem with studying aging in miniscule animals that can be kept in the laboratory by the millions is that it is difficult to assess the physical condition of old individuals or ask such questions. They obviously cannot be interviewed, and observable worm behavior is rather rudimentary. However, from what little we can see, the worms seem more Ganymede-like. Two bits of worm behavior that typically decline with age are the rate at which they pump food into their stomach and the speed at which they swim. Most (although not all) worm mutations that extend life, including the two mentioned above, also rescue to some extent the typical decline in food pumping and swimming speed. But wouldn't it be nice if we had more subtle and sophisticated measures of health and vitality?

And so we come full circle back again to the Ames dwarf mouse. Although simple genetic mutations that dramatically extend life had become commonplace in worms by 1996, nothing of the sort had been reported in a mammal such as a mouse. Not only was a mouse more complex by many measures than a worm or a fly, we could observe a lot about mice. No one knew (or knows) exactly why the worms or flies die. Maybe they were all dying of the same thing, because we did not know how to take proper care of them in the laboratory. In that case, it would have been possible that something in worm or fly husbandry made them sick, and somehow we got around that problem with these mutations. However, mice were larger, more complex, consisting of billions of cells, not one or a few thousand. Also, we knew a lot about how to take very good care of a mouse. Over the decades that mice had been used for laboratory research, we had developed a superb, well-defined diet for them and knew the best temperature and humidity to raise them. We knew how to isolate them from infectious diseases and could watch them behave and could determine when they were sick. Best of all, we often did know why they died. If the mutation simply cured a single disease that somehow affected a disease that nearly all laboratory mice got, we would know it. Finally, we were surprised that the Ames dwarf lived so long because you can never underestimate human hubris. Mice are mammals just like humans, have a genome of about the same size (some 16-fold larger than a fruit fly genome and 30-fold larger than the worm), and possess about 99% of the same genes as humans. By comparison, only about 50% of human genes have identifiable counterparts in flies or one third of such counterparts in worms (Austad & Podlutsky, 2006). How could something so similar to us, nearly as complex by many measures, live so much longer with just a single genetic change? The longevity increase seen in the Ames dwarf, although not overly impressive by worm standards, was huge—bigger than caloric restriction—by mammalian standards.

Now comes a key question. Are these mice experiencing a Tithonus-like extended life of increasing decrepitude or a Ganymede-like extended youth? For many traits, the dwarfs seem to be experiencing extended youth. For instance, unlike normal mice, old dwarfs do not move around in their cages less as they age. They also do not show the same age-related decline in spatial memory (Kinney, Meliska, Steger, & Bartke, 2001). Dwarf animals also make new nerve cells at a higher rate in a critical brain region, the hippocampus, known to be involved in spatial memory. This is a brain region particularly hard hit in Alzheimer's disease. Dwarfs get cancer later in life and have a lower overall incidence of some cancer types (Ikeno, Bronson, Hubbard, Lee, & Bartke, 2003). Dwarfs' collagen, the material that forms tendons and ligaments, ages more slowly, as do several aspects of their immune system (Flurkey, Papaconstantinou, Miller, & Harrison, 2001). All in all, it does seem possible to slow aging, at least in a mouse, by disabling one gene.

Two more issues need to be briefly addressed to complete a thorough analysis of the Ames dwarf. First, could it be that the mutation has its effect by simply reducing the amount animals eat? Is this just another manifestation of the caloric-restriction effect? Such a phenomenon beset numerous studies of the effect of dietary supplements on longevity during the 1970s and 1980s. The canonical case is that a researcher hypothesizes that a certain food additive, say, a novel antioxidant, will slow aging. He adds the substance to the food of his laboratory animals, and sure enough, the animals live longer. The researcher now dreams of untold wealth, imagines that telephone call from Stockholm informing him of his well-deserved Nobel Prize, until someone asks if he measured how much the animals ate during his experiment. The problem with many such experiments has been that the additive makes mouse or rat chow less palatable. Consequently, the animals eat less, so of course they live longer because of the caloric-restriction effect. The supplement had nothing to do with the result other than making their food taste bad.

Fortunately, food intake has been measured in Ames dwarf mice. Because they are only one third the size of a normal adult mouse, they eat less. However, when corrected for size, they eat slightly more than a normal mouse. To prove the point experimentally, if you restrict the caloric intake of a dwarf mouse, it lives even longer. A food-restricted dwarf mouse lives about 75% longer than a fully fed normal mouse (Bartke et al., 2001).

The final question to ask about the dwarf mouse and the other life-extension mutants (as well as the calorie-restricted animals) is whether the life-extension effect is free. That is, do the treatments that extend life have unwanted side effects that might affect how humans view such treatments if hypothetically available to them? Might these side effects explain why one doesn't find longevity mutations in wild animal populations? Put another way, why do genes that seem to shorten life occur in nature?

Well, yes, there are side effects that may or may not seem detrimental, depending on your point of view. All treatments, genetic, dietary, or environmental, that extend life and health and have been studied with care have side effects. Sometimes the effects are obvious. Ames dwarf mice are small and sterile. That is, neither sex is capable of reproducing because of hormone deficiencies. In nature, the small size of Ames dwarfs would likely make them especially sensitive to cold, and even if they were fertile, males would not be able to compete for mates with the other larger males in the population. Several long-lived fruit fly mutants are similarly small and sterile.

Caloric restriction has similar effects. In rodents, it causes sterility or at least reduced fertility. If started prior to adulthood, it leads to much smaller size and causes as much as a 6-fold delay in puberty. Calorie-restricted rats have smaller muscles and thus less physical strength than fully fed animals, although their muscles seem to deteriorate more slowly.

There have been a few high-profile reports of mutations that have no obvious side effects. However, when these cases were examined carefully, the effects have always (to date) turned out to be there, even though they can be very subtle. For instance, the *daf-2* mutation in worms, which increases life expectancy by 2 to 6 times, has no obvious effect on age at maturity or fertility (Dillin, Crawford, & Kenyon, 2002). However, when researchers placed these mutants in the same petrie dish with normal worms, the mutants all disappeared within seven generations (Jenkins McColl, & Lithgow, 2004). The competitive disadvantage of the mutation turned out to be a very small difference in reproductive rate early in life. However, in the petri dish crucible of competition, this small difference proved decisive. An even more subtle case is illustrated by the worm mutation *age-1*, which extends life by about 50% and has no apparent effect on development rate, fertility, or any other obvious trait. When competed directly against a normal worm under standard laboratory conditions, the *age-1* mutant held its own. However, when a more "natural" dietary regime was imposed with food abundance that fluctuated erratically, the mutant soon disappeared (Walker, McColl, Jenkins, Harris, & Lithgow, 2000). The longevity genes we find in the laboratory all have side effects that make them less suited for competitive superiority in the wild.

This last example, in which a particular gene is beneficial under certain conditions but becomes evolutionarily disadvantageous under other conditions, brings up a point often overlooked by laboratory scientists. Genes do not have their effects in a vacuum, but in specific environments. A gene may have one effect in environment A and a completely different effect in environment B. Evolutionary biologists are well aware of this, but because many laboratory researchers are not used to thinking in evolutionary terms, and because they typically do all their experiments under some standard condition, the context specificity of gene action is not sufficiently appreciated. The best illustration of this point is from a study of fruit flies, which sought to identify genes associated with fly life span under five different environmental scenarios (Vieira et al., 2000). The flies (of both sexes) were reared in one of five conditions: Standard condition, high temperature, low temperature, brief blast of heat, or starvation. There was no lack of genes found affecting longevity. However, the effect of any particular gene depended on the environment. A gene that extended life in one environment might shorten life in another environment and have no effect in a third environment. A gene that lengthened life in males might shorten life in females. You might have thought that this finding would cause lots of soul searching and a questioning of experimental design in the aging research community, but you would be wrong. Most experiments are still carried out only under a single condition. Even one of the celebrity worm mutations was called into question. The *daf-2* mutation, which causes worms to live 2 to 6 times longer when the worms live on agar, has no effect when the worms live in soil, their natural habitat (Van Voorhies, Fuchs, & Thomas, 2005). The implication of these findings, if they are relevant to humans, and no one knows whether or not they are, is that a drug that retards aging in one person, say, a female vegetarian of British ancestry living in Massachusetts, might not be effective or might actually be harmful in a Hispanic male omnivore from Texas. Of course, individual differences in response to drugs are a common medical problem already. But unless research is specifically directed at understanding the nature of these differences for future antiaging medications, you could take a drug for years only to find out too late that it was not the right drug for you.

Animal studies tell us that it is possible to create animals by genetic or environmental manipulation, even complex animals like mammals, which have extended youth, health, and a longer life in specifically defined environments. Creating these animals does cause some side effects, some subtle, others striking. However, there seems to be no obvious biological reason to think that similarly extending life in humans living in a benign environment will in the future be impossible.

THE AMES DWARF GENE

So what does the gene that is disabled in the Ames dwarf do? What might it mean for the future of human longevity? The gene, it turns out, is critical for the normal development of the pituitary gland. This gland, located at the base of the brain, produces a cocktail of hormones that affect reproduction, growth, metabolism, stress, and virtually every other bodily function. For this reason, the pituitary has been called the body's "master gland." The Ames dwarf mutation interferes with the fetal development of the pituitary, so that it cannot make three of its usual hormones: prolactin, which is involved in reproduction; thyroid-stimulating hormone (TSH), which is involved in controlling metabolic rate; and growth hormone, which is involved in growth and a variety of other functions. Any or all of these hormones could be involved in retarding aging in the Ames dwarf, but most attention has fallen on growth hormone as the key player.

Hormones with their manifold effects on many parts of the body have been suspected to modulate aging and longevity at least since the 1880s, when the elderly endocrinologist Charles Brown-Séquard injected himself with macerated dog testicles and felt immediately rejuvenated (Gosden, 1996). The intuitively plausible idea is that if something in our body declines as we age, then maybe that decline is causing the aging. If so, topping the hormones back up might be expected to help retard the aging process. Ever since Brown-Séquard, people have been seeking rejuvenation via hormone injections. The day before yesterday it was testicular hormones, yesterday it was melatonin, today it seems to be growth hormone.

That declining hormones contribute to aging is not the only possible interpretation, however. It could be that hormone production declines with age because aging itself interferes with the processes that make hormones. In other words, aging causes hormone decline rather than hormone decline causing aging. A third interpretation is that hormones decline with age because continuing production at youthful levels is harmful. Growth hormone, for instance, can stimulate cancer growth, an issue that may be significant in later life. The irony about the Ames dwarf mice is that they likely live longer because they never produce any growth hormone. We do know that if mice or people are given lots of extra growth hormone throughout life, they become enormous and are short-lived (Pendergrass, Li, Yiang, & Wolf, 1993; Sacca, Cittadini, & Fazio, 1994). In the human case, lots of extra growth hormone causes gigantism and acromegaly. Famous acromegalics include Andre, the Giant, a 7-foot-4-inch, 500-pound professional wrestler-turned-actor; and Ted Cassidy, who played Lurch on *The Addams Family* television show. Both died, as acromegalics often do, from heart disease in their late 50s. Smaller doses of medically administered growth hormone have improved some measures of functional decline in rats, such as muscle mass and memory, but properly controlled human studies, despite what hucksters, cranks, and con men claim, have had much more limited success when given to the elderly and at the same time elicited unwanted side effects like carpal tunnel syndrome, joint pain, and diabetes (Blackman, Sorking, & Munzer, 2002).

Why has attention focused on the loss of growth hormone for the Ames dwarf effect and not on the other missing hormones, prolactin and TSH? The answer is primarily because of worm research, believe it or not, even though worms do not have a pituitary gland and do not make growth hormone. The connection takes a bit of explaining. Growth hormone level affects growth, of course. It also affects muscle mass and strength, influences body composition, helps regulate nutrient metabolism, and likely has a host of other effects we are still in the process of uncovering (Sacca et al., 1994). Growth hormone appears to have most of its effects indirectly by stimulating the production of another hormone: insulin-like growth factor-1 (IGF-1). As its name implies, IGF-1 is quite similar to insulin, a hormone that also has multiple effects, the best known one being the removal of sugar from blood into cells, where it can be broken down to make energy. Insulin is produced in the pancreas, but IGF-1 is produced nearly everywhere—liver, intestines, muscles, bone, brain, and gonads. In order to have their appropriate effects, most hormones must bind to receptors on the surface of cells. There are dedicated specific growth hormone receptors, insulin receptors and IGF-1 receptors. Without properly functioning cell surface receptors, no matter how much hormone is in the blood, it will not have an effect. For instance, type 2 diabetes mellitus, the type that strikes in adulthood, is not due to a lack of insulin, as is most juvenile diabetes, but to a lack of functioning insulin receptors.

To clarify the worm connection, recall that a partially disabling mutation in a gene called daf-2 makes worms live 2- 6-fold longer. Daf-2 turns out to be the worm equivalent of an insulin or IGF-1 receptor. Although worms have lots of different proteins that look like insulin or IGF-1, they only have one receptor—DAF-2—so we are not sure whether it acts mainly like insulin, mainly like IGF-1, or some combination of both. What's more, fruit flies have a similar receptor. Partially disabling that receptor also leads to long-lived fruit flies. What this means is that reducing the activity of worm or fly insulin or IGF-1 lengthens life. Ames dwarf mice do not produce growth hormone. Because growth hormone is a potent stimulator of IGF-1 production, the Ames dwarf mouse has to have very low levels of IGF-1 (and insulin). This explains why researchers were most interested in growth hormone from almost the very beginning.

One of the key features of modern biomedical research is the ability to disable specific genes in experimental animals and thus identify the gene's function by assessing what the animals lacking it are like (Silver, 1995). The easiest way to try to understand the precise role of growth hormone in mouse longevity, then, was to genetically disable its receptor. The first report on animals lacking growth hormone receptor indicated they were, not surprisingly, small (less than half the weight of normal mice), had roughly one tenth as much IGF-1 in their blood due to the lack of growth hormone stimulation, and, to answer the big question, lived 40% to 50% longer (Coschigano, Clemmons, Bellush, & Kopchick, 2000). Subsequent research indicated that these mice had less age-related decline in memory than normal mice as well (Kinney, Coschigano, Kopchick, Steger, & Bartke, 2001). Information came pouring in from other related studies. A miniature mouse was discovered that had undergone a spontaneous mutation that reduced growth hormone levels to about 1% of normal. It also had only one fifth of normal levels of IGF-1. That mouse lived 25% longer than normal mice (Flurkey et al., 2001). Some IGF-1 is critically needed for normal development, so if you completely disable the IGF-1 gene or its receptor, the mice die long before reaching adulthood. However, Holzenberger et al. (2003) created mice that had only half the normal number of IGF-1 receptors. Those mice lived 25% longer as well. One thing shared by most of these genetically manipulated mice as well as calorie-restricted animals is lower blood insulin level. Given the similarity between insulin and IGF-1 and the well-known deleterious effects of too much insulin, it would not seem too surprising if lowering insulin activity somehow also extended life. One research group tried genetically disabling the insulin receptor only in fat cells of mice. These mice were leaner, despite eating more, than normal mice and had less than half as much body fat. They also had about one-third less blood insulin and lived 18% longer (Blüher et al., 2002; Blüher, Kahn, & Kahn, 2003). This may not seem like much of an effect, given the more spectacular results of other experiments, but consider that altering only one gene's activity in only one tissue (fat) had a longevity effect equivalent to changing human life expectancy from 80 to about 95 years, or as much a change as we would see if we cured all cardiovascular disease, diabetes, and cancer, which make up more than two thirds of all causes of death currently (Olshansky & Carnes, 1990).

In total, do these experimental results mean that all humans have to do to live longer, healthier lives is somehow reduce the insulin or IGF-1 activity in some critical tissue in their bodies? Maybe, maybe not. Humans exist, although they are very rare, who lack functional receptors for growth hormone. They are called Laron dwarfs, or are said to be afflicted with Laron syndrome. They are small, as you might expect, about 4 feet tall as adults. They are typically obese, with reduced muscle mass, strength, and thin, brittle bones. Because people with Laron syndrome are found most frequently in less-developed areas of the world, where life expectancy is short and birth records rudimentary, there is little good information on how long they live relative to others living in the same areas (Laron, 1999, 2004). However, even in these areas where early deaths are common in the general population, the dwarfs are often found living into their 70s. So, if they lived in societies with modern standards of hygiene and medical care, they might, just might, be longer lived than most of us.

The important point to be gleaned from our accelerating success rate at making laboratory animals live longer, and understanding why they live longer, often healthier lives, is not just that equivalent dietary treatments or genetic mutations might extend life and health in humans, but that these studies are rapidly increasing our understanding of the fundamental processes underlying aging. No one (almost no one, see Stock, 2003) is advocating human gene therapy to slow aging. The ongoing genetic research is helping to identify molecular targets at which pharmaceuticals can be directed. Growth hormone and IGF-1 are by no means the only leads we have. I have concentrated on that particular biochemical pathway only because we know it is conserved in very distantly related groups of animals (worms, flies, and mice), and it has been demonstrated repeatedly to alter longevity and vigor in these diverse species. It has therefore been the focus of a great deal of recent research. That research indicates quite clearly that a Ganymede-like future for humans is possible. Ultimately, we will be able to design pharmaceuticals specifically to slow our own aging rate. There are likely to be side effects of these pharmaceuticals, although no one knows if these effects will be subtle or striking, and different people may need to take different drugs. In the worst case, the new life-extending pharmaceuticals may make us smaller, thinner, and less likely to have children, but they should keep us alive, healthy, and mentally alert into a second century of life. Whether or not the side effects outweigh the benefits will in the best case be each person's individual decision to make.

PUBLIC CONCERNS ABOUT LIFE EXTENSION RESEARCH

Given the enormous promise of the animal research I just described to lead to therapies that will extend life and health span in humans, the public remains decidedly ambivalent about the endeavor. This comes as a surprise to most scientists working on the aging problem, because it is biologically so interesting However, I have begun interrogating audience members when I give public lectures on the current state of aging research about their attitudes. I usually ask my audience to imagine that we have developed a pill, call it Longisin, which halves the rate at which humans age. That is, those who take the pill live twice as long and remain healthy for twice as many years as if they had not taken the pill. To make this imaginary example as clear and straightforward as possible, I say that the pills are as cheap as aspirin and have no side effects. I then ask whether such a pill should be released on the market. What I find to my continuing amazement is that somewhere between one third and two thirds of people who have chosen to come to a lecture on progress in aging research think that releasing this pill is a bad idea. The proportion who believe this must be even higher in the public at large.

The ambivalence of the general public toward our collective research goal may be one reason that federal funding for aging research continues to lag behind that for specific diseases of aging, such as diabetes, cancer, and atherosclerosis, even though retarding aging would simultaneously mitigate these and a host of other late-life diseases (Miller, 2002). For instance, in the 2004 fiscal year budget, President George W. Bush requested only 3.6% of funding for the National Institutes of Health to be allocated to the National Institute on Aging, compared with more than 15% for the study of infectious diseases and more than 17% devoted to cancer.

What accounts for this ambivalence, and how can we as scientists best state our case that our research goal—extending healthy human life—is not only worthy of public support, but worthy of more public support than much disease-based scientific investigation?

It would be easy to attribute objections to life-extending research to simple ignorance about, or fear of, science. Some instinctive suspicion about the value of scientific progress probably does play a role in public ambivalence, as it does in resistance to the use of genetically modified food. However, it would also be a considerable oversimplification. There are at least three philosophical objections to extending life that warrant our serious attention, even if ultimately we decide to reject them. Explaining publicly the reasons that they should be rejected becomes important if we wish to increase societal support for our research. These arguments can be called the objection of natural law (Are we unwisely interfering with nature?), the fairness argument (Who will have access to antiaging drugs?), and the Malthusian problems (Won't all kinds of resources become more scarce, creating more human suffering?).

The "Natural" Human Life Span

Natural law theorists place moral value on human nature as we know it (Post, 2004). The folk version of this argument is that humans should not interfere with nature—the Frankenstein error, hubris. Its subtext is that nature as arranged by a Supreme Being should remain inviolate. Leon Kass, chairman of the President's Council on Bioethics, draws heavily on this tradition to argue that tinkering with the length and arc of decline inherent in human life is likely to negatively affect ambition, commitment, and engagement in the present, attitudes toward reproduction, relations between the generations, innovation and creativity, and a host of other central facets of human life (President's Council on Bioethics, 2003).

A clear indication of the natural law position is any reference to the "natural" human life span, as was found in the briefing book for the President's Council on Bioethics meeting on age-retardation in December 2002. The argument that what is, is right (e.g., the natural human life span should continue to be the biblical three score and ten) has been called by philosophers the naturalistic fallacy (Moore, 1903). An assumption of this argument is that something like a natural human life span is knowable, and that if such a thing exists, it is what ought to exist. Major parts of Leon Kass's objections to the development of life-extending therapies fall under this category of argument. Of course, now that nature in general has been much more thoroughly studied than previously, it is apparent that virtually all vile acts (in human terms) of murder, cruelty, or treachery can be found in some circumstances in nature. Infanticide, to pick one example, is routine in nature among species from chimpanzees to lions to spiders (Hausfater & Hrdy, 1984). Does that make it right for humans?

Another problem with the idea of a natural human life span is that the best available information tells us that for most of the 100,000 or so years of the history of modern humans (*Homo sapiens*), half of children died before the age of 10, and less than 5% of people lived to the age of 60 (Gage, 1988). That state of affairs was happily long gone by 1900, and good riddance to it. No one has suggested to my knowledge that Londoners in 1700 should have worried about how parent–child relations might be negatively affected if new technology allowed almost all children born to live to the age of 10. Should they have shunned advances in hygiene because if so many children survived, children might be devalued by parents because they could be so easily replaced?

An interesting argument that it would be immoral not to pursue life- and health-extending therapies has been put forward by John Harris (2004). He points out that we universally laud and admire people who save or improve lives. We give such people awards for heroism or Nobel Prizes. Yet "saving a life," whether by rescuing someone from a burning building or giving sustenance to a starving person, is only postponing death, because whoever is saved will ultimately die anyway. Thus whatever social or ethical value we attribute to saving a life ought to also apply to postponing death by other means, such as developing longevity-extending therapies, as long as the quality of the remaining life is acceptable.

Fairness

I try to avoid the fairness, or equal access, issue when I poll my lay audiences as to their level of enthusiasm for the medical retarding of senescence. It complicates the issue. The hypothetical case I present to them is that the therapy costs very little or nothing. Of course, in reality, new and effective medical therapies are often quite costly or not readily available for other reasons. Organ transplants are not available to anyone who needs one, because the supply of suitable organs is limited. Also, kidney dialysis machines were at one time rare, so that many people died who would have lived with access to a machine. An acquaintance of mine in high school died when his insurance coverage for dialysis lapsed, and his doctor took him off the machine. "There's always the next world, Buck," he told me his physician said to him. Today, the best drug cocktails for combating human immunodeficiency virus (HIV) infections are too expensive for most Africans, and so they die in droves. Yet we do not forbid or inhibit research into new and better HIV-combating drugs because they will not be available to all. Philosophers generally agree that making some people worse off (by forbidding or inhibiting promising age-retarding research) cannot be justified when doing so does not improve the lot of anyone else (Davis, 2004). Perhaps money not spent on senescence-retarding research would be redirected to help solve hunger and disease in the developing world, but is that really likely to happen? Socially, we have tacitly accepted that therapies, even those developed with public money, may not be accessible to everyone, at least initially. The hope is that, ultimately, the cost will drop, and availability will spread. In fact, probably the most rapid way to hasten the progress of aging-retardation research is likely to convince people with very deep pockets that they can make money from the development of these therapies. Many quacks and charlatans have enriched themselves with bogus therapies over the years; I see no reason legitimate scientists might not benefit as well (Haber, 2004).

Malthusian Concerns

There are a host of very real Malthusian or resource shortage issues associated with slowing our aging rate. For instance, the human population would grow at a faster rate, leading potentially to a greater strain on the environment, social services, and food production resources. This is probably the number one objection I hear to medically retarding aging.

Increasing numbers of old people would further strain the already strained Social Security and Medicare systems. If tenured professors died or retired even less frequently than they do now, there would be no room for newly fledged assistant professors. A more subtle incarnation of Malthusian arguments is to suggest that resources would be, to some extent, wasted on the newly numerous elderly, because they will be less productive in their chosen endeavors than younger people. Concentration of the elderly in positions of power, an emerging gerontocracy, would have a stultifying effect on ideas, attitudes, and innovation. Progress in many fields would stall as a consequence.

Several points need to be made about these types of arguments. First, most, if not all, of the problems stated as arising from increasing longevity are very real. However, they may not be as problematic as we think. Demographer Jay Olshansky points out that even if we achieved immortality tomorrow—that is, death ceased to exist in the United States—our low reproductive rate would increase population growth rate only to a fraction of what it was during the baby-boom years following World War II (Olshansky, personal communication, December 2, 2002). Second, some of the Malthusian problems will be as bad as we think, for example, increasing strain on the environment and government entitlements, whether we succeed in slowing aging or not, but we are going to have to deal with them, as attested to by the current ideological battle over Social Security reform. Binstock (2004) has advocated what he calls "anticipatory deliberation" about the social, policy, and economic consequences of antiaging interventions. I agree, but would expand the notion to suggest that we need these deliberations even in the absence of antiaging interventions. Traditional medical progress will create sufficient Malthusian difficulties on its own.

Admittedly, some of the Malthusian problems might be somewhat worse if we lived substantially longer, but on the other hand, they might not. The above Malthusian arguments assume that an 80-year-old in an age-retarded society will be like an 80-year-old today. But remember we are talking about retarding aging itself. An 80-year-old that has been aging more slowly might be as healthy and vigorous—Ganymede-like—as a 40-year-old today. People living longer, healthier, more vigorous lives would not be so likely to wish to retire at the youthful age of 65. Or, if they retired from one job, they might feel like starting a new career in another field. Who knows what would happen to patterns of reproduction? Women might routinely put off childbearing until they were in their 60s.

A little historical perspective might be useful. Worries about the drain supporting the aged would put on society were rife at the beginning of the 20th century. In 1908, Nobel Prize–winning physiologist Elie Metchnikoff, living in Paris, worried that France was supporting so many old people. "Already it is complained," he wrote, "that the burden of supporting old people is too heavy, and statesmen are perturbed by the enormous expense which will be entailed by State support of the aged" (Haber, 2004). If people worried about these Malthusian problems in the early 20th century when life expectancy was only 50 years, how did we make it through the rest of the century without economic and social collapse? Would we say things are worse now than they were in 1900? Also, if we as a society were really interested in preventing a Malthusian crisis, we should encourage smoking, renounce antibiotics and vaccines, destroy insulin supplies, reward drunk driving, and refuse to treat heart attack victims. Because we do not do these things, we have already made a tacit decision that preserving life (assuming it is of sufficient quality) is worth a considerable investment of economic and scientific resources. The mission statement of the U.S. National Institutes of Health specifically states that "[our] . . . mission is science in pursuit of fundamental knowledge about the nature and behavior of living systems and the application of that knowledge to *extend healthy life and reduce the burdens of illness and disability*" (emphasis added) (www.nih.gov/about/almanac/2002/). Senescence-retarding research is simply a smarter way of investing those resources than working at curing one disease at a time (Miller, 2002).

HOW THE SCIENTIFIC COMMUNITY CAN BEST MAKE ITS CASE

Given the above arguments, it seems evident to me that pursuing, preferably at an accelerated rate, antiaging therapies is a worthwhile endeavor. However given public ambivalence or even resistance to this idea, we in the research community have a marketing problem. How can we convince a doubting public about the value of our research?

I think one answer may be to quit putting the goal of our research in terms of life extension but instead put it in terms of improved health and vigor. The wish for longer and longer life with little emphasis on the quality of that life is easily interpreted as a species of greed, manifested by people with little concern for the social consequences. As philosopher Daniel Callahan points out, just because something is wished for by most individuals does not necessarily mean it is good for society as a whole (Stock & Callahan, 2004). The nearly universal wish to avoid paying taxes is a prime example. However, it is difficult to argue that improving everyone's health is not a laudable goal. If an inadvertent consequence of improving everyone's health turns out to be lengthening everyone's life as well, then that is just a happy accident. It is probably worth pointing out that in the few experiments for which we have some independent indicator of health and in which dietary or environment or genetic treatments increased longevity, the animals have also experienced longer health. Tithonus may be nothing more than a figment of the Greek imagination.

Focusing on improving health rather than simply lengthening life seems to me a good idea from a scientific perspective, not just from a crass marketing standpoint. The ultimate goal of virtually all researchers in the field really is to increase healthy life span. The only reason that virtually all studies now focus on length of life rather than health is that it is the easiest indicator of health we have. For humans, mortality data are the easiest to extract from the historical record. It is also easier to tell if an experimental animal, particularly in a laboratory, where to survive it only has to be capable of walking or crawling over to the food dish or water bowl, is alive or dead than whether it can still see, hear, jog, or solve a tricky mental problem. Moreover, if life span is the only indicator of health span we typically use, and if we rarely if ever examine health span itself, we will never really be sure how good an indicator life span is.

I issue a challenge to the community of biogerontologists who work on retarding aging. It is time to talk about our work as improving health, not merely lengthening life. It is also time to develop reliable indicators of health, which should be integrated into our experiments, whether our research subjects are worms, flies, mice, dogs, or humans. This will allow us to state with authority that the diet or drug we developed, or the gene we discovered, has improved health at any or all ages, regardless of its effect on life span.

ACKNOWLEDGMENTS

I gratefully acknowledge the financial support for my own aging research over the years to the National Institute on Aging, the National Science Foundation, The Ellison Medical Foundation, and the American Federation for Aging Research.

REFERENCES

Accord Jacobson vs. Massachusetts 191, U.S. *11*, 25–29 (1905).

Apfeld, J., & Kenyon, C. (1999). Regulation of lifespan by sensory perception in *Caenorhabditis elegans. Nature, 402,* 804–809.

Austad, S. N., & Podlutsky, A. (2006). A critical evaluation of nonmammalian models for aging research. In E. J. Masoro & S. N. Austad (Eds.), *Handbook of the biology of aging* (6th ed.). San Diego: Academic Press, in press.

Bartke, A., Wright J.,C., Mattison, J. A., Ingram, D. K., Miller, R. A., & Rosth, G. S. (2001). Extending the lifespan of long-lived mice. *Nature, 414,* 412.

Bazin, J. (2000). *The eradication of smallpox*. San Diego, CA: Academic Press.

Binstock, R. H. (2004). Anti-aging medicine and research: A realm of conflict and profound societal implications. *Journal of Gerontology: Biological Sciences, 59A,* 523–533.

Blackman, M. R., Sorkin, J. D., & Munzer, T. (2002). Growth hormone and sex steroid administration in healthy aged women and men: A randomized controlled trial. *Journal of the American Medical Association, 288,* 2282–2292.

Blüher, M., Michael, M. D., Peroni, O. D., Ueki, K., Carter, N., Kahn, B. B., et al. (2002). Adipose tissue selective insulin receptor knockout protects against obesity and obesity-related glucose intolerance. *Developmental Cell, 3,* 25–38.

Blüher, M., Kahn, B. B., & Kahn, C. R. (2003). Extended longevity in mice lacking the insulin receptor in adipose tissue. *Science, 299,* 572–574.

Brown-Borg, H. M., Borg, K. E., Meliska, C. J., & Bartke, A. (1996). Dwarf mice and the ageing process. *Nature, 384,* 33.

Butov, A., Johnson, T., Cypser, J., Sannikov, I., Volkov, M., Sehl, M., et al. (2001). Hormesis and debilitation effects in stress experiments using the nematode worm *Caenorhabditis elegans*: The model of balance between cell damage and HSP levels. *Experimental Gerontology, 37,* 57–66.

C. *elegans* Sequencing Consortium. (1998). Genome sequence of the nematode C. *elegans*: A platform for investigating biology. *Science, 282,* 2021–2018.

Chapman, T., Hutchings, J., & Partridge, L. (1993). No reduction in the cost of mating for *Drosophila melanogaster* females mating with spermless males. *Proceedings of the Royal Society of London B, Biological Sciences, 253,* 211–217.

Cheng, A. W., Miller, M. L., & Morris, M. et al. (2004). A stochastic model of the long-range financial status of the OASDI Program. *Actuarial Study No. 117* (SSA Publ. No. 11–11543) U.S. Government Printing Office.

Coschigano, K.T., & Clemmons, D., Bellush, L. L., & Kopchick, J. J. (2000). Assessment of growth parameters and life span of GHR/BP gene-disrupted mice. *Endocrinology, 141,* 2608–2613.

Davis, J. K. (2004). Collective suttee: Is it unjust to develop life extension if it will not be possible to provide it to everyone? *Annals of the New York Academy of Science 1019,* 535–541.

Davis, M. P., & Srivastava, M. (2003). Demobraphics, assessment and management of pain in the elderly. *Drugs Aging, 20,* 23–57.

De Costa, C. M. (2002). The contagiousness of childbed fever: a short history of puerperal sepsis and its treatment. *Medical Journal of Australia, 177,* 668–671.

Diamond, J. (1997). *Guns, germs, and steel: The fates of human societies*. New York: W. W. Norton.

Dillin, A., Crawford, D. K., & Kenyon, C. (2002). Timing requirements for insulin-IGF-1 signaling in C. *elegans*. *Science, 298,* 830–834.

Effros, R. B., Walford, R. L., Weindruch, R., & Mitcheltree, C. (1991). Influences of dietary restriction on immunity to influenza in aged mice. *Journal of Gerontology, 46,* B142–147.

Everitt, A. V. (1973). The hypothalamic-pituitary control of aging and age-related pathology. *Experimental Gerontology, 8,* 265–277.

Everitt, A. V., & Burgess, J. A. (Eds.). (1976). *Hypothalamus, pituitary, and aging.* Springfield, IL: Charles C Thomas.

Faber, J. F. (1982). Life tables for the United States: 1900–2050. *Actuarial Study No. 87* (SSA Publ. No. 11–11534) U.S. Government Printing Office.

Finch, C. E., & Crimmins, E. M. (2004). Inflammatory exposure and historical changes in human life-spans. *Science, 305,* 1736–1739.

Flurkey, K., Papaconstantinou, J., Miller, R. A., & Harrison, D. E. (2001). Lifespan extension and delayed immune and collagen aging in mutant mice with defects in growth hormone production. *Proceedings of the National Academy of Sciences USA, 98,* 6736–6741.

Fogel, R. W., & Costa, D. L. (1997). A theory of technophysio evolution, with some implications for forecasting population, health care costs, and pension costs. *Demography, 34,* 49–66.

Friedman D. B., & Johnson T. E. (1988). A mutation in the *age-1* gene in *Caenorhabditis elegans* lengthens life and reduces hermaphrodite fertility. *Genetics, 118,* 75–86.

Gage, T. B. (1988). Mathematical hazard models of mortality: An alternative to model life tables. *American Journal of Physical Anthropology, 76,* 429–441.

Gosden, R.G. (1996). *Cheating time: Science, sex, and aging.* New York: W. H. Freeman.

Haber, C. (2004). Life extension and history: the continual search for the fountain of youth. *Journal of Gerontology: Biological Sciences, 59A,* 515–522.

Hamilton, J. B., Hamilton, R. S., & Mestler, G. E. (1969). Duration of life and causes of death in domestic cats: Influence of sex, gonadectomy, and inbreeding. *Journal of Gerontology, 24,* 427–437.

Hamilton, J. B., & Mestler, G. E. (1969). Mortality and survival: Comparison of eunuchs with intact men and women in a mentally retarded population. *Journal of Gerontology, 24,* 395–411.

Harris, J. (2004). Immortal ethics. *Annals of the New York Academy of Sciences, 1019,* 527–534.

Harrison, D. E., Archer, J. R., & Astle, C. M. (1984). Effects of food restriction on aging: Separation of food intake and adiposity. *Proceedings of the National Academy of Sciences USA, 81,* 1835–1838.

Hausfater, G., & Hrdy, S. B. (1984). *Infanticide: Comparative and evolutionary perspectives.* Chicago: Aldine.

Hayden, F. J. (1970). Maternal mortality in history and today. *Medical Journal of Australia, 1,* 100–109.

Holloszy, J. O. (1997). Mortality rate and longevity of food-restricted exercising male rats: A reevaluation. *Journal of Applied Physiology, 82,* 399–403.

Holzenberger, M., Dupont, J., Ducos, B., Leneuve, P., Géloën, A., Even, et al. (2003). IFG-1 receptor regulates lifespan and resistance to oxidative stress in mice. *Nature, 421,* 182–184.

Hsin, H., & Kenyon, C. (1999). Signals from the reproductive system regulate the lifespan of C. elegans. Nature, 399, 362–366.

Hy, L. X., & Keller, D. M. (2000). Prevalence of AD among whites: A summary of levels of severity. Neurology, 55, 198–204.

Ingram, D. K., Weindruch, R., Spangler, E. L., Freeman, J. R.,& Walford, R. L. (1987). Dietary restriction benefits learning and motor performance of aged mice. Journal of Gerontology, 32, 78–81.

Ikeno, Y., Bronson, R. T., Hubbard, G. B., Lee, S., & Bartke, A. (2003). Delayed occurrence of fatal neoplastic diseases in Ames dwarf mice: Correlation to extended longevity. Journal of Gerontology: Biological Sciences, 58, B291–96.

Jenkins, N. L., & McColl, G., & Lithgow, G. J. (2004). Fitness cost of extended lifespan in Caenorhabditis elegans. Proceedings of the Royal Society London B, Biological Sciences, 271, 2523–2526.

Johnson, T. E., Henderson, S. T., & Rea, S. (2006). Genetic manipulation of life span in C. elegans. In E. J. Masoro & S. N. Austad (Eds.), Handbook of the biology of aging (6th ed.). San Diego, CA: Academic Press, in press.

Kass, L. R. (1985). Toward a more natural science: Biology and human affairs. New York: Free Press.

Kenyon, C., Chang, J., Gensch, E., Rudner, A., & Tabtiang, R. (1993). A C. elegans mutant that lives twice as long as wild type. Nature, 366, 461–464.

Khazaeli, A. A., Tatar, M., Pletcher, S. D., & Curtsinger, J. W. (1997). Heat-induced longevity extension in Drosophila: 1. Heat treatment, mortality, thermotolerance. Journal of Gerontology: Biological Sciences, 52, B48–B52.

Kinney, B. A., Coschigano, K. T., Kopchick, J. J., Steger, R. W.,& Bartke, A. (2001). Evidence that age-induced decline in memory retention is delayed in growth hormone resistant GH-R-KO (Laron) mice. Physiology and Behavior, 72, 653–660.

Kinney, B. A., & Meliska, C. J., Steger, R. W., & Bartke, A. (2001). Evidence that Ames dwarf mice age differently from their normal siblings in behavioral and learning and memory parameters. Hormones and Behavior, 39, 277–284.

Lane, M. A., Mattison, J. A., Roth, G. S., Brant, L. J.,& Ingram, D. K. (2004). Effects of long-term diet restriction on aging and longevity in primates remain uncertain. Journal of Gerontology: Biological Sciences, 59A, 405–407.

Laron, Z. (1999). The essential role of IGF-I: Lessons from the long-term study and treatment of children and adults with Laron syndrome. Journal of Clinical Endocrinology and Medicine, 84, 4397–4404.

Laron, Z. (2004). Laron syndrome (primary growth hormone resistance or insensitivity): The personal experience, 1958–2003. Journal of Clinical Endocrinology and Metabolism, 89, 1031–1044.

Lee, C. K., Klopp, R. G., Windruch, R., & Prolla, T. A. (1999). Gene expression profile of aging and its retardation by caloric restriction. Science, 285, 1390–1393.

Lee, R. D., & Carter, L. R. (1992). Modeling and forecasting U.S. mortality. Journal of the American Statistical Association, 87, 659–671.

Lovejoy, C. O., Meindl, R. S., Pryzbeck, T. R., Barton, T. S., Heiple, K. G., & Kotting, D. (1977). Paleodemography of the Libben Site, Ottawa County, Ohio. *Science, 198,* 291–293.

Magnusson, K. R. (2001). Influence of diet restriction on NMDA receptor subunits and learning during aging. *Neurobiology of Aging, 2,* 613–627.

Manton, K. G.,& Gu, X. L. (2001). Changes in the prevalence of chronic disability in the United States black and nonblack population above age 65 from 1982 to 1999. *Proceedings of the National Academy of Sciences USA, 98,* 6354–6359.

Manton, K., Stallard, E.,& Tolley, H. D. (1991). Limits to human life expectancy: Evidence, prospects, and implications. *Population and Development Review, 17,* 603–637.

Masoro, E. J. (2002). *Caloric restriction: A key to understanding and modulating aging.* Philadelphia: Elsevier Science..

Maternal mortality—United States, 1982–1996. (1998, September 4). *Morbidity and Mortality Weekly Report,* pp. 705–707.

McCarter, R. J., & Palmer, J. (1992). Energy metabolism and aging: A lifelong study of Fischer 344 rats. *American Journal of Physiology, 263,* E448–E452.

McCarter, R. J., Shimokawa, I., Ikeno, Y., Higami, Y., Hubbard, G. B., Yu, et al. (1997). Physical activity as a factor in the action of dietary restriction on aging: Effects in Fischer 344 rats. *Aging (Milano), 9,* 73–79.

Miller, R. A. (2002). Extending life: Scientific prospects and political obstacles. *Milbank Quarterly, 80,* 155–174.

Moore, G. E. (1903). *Principia ethica.* Cambridge: Cambridge University Press.

Oeppen, J., & Vaupel, J. W. (2002). Broken limits to life expectancy. *Science, 196,* 1029–1030.

Olshansky, S. J., & Carnes, B. A. (1990.) In search of Methuselah: Estimating the upper limits to human longevity. *Science, 250*(4981), 634.

Olshansky, S. J., Carnes, B. A., & Désesquelles, A. (2001). Prospects for human longevity. *Science, 291,* 1491–1492.

Partridge, L., & Gems, D. (2002). Mechanisms of ageing: Public or private? *Nature Reviews: Genetics, 3,* 165–175.

Pendergrass, W. R., Li, Y., Yiang, D., & Wolf, N. S. (1993). Decrease in cellular replicative potential in "giant" mice transfected with the bovine growth hormone gene correlates to shortened life span. *Journal of Cell Physiology 156,* 96–103.

Post, S. G. (2004). Establishing an appropriate ethical framework: the moral conversation around the goal of prolongevity. *Journals of Gerontology: Biological Sciences, 59A,* 534–539.

President's Council on Bioethics. (2003). *Beyond therapy: Biotechnology and the pursuit of happiness.* New York: Regan Books.

Rose, M. R. (1991). *Evolutionary biology of aging.* Oxford: Oxford University Press.

Sacca, L., Cittadini, A., & Fazio, S. (1994). Growth hormone and the heart. *Endocrine Reviews, 15,* 555–573.

Silver, L. (1995). *Mouse genetics: Concepts and applications.* Oxford: Oxford University Press.

Stock, G. (2003). *Redesigning humans: Choosing our genes, changing our future.* New York: Mariner Books.

Stock, G., & Callahan, D. (2004). Point-counterpoint: Would doubling the human life span be a net positive or negative for us either as individuals or as a society? *Journal of Gerontology: Biological Sciences, 59A,* 554–559.

Sun, D., Muthukumar, A. R., Lawrence, R. A., & Fernandes, G. (2001). Effects of calorie restriction on polymicrobial peritonitis induced by cecum ligation and puncture in young C57BL/6 mice. *Clinical and Diagnostic Laboratory Immunology, 8,* 1003–1011.

Tatar, M., Kopelman, A., Epstein, D., Tu, M.-P., Yin, C.-P., & Garofalo, R. S. (2001). A mutant *Drosophila* insulin receptor homolog that extends life-span and impairs neuroendocrine function. *Science, 292,* 107–110.

Tomalin, C. (2003). *Samuel Pepys: The unequalled self.* London: Penguin Press.

Tuljapurkar, S., Li, N., & Boe, C. (2000). A universal pattern of mortality decline in the G7 countries. *Nature, 405,* 789–792.

U.S. Census Bureau. (2004). International data base (IDB). Washington, DC: Population Division, International Programs Center.

University of California, Berkeley & Max Planck Institute for Demographic Research. (2004). *Human mortality database.* Retreieved December 2004 from www.mortality.org and www.humanmortality.de

Van Voorhies, W. A., Fuchs, J., & Thomas, S. (2005). The longevity of *Caenorhabditis elegans* in soil. Biological Letters of the Royal Society, *1,* 247–249. *Proceedings of the Royal Society of London.*

Vieira, C., Pasyukova, E. G., Zeng, Z.-B., Hackett, J. B., Lyman, R. F., & Mackay, T. F. C. (2000). Genotype–environment interaction for quantitative trait loci affecting life span in *Drosophila melanogaster. Genetics, 154,* 213–227.

Walker, D. W., McColl, G., Jenkins, N. L., Harris, J., & Lithgow, G. J. (2000). Evolution of lifespan in *C. elegans. Nature, 405,* 296–297.

Weindruch, R., & Walford R. L. (1988). *The retardation of aging and disease by caloric restriction.* Springfield, IL: Charles C Thomas.

Wilmoth, J. R., Deegan, L. J., Lundström, H., & Horiuchi, S. (2000). Increase of maximum life-span in Sweden, 1861–1999. *Science, 289,* 2366–2368.

Yanai, S., Okaichi, Y., & Okaichi, H. (2004). Long-term dietary restriction causes negative effects on cognitive function in rats. *Neurobiology of Aging, 25,* 325–332.

CHAPTER 3

New Avenues, New Questions, and Changing Perspectives in Geriatric Medicine

Kenneth Brummel-Smith

The provision of medical care to older persons will face significant challenges, and experience major changes, in the next half-century. These changes will involve modifications in the doctor–patient relationship, new ways in which medicine is practiced, and an increased need for sociopolitical decisions regarding the provision and cost of health care. Furthermore, advances in medical science will extend the role of technology in health care, bringing into play a collision between high-tech interventions and a growing desire for holistic and alternative approaches. Medicine will increasingly focus on chronic conditions and preventive care. Health promotion activities will become the purview of other health care providers, such as nurse-practitioners, physician assistants, and exercise and nutrition specialists. Finally, there will likely be a deepening conflict between what consumers of health care services want and what they are willing to pay. A national health insurance program and health care rationing will become necessary for controlling health care costs.

THE BABY-BOOM GENERATION AND THE CHANGING DOCTOR–PATIENT RELATIONSHIP

The first members of the baby-boom generation (BBG) will begin to turn 65 in 2011 and affect all aspects of medical care. Geriatric medicine as a discipline was established at a time when patients served were primarily from the World War II generation, and that generation's view of doctor–patient relationships, control of health care decisions, the role of science in health care, and authority are markedly different than the views held by many in the BBG. Many, if not most, in the World War II age group continue to view physicians as authority figures. Older patients have been accustomed to receiving the information they need regarding health care from their physicians. The present older generation grew up at a time when the extent of medicine's advances was almost inconceivable. The eradication of certain diseases, such as smallpox, was attended by more personal experiences, like seeing the benefits of polio vaccines and other childhood immunizations. Antibiotics changed the perception that death was just around the corner, if one was sick enough. Health care focused on developing solutions to common, acute problems presented most frequently. Reaching old age was seen as an uncommon occurrence and not part of an anticipated pattern.

The type of relationship that baby boomers expect of their physicians will be different than patients of the past. Instead of the paternalistic doctor advising the patient of a certain choice, the BBG will want to participate and be engaged in decision making. Studies have shown that a significant portion of BBG patients want direct advice but still seek out additional health-related information by "researching" it themselves online (Institute for the Future, 2000). The widespread use of computers, the Internet, and consumers' access to health information is driving a far-reaching change in the nature of the doctor–patient relationship. The advent of pervasive consumer awareness will extend to the area of health care as well.

The BBG will no doubt use all available resources in the maintenance of health, care of illness, and management of health services. The use of information resources will become increasingly important as the shift of attention from acute medical conditions to a focus on management of chronic diseases continues (Wagner, Austin, & Von Korff, 1996). Chronic disease self-management techniques have been demonstrated to be cost-effective and lead to better health outcomes (Lorig et al., 1999). Patients can learn, from lay health care trainers, how to manage their conditions, when to use physicians, and how to take charge of there own health care. Using this model, persons with chronic conditions can learn more about their diseases, how to practice preventive techniques, how to monitor their own health status, and how to best make use of various health care providers.

Already some physicians are incorporating advanced methods of sharing information, using e-mail to answer questions, and guiding patients in their own searches of the literature (Scherger, 2004). The geriatrician of the future will need to be an expert information manager and provide "information therapy" (Kemper & Mettler, 2002). Information therapy moves beyond the traditional role of information and referral to use information to facilitate the practice of evidence-based care, provide more autonomy and control to patients, and help achieve better decisions.

With the increased use of electronic medical records (EMRs), physicians will be able to use e-mail to automatically provide educational materials, references or referrals to community resources, and links to self-care materials to the patient. The EMRs of the future will link an office visit–generated diagnosis with an electronically signed prescription (thereby decreasing the risk of a medical error caused by illegible handwriting), an educational e-mail to the patient, all generated automatically based on the billing code for that visit. For instance, a patient seen with hypertension and needing a modification of her medication treatment would receive an e-mail after the visit discussing the medication use and potential side effects, describing exercise measures that would be beneficial, and giving links to senior-friendly health clubs in her area. Although large-scale studies of the outcome of these changes have not been completed, initial evidence is that they are effective at improving the quality of care and reducing health care costs.

Decision support services will also become increasingly important to those with chronic conditions. One such example, Health Dialog (www. healthdialog.com), is operating at this time with over 13 million members. This program, which works in collaboration with health plans and physicians' offices, offers "Collaborative Care Health Coaching." This service is a source of information and support that individuals can turn to for a broad spectrum of health care concerns. Participants have access to tools and information that teach self-management and decision-making skills, enabling them to assume a more active role in the management of their medical conditions in concert with their physicians. Studies are under way to determine outcomes and cost-effectiveness.

In some practices, patients are already able to view portions of their own EMR to review problem lists and recommendations, medication lists, and correct errors (www.medicalogic.com/products/aboutmyhealth). Many programs allow the patient to schedule or check appointments. The difficulties in implementing these innovations are large, however, due to differences in computer systems and other technical issues (Winkelman & Leonard, 2004). As in all areas of information technology, these problems will be resolved. The geriatrician will focus on those with chronic conditions, helping the patient to manage his or her own condition with frequent, asynchronous communications and advice.

What is unknown about the future use of electronic information systems is how an aged user base will affect development. Older people have adapted to the information age fairly rapidly, though the present cohort does not use the Internet or e-mail as much as younger cohorts. A recent study found that 22% of the older population uses the Internet, and of these users, 60% are online daily (Pew Internet and American Life, 2004). Of course, the BBG is significantly more familiar with the use of computers in both work and daily life. Physicians are somewhat slow to adopt computer innovations when compared with other professionals (Institute of Medicine, 2001). The reasons for this are numerous: Physicians may fear the computer will interfere with the doctor–patient relationship, have privacy concerns, lack experience with personal computers, or some simply cannot afford the high cost of the technology. Still, an increasing number of physicians are adopting handheld and tablet computers in their medical practice. If the predictions of some experts come to pass, complete integration of computers into daily life is inevitable (Kurzweil, 1999).

These changes are facilitated by the growing emphasis on evidence-based medicine, in which medical decision-making is based on the latest research trials (Sackett, Straus, Richardson, Rosenberg, & Haynes, 2000). Meta-analysis, where the results of a large number of studies on a particular issue are compiled and analyzed, is an increasingly important method of evaluating the effectiveness of a diagnostic process or treatment. Evidence-based medicine incorporates evidence from controlled medical studies, the patient's values, and the physician's clinical expertise into the decision-making process (see Fig. 4.1). Physicians can use handheld personal digital assistants to quickly find the latest evidence on the Web, and can review that information with the patient. InfoRetriever (www.infopoems.com), FirstConsult (www.firstconsult.com), and DxPlain (www.lcs.mgh.harvard.edu) are but a few examples of such resources. Well-equipped offices oriented to providing information therapy have computers easily accessible to physicians, staff, and patients. With easy access to information technology, physicians will be able to use decision-support programs that take into account the prevalence of the disorder in the community, the current evidence, and even the patient's values to inform a recommendation for the patient. The use of patient-directed, decision-support tools has also been shown to be effective. In a study of patients with breast cancer, the subjects were randomized into two groups; one group used a computer-assisted decision aid to help with decision making regarding treatment, and the other received the usual method of aid in decisions: talking it over with a physician. The patients who used the computer system chose breast-conserving surgery more frequently and were more knowledge-

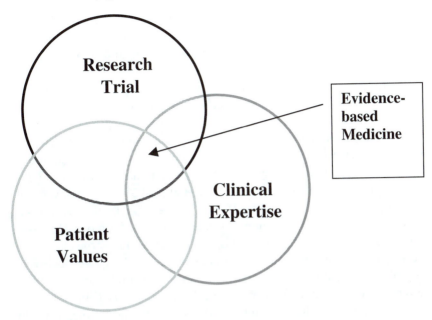

FIGURE 4.1 Evidence-based medicine. The practice of evidence-based medicine requires the provider to integrate information gained from clinical trials with his or her own experience and the patient's values. (Adapted from Sackett, Straus, Richardson, Rosenberg, & Haynes, 2000.).

able about their disease, satisfied with their decision, and felt less conflict about their treatment (Whelan et al., 2004).

The Institute of Medicine published in *Crossing the Quality Chasm* 10 rules to guide the redesign of the health care system, five of which are directly applicable to information systems (Institute of Medicine, 2001):

1. *Care based on patient needs and values.* Patients receive care when they need it and in a variety of forms. Access to care can be through visits, by telephone, or over the Internet.
2. *Customization based on patient needs and values.* Not only should the system be designed to meet the most common needs, but attention to special needs and values is also required.
3. *The patient as the source of control.* The ethical principle of autonomy requires that patients be given all the information they need to be able to make informed health care decisions. It is not up to the health care provider to decide which patient needs what information.

4. *Shared knowledge and free flow of information.* Patients should have access to their own medical information and to clinical knowledge. Providers need to be able to share information and communicate effectively.

5. *Evidence-based decision making.* Care should be provided that is based on the best and most up-to-date scientific knowledge.

Access to up-to-date information is particularly important to physicians as patients increasingly make their own health care decisions regarding interventions. For instance, complementary and alternative medicine (CAM) is practiced by 25% of patients (Eisenberg et al., 1993) and as many as 39% of older patients (Cook, Frighetto, Marra, & Jewesson, 2002). Evidence suggests that over 60% of ethnic minority elders use some form of CAM (Najm, Reinsch, Hoehler, & Tobis, 2003). Physicians need to know the effects, side effects, and possible interactions of CAM interventions. Resources such as the Natural Medicines Comprehensive Database (www.naturaldatabase.com) can be very useful in discussing the patient's self-care decisions. CAM, a desire to be involved, if not in charge of, medical decisions, and the use of information therapy will all change the nature of the doctor–patient relationship over the next 25 to 50 years.

TRAINING PHYSICIANS IN GERIATRIC MEDICINE

Geriatric medicine emerged as a discipline in 1942, when a group of internists and family physicians interested in advancing medical care for older adults met with the intention of forming a specialty society, the American Geriatrics Society (AGS). Among those physicians were Ignatz Leo Nascher, who coined the term *geriatrics*; Malford W. Thewlis, who was named first executive secretary of the society; and Lucien Stark, who was appointed the first president. However, it was not until the 1970s that the looming demographic imperative brought wider interest in geriatrics. Full status as a specialty in medicine was recognized with the development of the first certifying examination in 1988 and the establishment of an accreditation mechanism for fellowship training. This certifying exam was the first that was accessible through two different primary specialties: internal medicine and family practice. Those with formal fellowship training, as well as physicians who had a significant amount of experience practicing or teaching geriatrics, were eligible to sit for the exam. The vast majority of those that completed the exam in the first 6 years were "grandfathered," based on their own practice-based experience and not fellowship training.

In the initial years (1988–1994) after the creation of the certifying exam, 8,252 physicians successfully passed the test and were recognized as geriatricians (Warshaw, Bragg, & Shaull, 2002). After 6 years, the practice pathway for certification was closed, and only graduates of accredited geriatric medicine fellowship programs were permitted to sit for the certifying exam. Although an average of 2,068 physicians passed the test each time it was offered during the "grandfathering" years, since that track closed only about 326 physicians have been certified each time the test has been offered. From its inception, recertification every 10 years has been required. The number of physicians seeking recertification has been low. It has been estimated that from 1998 to 2004 there was a 34% reduction (from 9,256 to 6,137) of certified geriatricians in the United States (Warshaw et al., 2002).

Geriatric medicine fellowship training is open to graduates of family medicine and internal medicine training programs. When the first programs were established, a 2-year fellowship was required. The early aim of fellowships was to train geriatricians who would be the teachers and researchers in geriatrics. In 1995 the boards of family medicine and internal medicine decided to reduce the fellowship to 1 year, with the hope that a significant increase in applicants desiring clinical practice in geriatrics would be seen. There has been a slight increase, with an average of 215 fellowship graduates each year before 1995, and an average of 299 graduates per year since. Since 1994 only 535 family physicians and 1,737 internal medicine physicians have been certified in geriatrics (Warshaw et al., 2002).

From its inception, the discipline has walked a fine line between declaring itself a primary care specialty and a consultative specialty (Reuben et al., 1993). During the 1990s there was a gradual and continuous decline in the number of medical school graduates choosing residencies in the primary care fields, while an increasing number were choosing specialty and subspecialty areas of practice. The decreasing number of primary care trainees limits the number of residency graduates available for fellowship training slots. The number of internal medicine, family medicine, and psychiatry graduates entering fellowships has leveled off in the last few years. With the expected retirement of many of the geriatricians who received the first wave of certificates and the low number of primary care residents, the number of geriatricians projected to be trained is significantly lower than what will be needed. It has been estimated that at least 9,000 geriatricians were needed in 2000 (Reuben & Solomon, 1997). Although the total number of physicians certified exceeded that number, few were in positions of teaching and conducting research, and many were withdrawing from practice due to retirement or difficulties in conducting a primary care geriatric practice.

Currently, the national average of geriatricians is 5.5 per 10,000 persons over the age of 75. Individual areas range widely from 2.2 (Oklahoma) to 15.9 (Washington, DC). Some of the states with the highest percentage of older persons have the lowest percentage of geriatricians. Florida has only 3.4 geriatricians per 10,000 elders, and Arizona only 4.0.

THE PRACTICE OF *GERIATRICS*

The central goal of *geriatric medicine* is maintenance of functional independence into late life. *Geriatric medicine* deals mostly with persons who have multiple chronic illnesses. The management of chronic conditions requires a different approach than standard, office-based medical care (Wagner et al., 1996). Attention is paid not just to disease management, but, more importantly, to the person's adaptation to functional problems that accompany those conditions. The geriatrician's goal in chronic care is to maximize the older adult's productivity, well-being, and quality of life (William, 1994).

The provision of geriatric care occurs not only in the traditional sites of the hospital and office, but also in nursing homes, assisted living facilities, retirement homes, day care, hospice, and the patient's home. *Geriatric medicine* incorporates the general knowledge of internal medicine and family practice, as well as neurology, psychiatry, and rehabilitation. In addition, geriatricians focus on common geriatric syndromes that do not fit neatly into a diagnostic category (or billing code). Problems such as falls and instability, confusion, incontinence, immobility, sensory impairment, chronic pain, and end-of-life care are commonly addressed in geriatric medical care settings.

Geriatric medicine uses a multidisciplinary approach that focuses not only on medical problems, but also on psychological, functional, social, and economic issues. In collaboration with other disciplines, especially nurses, social workers, and allied health professionals, geriatricians use comprehensive geriatric assessment (CGA) (Solomon et al., 1988). Through CGA, the geriatric team identifies an elder's strengths and weaknesses, diagnoses, conditions, assesses the psychological state and the support system, and develops a comprehensive care plan. Geriatricians recognize that frail elders are at greater risk for iatrogenic (problems caused by health care) complications and medical errors, and seek to balance the benefits of treatment with inherent risks.

A variety of methods for optimizing geriatric care have been designed that involve geriatricians. The Acute Care of the Elderly (ACE) unit has been implemented in many hospitals as a means for ensuring high-quality inpatient care while reducing the risks involved in hospitalization, such as the development of delirium, loss of function, falls, or pressure sores (Palmer, Landefeld, Kresevic, & Kowal, 1994). An alternative approach that is not unit-based uses a multidisciplinary team (Hospital Elder Life Program) to reduce the risk of delirium (Inouye, Bogardus, Baker, Leo-Summers, & Conney, 2000). A subacute model for medical and rehabilitation care has been tried (von Sternberg et al., 1997). Perhaps the largest demonstration of a new model is the Program of All-inclusive Care for the Elderly (PACE). The program was designated a permanent Medicare provider in 1997 and now has been implemented in some 30 programs around the country. The PACE multidisciplinary team receives capitated payments from Medicare and Medicaid to care for frail elders certified as needing nursing home care. The goal of PACE is to keep participants living in the community for as long as possible (Eng, Pedulla, Eleazer, McCann, & Fox, 1997). A 1998 evaluation of outcomes reported that PACE participants had lower rates of nursing home and hospital use, higher utilization of ambulatory services, better health status and quality of life, and a lower mortality rate when compared with matched controls (Chatterji, Burstein, Kidder, & White, 1998). Unfortunately, the program remains relatively small, serving only about 10,000 members nationally.

Though the development of these model programs has advanced our knowledge of what can be done to improve geriatric practice, the reality is that most medical care for older adults is still provided in traditional ways, with the usual specialties providing the care. One reason for this state of affairs is that there are too few geriatricians to meet the needs of the population; also, as noted above, the number of geriatricians is declining.

What are the reasons behind the incongruous state whereby the general population is aging dramatically, but the number of geriatric-trained physicians is declining? Unfortunately, a large part of the problem is the design of Medicare reimbursement. Medicare reimbursement for physicians is modeled on older, traditional primary care medical practices. In such practices physicians have a small percentage of older patients (20% for family physicians and 39% for general internists). The balance of patients in these practices is younger, healthier, takes less time to see, and has better reimbursement with commercial insurance. Essentially, care for Medicare patients is subsidized by fee-for-service and insurance patients.

Geriatric medicine practices tend to be predominantly, if not completely, Medicare reimbursed. The patients are more complex, take more time, and often require involvement of family members during visits. In addition, whereas many primary care physicians have relinquished hospital care to hospitalists and nursing home care to other physicians, geriatricians typically remain involved in these aspects of care. Finally, because many of a geriatrician's patients are in long-term care facilities, there is a large amount of work that is done by phone or fax, both of which are not reimbursed. This is why geriatricians are the lowest paid specialty of all physicians, including pediatrics, internal medicine, and family practice (Warshaw et al., 2002). Although interdisciplinary care is the hallmark of *geriatrics*, much of it is not reimbursed as well. CGA is not reimbursed by Medicare. Specialized evaluations by nurses and social workers, as part of CGA, are also not reimbursed. In an informal survey of leaders in *geriatrics*, concerns over the very survival of the specialty were widespread. Many of those surveyed wondered whether the disciplines of family medicine and general internal medicine would eclipse geriatrics and render the specialty obsolete, and others were concerned whether primary care specialties would even survive.

It is uncertain whether full-time geriatric medical practice will ever be economically viable, at least under the present concepts of private practice and Medicare reimbursement. Most geriatricians serve in a variety of roles in order to succeed in practice, including medical directorships for nursing facilities and health system administrator roles of various types. The fee-for-service practice environment is particularly difficult for geriatricians, as noted above. Geriatricians have functioned well, however, in health system positions, particularly in health maintenance organizations (HMOs). In this setting, the geriatrician's role in designing coordinated care and age-sensitive disease management programs and in caring for high-risk, frail elders has been very useful. In prepaid or capitated programs, the goals of prevention of illness and limiting unnecessary utilization are closely aligned with the traditional goals of *geriatrics*.

Potential solutions to Medicare reimbursement issues abound, but so far we have lacked the political will to implement them. Mixed fee-for-service and capitated programs are being piloted by the Centers for Medicare and Medicaid Services. Risk-adjusted capitation payments are being instituted in Medicare HMOs. Reimbursement codes and payment schedules have been proposed for comprehensive geriatric assessment, physician case management, and asynchronous e-mail communications. Ideally, all activities leading to the improved use of information therapy practices would be valued and considered worthy of reimbursement. This would include reimbursement for e-mail communications, provision of provider-reviewed information resources, and education in self-management skills.

ROLE OF OTHER PROVIDERS

Geriatric medicine has always been interdisciplinary, and if it does survive, it will become increasingly so. Preventive care and health promotion activities will be managed less by the physician and coordinated more by other team members, such as nurse-practitioners, physician assistants, nutritionists, and exercise consultants. Persons with chronic conditions will have access to a health care team in which the geriatrician is an important, though not always central, member. Nurse-practitioners are likely to be main providers of routine services, while the geriatrician focuses on more complex cases and situations where coordinating the work of multiple medical specialists is needed. The geriatrician will also play a major role in assisting patients and caregivers in making decisions about the appropriateness of intensive interventions. Nurses, social workers, rehabilitation therapists, and others will coordinate services to promote independence and prevent unnecessary decline. This approach will be economically necessary (to prevent expensive hospitalizations or admissions to long-term care) but also highly desired by the BBG.

In their brilliant article, Christensen, Bohmer, and Kenagy (2000) describe the role that "disruptive innovations" play in changing health care. Disruptive innovations are "cheaper, simpler, or more convenient products or services that start by meeting the needs of less demanding customers" (p. 104). Within the Medicare population, there are large numbers of healthy persons. The percentage of such persons is increasing and will continue to do so as the BBG matures. The so-called 80–20 rule plays out in geriatrics—80% of elders are reasonably healthy and have low rates of health care utilization and costs. Twenty percent of elders, however, are very high utilizers and have huge health care costs. Medical schools have dedicated tremendous resources to train primary physicians, and even geriatricians, to care for all levels of need, but it is increasingly clear that many patients do not need such highly trained, and expensive, providers. Instead, a system is needed in which the clinician's skill is matched to the difficulty of the medical problem.

As noted by Christensen et al., the entrenched institutional forces usually respond negatively to disruptive innovations. Although over 20 states allow independent practice by nurse-practitioners, the American Academy of Family Physicians policy on nurse-practitioners states that they "should not function as an independent health practitioner" (American Academy of Family Physicians, 2003). Likewise, the professional organization for internal medicine, the American College of Physicians/American Society for Internal Medicine, does not approve of independent practice by nurse-practitioners (American College of Physicians/American Society for Internal Medicine, 2000). In spite of this disapproval, the number of nurse-practitioners and physician assistants continues to grow. However, as in medicine, relatively few of them have chosen training or careers in *geriatrics*.

Given the unprecedented growth in the aging population, it is likely that improvements in training and access to all four levels of geriatric care providers will be needed (Fig. 4.2). In the future, the vast numbers of healthy aged baby boomers will need to develop skills in self-management and information retrieval. They will need quick access to providers who can help in dealing with common, non-life-threatening conditions, such as routine infections and preventive medicine interventions. They will occasionally require assistance from general internists and family physicians for more complex medical conditions. And a small percentage of the older population will need access to geriatricians, primarily those with multiple chronic conditions and problems that affect their daily functional independence.

CHRONIC DISEASE CARE

Chronic disease is and will continue to be the primary focus of geriatric medical care. Health plans and the Centers for Medicare and Medicaid Services have begun to recognize this fact. However, the approach most commonly used at this time is "disease management" (Ahmed, 2002). In disease management programs, a variety of mechanisms are used to optimize care. First, the population at risk is identified. This is often accomplished either by having enrolled patients complete surveys designed to detect high risk, or by analyz-

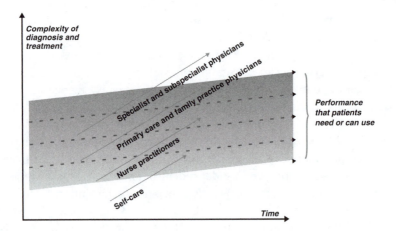

FIGURE 4.2 Disruptive innovations. Over time, and as the complexity of care increases, the types of problems managed by persons of different skill levels increases, used with permission. (Christiansen, 2000.).

ing administrative data for diagnoses or encounters that indicate the presence of a chronic condition. Once the "registry" of members with a chronic condition is developed, interventions targeted at reducing risk are made available to those members. Specialized clinics, targeted educational interventions, group visits, and telephone monitoring may be used to help the person with the chronic condition manage his or her own disease or get help early to avert crises. Sometimes chronic disease management programs are married to educational or reimbursement interventions to physicians in order to improve the quality of care, so-called academic detailing. In academic detailing, physicians in practice are visited by health educators and provided training in disease management. The physicians are paid for their time, so there is no lost productivity. It has been shown to be an effective way to modify physician behavior (Soumerai & Avorn, 1990).

There are problems with chronic disease management programs in *geriatrics*. First, many of the highest risk older patients have multiple chronic conditions. For instance, the average number of medical conditions among PACE participants is eight. It is not feasible, and probably inhumane, to subject a patient to eight different disease management programs. Second, it is possible that applying multiple disease management programs to an individual could actually worsen that person's health status. For instance, too stringent attention to diabetes "control" could lead to an increase in the number of hypoglycemic episodes, a complication particularly worrisome in older patients. Third, disease management programs typically focus on biomedical interventions. For instance, Ellrodt and colleagues (1997), in a review of evidence-based disease management stated, "Management of patients with diabetes is composed of primary prevention and diagnostic, treatment, and rehabilitative strategies for the macrovascular and microvascular sequelae." Notice that there is no mention of psychosocial interventions, or, although diabetes is the sixth leading cause of death in the United States, end-of-life care in diabetes management. Fourth, most disease management programs do not address the critically important issue of function. Maintenance of activities of daily living, mobility, transportation, and a host of other aspects of geriatric care are ignored. Disease management targeted to older adults is largely unstudied. In one recent review of disease management for heart failure in elders, the results were mixed (Ahmed, 2002). In 11 studies, most showed no effect on hospitalization or mortality. The only two that were successful used a team approach, patient education, medication management, diet consults, social services, and home visits, all activities that are central to *geriatrics* and usually not included in proprietary disease management programs. Unfortunately, team approaches to care are not commonly used in traditional medical settings. Hence, it is unknown whether disease management will be beneficial in geriatric populations.

Similar to disease management, clinical guidelines have been offered as solutions to the problem of widespread variance in quality of care. The Dartmouth studies have shown that quality outcomes vary widely across the United States. In addition, there is little evidence that cost of care and quality are directly linked. Some of the areas in America with the highest costs have the lowest quality measures, whereas others known for low cost of care have high-quality outcomes (Fisher et al., 2003). Part of the problem is the traditional approach to care where "experts" have made recommendations that are directly opposed by another group of experts. For instance, the U.S. Preventive Task Force has determined that routine screening of all men using the blood test for prostate-specific antigen (PSA) is not recommended (a level D rating). However, the American Urological Association (AUA) has recommended PSA for routine screening. Advocates for improved cancer care will argue that the more liberal recommendation will help control a potentially lethal disease, whereas health care skeptics consider the AUA recommendation to be a wanton attempt to increase business (urologists are the specialists who perform prostate biopsies and surgeries should the PSA test be elevated). As a result of these kinds of situations, many organizations have attempted to develop clinical practice guidelines to foster evidence-based care.

Clinical practice guidelines are used to provide guidance to practicing physicians and their patients, to summarize evidence-based knowledge, and for continuing education. More recently, they have been used by health plans to set or determine benefit coverage and reimbursement decisions. Perhaps most disturbingly, they have also been entered into testimony in malpractice suits as indicators of the "standard of care." However, when properly used, they are most helpful to the busy clinician or the interested health care consumer. The Agency for Healthcare Research and Quality (AHRQ) maintains a Web site dedicated to clinical practice guidelines (www.guidelines.gov). The National Guideline Clearinghouse had 1,159 published guidelines as of 2004.

Unfortunately, there is little evidence that simply developing and disseminating a set of guidelines has any effect on the quality of medical care (Bland et al., 2003). Even when guidelines are required through regulation, there does not seem to be much improvement. It is only when guidelines incorporate patient feedback and reminders (again, using the principles of information therapy) that they appear to work.

A further problem with current clinical guidelines is that they are rarely developed with specific geriatric issues in mind, such as comorbidity or functional problems. For instance, a guideline developed by the American College of Cardiology/American Heart Association (2001) on heart failure (the most common cause of hospitalization among older persons) included 21 recommendations for assessment, but only one addressed functional status. Out of 17 recommendations for treatment, only one addressed enhancement of function, and none addressed end-of-life care, even though heart conditions are the leading cause of death in older persons.

Recently, organizations dedicated to care of older persons have begun to develop clinical practice guidelines. These guidelines address key geriatric topics such as risk-benefit considerations in treatment, the effect of the patient's functional status and life expectancy on recommendations, and end-of-life care. A good example is the guideline on heart failuare published by the American Medical Directors Association (2002), the association of nursing home medical directors. They include issues like whether to work up the patient's heart failure or attempt to control risk factors, as affected by the patient's personal desires or life expectancy. They also specifically address end-of-life care. Another example is the diabetes care guideline published by the American Geriatrics Society (2003). Unlike the guidelines published by the American Diabetic Association, these address treatment of geriatric conditions, such as falls and incontinence, the importance of incorporating the patient's or caregiver's values, and managing pain.

Finally, there is the problem of implementing clinical practice guidelines for patients with multiple conditions. In an interesting study by Boyd and colleagues (Boyd, Darer, Fried, Boult, & Wu, 2003), a hypothetical geriatric patient with chronic obstructive pulmonary disease, diabetes, osteoporosis, hypertension, and osteoarthritis was envisioned. The most respected guideline for each condition was applied. Boyd et al. found that the majority of the guidelines failed to address comorbid conditions, end-of-life care, quality of life, patient preferences, or short- and long-term goals. If all the guidelines were applied simultaneously to the patient, he or she would receive 13 medications in 21 doses per day, see a primary care provider plus six specialists, experience frequent adverse drug events, and incur medication costs of $411 per month in 2003.

In order for disease management and clinical practice guidelines to be useful in the care of frail older persons, significant review and modification of their design will be needed. This includes more attention to patient values and recognition that there is no time in life when clinical variability is larger than in advanced ages, as well as awareness that both maintenance of function and end-of-life care need to be addressed.

THE ROLE OF THE HEALTH CARE SYSTEM IN *GERIATRICS*

The system of care is as important to achieving desired outcomes as the quality of the care provided within the system. Fragmented, uncoordinated care is unlikely to result in acceptable outcomes, from the patient's view, even if the specific care provided in one part of the system is acceptable. Geriatric care always involves at least two care settings: where the patient lives and where he or she gets care. The vast majority of elders will experience care provided for the same condition (e.g., chronic heart failure) over the long run in a physician's office, during admissions to a general hospital bed for minor exacerbations, occasionally in an intensive care unit, sometimes in a nursing home for convalescence after a hospital admission, perhaps while living in an assisted living facility, and, all too often, finally during a long-term nursing home displacement. In addition, if the patient is fortunate, hospice care will be delivered as he or she nears death, in many of these settings. Multiple providers, multiple assessments, multiple facilities, separate charts, and little or poor communication between each of them are the rule.

The field of quality assurance has taught us that errors are most likely to occur during "pass–offs"—when a work process is passed from one party to another. In order for modern geriatric care to be successful, particularly that care focused on chronic conditions, there will need to be significant improvements in what is called "transitional care" (Coleman & Boult, 2003). Transitional care is defined as a set of actions designed to ensure the coordination and continuity of health care as patients transfer between different locations or different levels of care within the same location. This problem has been exacerbated by the growing trend for physicians to not follow their patients across different health care settings. Although the use of hospitalists may be beneficial for the unusual case of a patient admitted with a rare condition or unexpectedly, the benefit for frail elders has yet to be demonstrated.

Care transitions are all too common (Coleman, 2003). An older person with one or more chronic conditions is likely to see eight different physicians over the course of a year. Twenty-three percent of hospitalizations of older persons end in a transfer to another health care institution, and 11.6% are discharged with home care. Nineteen percent of residents in skilled nursing facilities are transferred back to the hospital in 30 days, and 42% return to the hospital in 24 months. The American Geriatrics Society has recommended a number of steps that can be taken to ensure high-quality transitional care, including the following:

1. Prepare patients and their caregivers for transitions, and involve them in the planning of care.

2. Use bidirectional communication to complete the transition.
3. Develop policies that promote high-quality transitions.
4. Educate all involved health care professionals in the principles of quality transitional care.
5. Conduct research to improve transitional care.

Clearly, the second recommendation would be facilitated by increased use of electronic medical records. To develop a shared electronic record, there will need to be closer collaboration between hospitals, medical groups, long-term care providers, and third-party payers. Information systems need to be developed to conduct safe and effective transitions in care.

Another critically important process that will be needed to care for the frail elders of the future is risk identification and targeted interventions, based on scientifically sound quality indicators. An example of prospective risk identification is the use of the probability of repeated hospitalization measurement in Medicare health plans (Boult et al., 1993), and an example of frailty-specific quality indicators is the Acute Care and Vulnerable Elderly (ACOVE) project (Wenger & Shekelle, 2001). Other health plans have developed similar tools. Some geriatric practice groups have initiated risk screening as part of their enrollment process (PeaceHealth in Eugene, OR; Ron Stock, MD, personal communication 06–01–2005). Center for Medicare and Medical Services now requires health risk screening upon enrollment in a Medicare HMO. Ideally, health plans can use these data to target interventions designed to prevent frail elders from declining. Recent studies have shown that risk identification followed by targeted interventions is cost-effective and leads to better outcomes (Clark et al., 2001).

The RAND Corporation's work on advancing quality of care indicators for frail elders is another important step in the right direction. In the ACOVE project, geriatric experts analyzed evidence available on care of geriatric conditions in multiple settings (Wenger & Shekelle, 2001). Using systematic literature reviews, expert opinion, and the guidance of expert groups and stakeholders, the project developed a set of evidence-based, quality-of-care indicators that are relevant to vulnerable elders. The Medicare Current Beneficiary Survey was used to determine that functional status is a more important predictor of death and functional decline than are specific clinical conditions. The team produced a set of factors that could be asked about in a brief interview, including age, self-rated health, and functional disabilities and limitations, which predict functional decline and death. Using these factors, a scoring system was developed that identified 32% of a nationally representative sample as vulnerable: This group had more than 4 times the risk for death or functional decline over a 2-year period compared with the lower-scoring majority of the sample. When the researchers applied this definition to a random sample of persons 65 years of age and older enrolled in managed care plans, 21% of elders were classified as vulnerable. It is with models like this that health plans of the future will need to target interventions aimed at limiting functional decline and enhancing the functional abilities of those with deficits.

To be both financially successful and promote positive changes in elders' lives, the health plan of the future will need a comprehensive approach that identifies at-risk elders upon enrollment, provides coordinated approaches to those with significant problems (using geriatric-sensitive disease management and clinical practice guidelines), supports primary care physicians in providing and coordinating care, assists with care management across transitions in care, and measures outcomes using frailty-sensitive quality indicators.

ETHICAL ISSUES

Ethical issues abound in geriatric care. The overriding issue for *geriatrics* will not be what we can do but what we should do. An ethical dilemma is involved in almost every important medical decision in *geriatrics*. Although the media have focused on dramatic issues such as end-of-life care and physician-assisted suicide, there are many issues that occur on a daily basis that receive little attention. These entail questions about the informed consent for treatments, safety concerns and "placement" in a facility, control over everyday affairs by residents in long-term care facilities, and artificial nutrition and hydration.

Most health care providers recognize that obtaining informed consent before a surgical procedure is both good medicine and legally required. However, many in the profession, including physicians, do not know what informed consent is or what is required to obtain it. Informed consent is the process by which a patient receives all the information he or she needs in order to make an informed decision. At a minimum the process should include a recommendation from the physician(s), along with risks and benefits, a discussion of alternative treatments and their risks and benefits, and a discussion of what is likely to happen if nothing is done. When considering that certain medications (e.g., high-potency antipsychotics) may have a higher rate of expected complications than many surgical procedures, it is distressing that complete informed consent for these drugs rarely occurs. Most predictions are that baby boomers as they age will demand more of the information they need to make decisions. New methods for providing the information, including interactive computer-based systems, will likely be the answer.

Although only about 5% of elders are in nursing homes at any single point in time, the risk of spending some time in a nursing home is about 25% during that period normally described as old age. Admission to a nursing home is one of the most dreaded events in an older person's life. In fact, 30% of older adults would rather die than go to a nursing home (Mattimore et al., 1997). The decision to move to a nursing home (often called "placement" in medical settings) is usually made by the children or spouse, rather than the patient. Given the antipathy to nursing homes, such a change in living should properly be called "displacement" (Jeffrey Spike, PhD, personal communication, 09–05–2004). One of the most common reasons for displacement is the caregiver's fear for the older person's safety, especially fear of injurious falls or wandering in the case of demented patients. However, the risk of a fall may increase after admission due to the resident not being familiar with the surroundings. A period of depression or sadness may follow admission, which is usually associated with less physical activity and increased risk of a fall. Although the use of physical restraints has diminished dramatically with regulations and quality improvement initiatives, the risk of being restrained in a health care facility is still higher than in the patient's home and brings additional risks (Parker & Miles, 1997). Hence, although caregivers may believe they are seeking placement to increase the safety of their loved ones, the risks may actually be greater following displacement (Kapp, 2003).

One of the reasons that older persons fear nursing home placement is the pervasive loss of autonomy that accompanies admission. Studies have shown that everyday matters, such as choices over bed and rise time, food, roommates, care routines, money, telephone, and initiating contact with physicians, are of great importance to persons living in nursing homes (Kane, 1997). Given the difficulty of providing residents with these choices, it is no wonder that there has been a tremendous growth of alternatives to nursing homes. Geriatricians of the future will need to be advocates for frail older persons to be able to make such choices based on their individual risk-benefit analysis.

As the population continues to age, an increasing number of elderly will develop dementia, most commonly caused by Alzheimer's disease. In the most advanced stage of this condition, neurological problems develop that interfere with normal swallowing function. Hence, many patients with dementia who live long enough will face the question of having a tube placed for providing artificial nutrition and hydration (ANH). Because Alzheimer's disease progresses over time, these choices need to be discussed early when the patient can still express his or her wishes. Unfortunately, end-of-life care is a subject that is usually avoided, and often by the time the medical decision is needed, the patient is no longer capable of participating in the decision. As many as 30% of patients consider living a long time with advanced dementia to be a "fate worse than death" (Patrick et al., 1997). Others, however, may want to live longer regardless of the interventions required. Still others may have mistaken beliefs that ANH prolongs life, reduces suffering, or is just ordinary care, all of which have been shown not to be true (Brummel-Smith, 1998). Many studies have shown that physicians, nurses, and social workers are unable to accurately predict which treatment the patient desires. The only way to clarify patient wishes is to discuss them directly with the patient.

Some patients and their families believe that they can protect their wishes by completing advance directives, sometimes called living wills or durable powers of attorney. Although these documents are clearly beneficial in assigning the legal authority to make medical decisions, they have not been as successful in ensuring outcomes as hoped. Part of the reason is that they are not considered "medical documents," and health care workers may question how they are used in hospital settings. Copies may not be available when needed. The Center for Ethics in Health Care in Portland, Oregon, has created a Physician Orders for Life-Sustaining Treatment (POLST) formis now used in over 90% of Oregon nursing homes and thousands of community-dwelling patients (Tolle & Tilden, 2002). Unlike the advance directive form, this is a medical order written by a physician or a nurse-practitioner and is honored by emergency medical technicians. In addition to including an order to resuscitate or not to resuscitate, it includes a section dealing with the level of care and whether to transfer the patient to the hospital or intensive care unit. It also includes orders regarding the use of antibiotics and artificial nutrition and hydration. It has been shown to significantly increase the chance that a patient's wishes for end-of-life care will be followed (Lee, Brummel-Smith, Meyer, Drew, & London, 2000). Four other states are using a variation or investigating using the POLST form. In order for a patient's wishes to be followed, all states will need to move beyond the traditional advance directive approach (Kass-Bartelmes, Hughes, & Rutherford, 2003).

A common theme in medical care of the future will be the conflict over costs and access. Technology will continue in its relentless progression. The replacement or augmentation of body components, either mechanical or through genetic engineering, will be commonplace. Computerized implantable hearing devices, visual augmentation devices, bladder control systems, and cardiac defibrillators are but a few that are or will be available to fight the common maladies of aging. When new devices are invented, they are often recommended for a restricted set of patients. Over time research studies are conducted on other populations that often show the potential for wider application. The ethics of "rescue" will lead some to recommend that the new devices be widely available, and part of the standard of care. At that point, the discussions begin about coverage of the device by Medicare or other insurance plans. Sometimes, the expensive intervention so widely praised as a savior for people in dire need is later determined to be of no value. Such was the case of bone marrow transplantation interventions for advanced breast cancer. HMOs were widely blasted in the media for withholding medical care "to save money," when in reality the decisions were based on a policy that limited payment for experimental treatments. In time, randomized trials indeed showed no benefits of the treatment, and the controversy has disappeared. But the negative view of HMOs withholding needed care lingers. However, other types of organ transplants continue to be better managed with better outcomes than previously seen. Transplants are being used in an increasing number of older persons. In 1988 there were 266 organ transplants in the United States in persons over age 65. In 2003 there were 2,414 (The Organ Procurement and Transplantation Network, 2004).

Research into the development of technological "cure" of a problem continues while attention to technology designed for ongoing management suffers. For instance, is it a wise use of societal resources to research implantable cochlear devices for elders with presbycusis, where the cost of the device and surgery may be in the range of $50,000 to $100,000 a person, or to research better hearing aid devices, where the ultimate cost will be $700 to $1,500? These decisions are not usually made by informed cost-benefit analyses that are population based and almost never decided based on a public discussion of priorities in health care expenditures. Such a discussion will necessarily include the need to balance cost considerations with the potential to improve quality of life, particularly if the intervention being considered is deemed "Medicare-covered."

Implantable cardiac defibrillators (ICDs) provide a challenging question. Heart disease is the leading cause of death among older people. An irregular heart rate precedes death in virtually every person who dies. There are approximately 400,000 sudden cardiac deaths in America each year. The incidence of this condition is so high that it is possible that all persons could conceivably be recommended for an ICD (Raj & Sheldon, 2001). In a recent review it was stated:

> Implantable [cardiac] defibrillators have proven to be invaluable in the primary and secondary prevention of sudden cardiac death. Incorporation of new technology in these devices has resulted in expanded indications

that improve survival and quality of life of new patient populations. (Rao & Saksena, 2003, p. 362)

Indeed, it does appear that the devices are extremely valuable in properly selected patients. However, what is universally missing from the discussion is the overall cost to society of the use of these devices. With a median survival improvement of only 1.3 years, and at over twice the annual cost of medical interventions ($78,500 vs. $37,200), the cost to society of ICDs in the reported incidence of 400,000 persons would be $16 billion annually (Agency for Healthcare Research and Quality, 2002). How does this expenditure stack up against other potential expenditures, such as covering the 47 million Americans without health insurance? These discussions need to be addressed at a national level. Other new technologies that have proven effectiveness in individual patients will be developed. The question will not be whether the technology works, but whether society believes that implementation of the technology that extends life or improves the quality of life for all patients in need is "worth the cost" and is willing to pay for it.

A related problem is the role of pharmaceutical development in *geriatrics*. Every major chronic condition seen in geriatric medical care has a number of pharmaceutical interventions. Major problems, such as Alzheimer's disease, diabetes, and arthritis, have large advocacy groups who often state that "cure" of the problem is the goal. I believe it is unlikely that there ever will be a cure for these problems. Almost all gains in health seen in the last few decades are related to prevention or early detection. For instance, in spite of a 30-year "war" on cancer, there is little evidence that the incidence of most cancers is declining (Brickley, 2003). Deaths from cancer have declined slightly, and longer survival is common (Wingo, Ries, Rosenberg, Miller, & Edwards, 1998). But these changes in outcomes are due to earlier detection and better management, not cure. Medications will play a major role in that management.

From a societal and ethical standpoint, there are two major problems with medication usage in the older population. The first is the high cost of medications, with the accompanying relative lack of benefits of many new medications developed for use in geriatrics. The second problem is that genetic research will develop an increasing number of very effective drugs that are incredibly expensive.

Newly developed drugs are often touted for their effectiveness directly to the public. For instance, one medical journal marketing campaign for donepezil (Aricept), a cholinesterase inhibitor drug used for Alzheimer's disease, shows an elderly grandmother reading to her grandchild, with the caption implying that Aricept enabled her to read again. Recovery of reading skills lost due to Alzheimer's disease has never been demonstrated in randomized trials. Numerous review articles in the medical journals state that anticholinesterase inhibitors are the "standard of care." The pharmaceutical company that manufactured the drug (Pfizer) conducted almost all the original research related to efficacy, and authors who receive payment from the companies for research or speaking fees usually write the review articles. Yet a recent large-scale, randomized trial conducted under government funding found that while Aricept led to small improvements in cognition and function, it did not reduce institutionalization and was not cost-effective (AD2000 Collaborative Group, 2004). Unfortunately, two "me-too drugs," drugs that have the same mechanism of action as the original product, are now on the market, and annual expenditures for cholinesterase inhibitors exceeds $1 billion. Of note, when searching the Internet for information that is easily accessible to the public regarding the study questioning the value of Aricept, I came across the About.com Web site dedicated to Alzheimer's disease (alzheimers.about.com) that had a banner ad touting that exact drug.

Genetic engineering allows for the creation of novel drugs that have very specific actions and limited side effects. For instance, the drug etanercept (Enbrel) is used for rheumatoid arthritis. Rather than simply treating pain or inflammation, it has been shown to modify the course of the disease. It costs over $2,000 per week. In the United States, decisions to use this drug are made on an individual case basis, most often based on the patient's ability to pay for it. Some have argued that it should be covered under insurance. Unlike the situation with breast cancer described above, there is no question as to the efficacy of the treatment. The science of developing drugs that are specific to a person's genetic makeup is just beginning but will grow dramatically over the next 25 years. Pharmacogenomics will match a patient's genetic structure to a particular drug. These drugs will be as expensive as Enbrel. Our society will increasingly face these issues as advancements in pharmaceutical development continue.

One might hope that physicians could play a "gatekeeper" role in these decisions. That is unlikely to happen, and I would argue that it is not the role of the physician to make such decisions anyway. Physicians face a difficult situation where patients often are demanding prescriptions for the newest drugs, in part due to direct-to-consumer advertising. They fear that if a prescription is not provided, the patient will choose to go elsewhere for medical care. Even more insidiously, many physicians who speak expertly on these subjects have received large subsidies in research funding or honoraria from the drug companies that market the medications (Angell, 2004). More importantly, these are decisions that have to with how our society should choose to fund health care, not a decision to be "made at the bedside."

CONTROLLING HEALTH CARE COSTS

Increased use of organ transplants, development of genetically engineered drugs, and technological interventions will continue to drive up the cost of health care. When the aging demographic changes are factored in, it is clear that the risk of health care consuming greater than the present 14% of the gross domestic product is real.

A number of approaches are likely to be needed to manage the rising costs of care, including a system for providing universal coverage, a process for creating a global budget for national health care expenditures, a system for funding health care that is tax-based rather than employer-based, and possibly, health care rationing.

The Physicians for a National Health Plan have promoted universal coverage, and the concept has been embraced by the Institute of Medicine, the American Academy of Family Physicians, the American College of Physicians, and numerous other professional organizations (Woolhandler, Himmelstein, Angell, & Young, 2003). A national health insurance (NHI) program would save $200 billion annually. It would cover the 47 million uninsured Americans and increase benefit coverage. Much of the savings would come from reductions in overhead that runs 12% to 37% in current HMOs and for-profit insurance plans. Such a plan would be paid for by ear-marked income taxes, payroll taxes, and dedicated employer contributions (Bodenheimer & Sullivan, 1997). Payments to hospitals would be capitated, while payments to providers could be established through fee-for-service or capitated arrangements.

A global budget is a central feature of an NHI program. The federal government would be responsible for the creation of the budget with input of health care experts and citizens. Budget-making processes would include attention to values-based decisions affecting benefit coverage. The issues discussed above regarding the payment for expensive new technologies and drugs would have a forum in which to be debated. That is not to say the process would be easy or without conflict, but at least there would be a process where differing opinions could be expressed.

Without such a change, we will not be able to afford the health care costs of the coming bulge in the geriatric imperative. The only other alternative will be some form of health care rationing (Callahan, 2000). Even with the change, it may be necessary to ration extremely high cost interventions.

Whereas explicit health care rationing for older persons is likely to raise significant outcry, less obvious rationing happens frequently at all levels of care. Health plan decisions regarding payment for various interventions, consumer demands (or lack thereof), differences in the way highly educated versus those with little education utilize services, the use of clinical practice guidelines to drive benefit decisions, and a host of other methods are recognized mechanisms for rationing health care (Kapp, 2002). Callahan (2003) has proposed a model for age-based rationing beginning at age 80 if a lengthy list of basic care needs have been met by society before implementing such a policy. It remains to be seen whether an open approach to health care rationing will be adopted in the United States, as it has in some European countries. But given the rising numbers of older persons and the growing use of treatments of chronic conditions with expensive technologies and drugs, there is little doubt that our society will need to find a solution.

REFERENCES

AD 2000 Collaborative Group. (2004). Long term donepezil treatment in 565 patients with Alzheimer's disease: Randomized double blind trial. *Lancet, 363,* 2105–2115.

Agency for Healthcare Research and Quality. (2002). Retrieved month, day, year, from www.ahrq.gov/research/aug02/0802RA4.htm

Ahmed, A. (2002). Quality and outcomes of heart failure and older adults: Role of multidisciplinary disease management programs. *Journal of the American Geriatrics Society, 50,* 1590–1593.

Alzheimer's disease. (2004). Retrieved September 2004 from http://alzheimers.about.com/od/research/a/aricept_doubts.htm

American Academy of Family Physicians. (2003). Policies on health issues/Nurse practitioners. Retrieved November 2004 from www.aafp.org/x6946.xml

American College of Cardiology/American Heart Association. (2001). Guidelines on heart failure. Available at National Guideline Clearinghouse, www.guideline.gov

American College of Physicians/American Society of Internal Medicine. (2000). Position paper on expanding roles of nurse practitioners and physician assistants. Retrieved November 2004 from www.acponline.org/hpp/pospaper/expand_roles.pdf

American Geriatrics Society. (2003) AGS guidelines for improving diabetes care in older persons. *Journal of the American Geriatrics Society, 51,* S265.

American Medical Directors Association. (2002). Heart failure guidelines. Available at National Guideline Clearinghouse, www.guideline.gov

Angell, M. (2004), *The truth about drug companies,* New York: Random House.

Bland D. R., Dugan, E; Cohen, S. J.; Preisser, J.; Davis, C. C.; McGann, P. E.; Suggs, P. K.; Pearce, K. F. (2003). The effects of implementation of the AHCPR urinary incontinence guideline. *Journal of the American Geriatrics Society, 51,* 979–984.

Bodenheimer, T. (1999). Disease management—promises and pitfalls. *New England Journal of Medicine, 340,* 1202–1205.

Bodenheimer, T., & Sullivan, K. (1997). The logic of tax-based financing for health care. *International Journal of Health Services, 27,* 409–425.

Boult, C., Dowd, B., McCaffrey, D., Boult, L., Hernandes, R., Krulevitch, H. (1993). Screening elders for risk of hospital admission. *Journal of the American Geriatrics Society, 41,* 811–817.

Boyd, C. M., Darer, J., Fried, L., Boult, C., & Wu, A. W. (2003). The challenge of following clinical practice guidelines in the care of older patients with multiple comorbid conditions. *Journal of the American Geriatrics Society, 51,* S220.

Brickley, P. (2003). The 21st century war on cancer. Retrieved from http://www.the-scientist.com/yr2003/sep/feature11_030923.html

Brummel-Smith, K. (1998). A gastrostomy in every stomach? *Journal of the American Board of Family Practitioners, 11,* 242–244.

Callahan, D. (2000). Rationing, equity, and affordable care. *Health Progress, 81,* 38–41.

Callahan, D. (2003). *Setting limits: Medical care in an aging society.* Washington, DC: Georgetown University Press.

Chatterji, P., Burstein, N. R., Kidder, D., & White, A. (1998, July). Evaluation of the Program of All-inclusive Care of the Elderly (PACE) demonstration. Retrieved, from http://www.cms.hhs.gov/researchers/reports/1998/chatterji.pdf

Christensen, C. M., Bohmer, H., Kenagy, J. (2000, September–October). Will disruptive innovations cure health care? *Harvard Business Review,* pp. 102–112.

Clark, C. M., Snyder, J. W., Meek, R. L., Stutz, L. M., Parken, C. G. (2001). A systematic approach to risk stratification and intervention within a managed care environment improves diabetes outcomes and patient satisfaction. *Diabetes Care, 24,* 1079–1086.

Coleman, E. A. (2003) Falling through the cracks: Challenges and opportunities for improving transitional care for persons with continuous complex care needs. *Journal of the American Geriatrics Society, 51,* 549–555.

Coleman, E. A., & Boult, C. (2003). Improving the quality of transitional care for persons with complex care needs: AGS position statement. *Journal of the American Geriatrics Society, 51,* 556–557.

Cook, T. F., Frighetto, L., Marra, C. A., & Jewesson, P. J. (2002). Patterns of use and patients' attitudes toward complementary medications: A survey of adult general medicine patients at a major Canadian teaching hospital. *Canadian Journal of Clinical Pharmacology, 9*(4), 183–189.

Eisenberg, D. M., Kessler, R. C., Foster, C., Norlock, F. E., Calkins, D. R., & Delbanco, T. L. (1993). Unconventional medicine in the United States: Prevalence, costs, and patterns of use. *New England Journal of Medicine, 328,* 246–252.

Ellrodt, G., Code, D. J., Lee, J., Cho, M., Avant, D. Weingarten, S. (1997). Evidence-based disease management. *Journal of the American Medical Association, 278,* 1687–1692.

Eng, C., Pedulla, J., Eleazer, G. P., McCann, R., & Fox, N. (1997). Program of All-inclusive Care for the Elderly (PACE): An innovative model of integrated geriatric care and financing *Journal of the American Geriatrics Society, 45,* 223–232.

Fisher, E. S., Wennberg, D. E., Stukel, T. A., Gottlieb, D. J., Lucas, F. L., & Pinder, E. L. (2003). The implications of regional variations in Medicare spending: 1. Content, quality, and accessibility of care. *Annals of Internal Medicine, 138,* 273–287.

Inouye, S. K., Bogardus, S. T., Baker, D. I., Leo-Summers, L., & Cooney, L. M. (2000). The Hospital Elder Life Program: A model of care to prevent cognitive and functional decline in older hospitalized patients. *Journal of the American Geriatrics Society, 48*(12), 1697–1706.

Institute for the Future. (2000). *Health and health care 2010: The forecast, the challenge.* San Francisco: Jossey-Bass.

Institute of Medicine. (2001). *Crossing the quality chasm: A new health system for the 21st Century.* Washington, DC: National Academy Press.

Kane, R. A. (1997). Everyday matters in the lives of nursing home residents: Wish for and perception of choice and control. *Journal of the American Geriatrics Society, 45,* 1086–1090.

Kapp, M. B. (2002). Health care rationing affecting older persons: Rejected in principle but implemented in fact. *Journal of Aging and Social Policy, 14,* 27–42.

Kapp, M. B. (2003). "At least Mom will be safe there": The role of resident safety in nursing home quality. *Qual Saf Health Care, 12,* 201–204.

Kass-Bartelmes, B. L., Hughes, R., & Rutherford, M. K. (2003). Advance care planning: Preferences for care at the end of life (AHRQ Pub. No. 03–0018). Rockville, MD: Agency for Healthcare Research and Quality.

Kemper, D. W., & Mettler, M. (2002). *Information therapy: Prescribed information as reimbursable medical science.* Boise, ID: HealthWise.

Kurzweil, R. (1999). *The age of spiritual machines: When computers exceed human intelligence.* New York: Penguin Books.

Lee, M. A., Brummel-Smith, K., Meyer, J., Drew, N., & London, M. (2000). Physician orders for life-sustaining treatment (POLST): Outcomes in a PACE program. *Journal of the American Geriatrics Society, 48,* 1219–1225.

Logician: Data health record systems for today's practices. (2004). Retrieved November 2004 from www.medicalogic.com/products/aboutmyhealth

Lorig, K. R., Sobel, D. S., Stewart, A. L., Brown, B. W., Bandura, A., Ritter, P., Gonzalez, V. M., Laurent, D. D., & Holman, H. R. (1999). Evidence suggesting that a chronic disease self-management program can improve health status while reducing hospitalization: A randomized trial. *Medical Care, 37,* 5–14.

Mattimore, T. J., Wenger, N. S., Desbiens, N. A., Teno, J. M., Hamel, M. B., Liu, et al. (1997). Surrogate and physician understanding of patients' preferences for living permanently in a nursing home. *Journal of the American Geriatrics Society, 45,* 818–824.

Najm, W., Reinsch, S., Hoehler, F., & Tobis, J. (2003). Use of complementary and alternative medicine among the ethnic elderly. *Alternative Therapies in Health and Medicine, 9*(3), 50–57.

The Organ Procurement and Transplantation Network. (2004). Data retrieved November 2004 from http://www.optn.org/latestData/rptData.asp

Palmer, R. M., Landefeld, C. S., Kresevic, D., & Kowal, J. (1994). A medical unit for the acute care of the elderly. *Journal of the American Geriatrics Society, 42,* 545–552.

Parker, K., & Miles, S. H. (1997). Deaths caused by bed rails. *Journal of the American Geriatrics Society, 45,* 797–802.

Patrick, D. L., Pearlman, R. A., Starks, H. E., et al. (1997). Validation of preferences for life-sustaining treatment: Implications for advanced care planning. *Annals of Internal Medicine, 127,* 509–517.

Pew Internet and American Life. (2004). Retrieved November 2004 from www.pewinternet.org/pdfs/PIP_Seniors_Online_2004.pdf

Raj, S. R., & Sheldon, R. S. (2001). The implantable cardioverter-defibrillator: Does everybody need one? *Progress in Cardiovascular Diseases, 44*(3), 169–194.

Rao, B. H., & Saksena, S. (2003). Implantable cardioverter-defibrillators in cardiovascular care: Technologic advances and new indications. *Current Opinion in Critical Care, 9,* 362–368.

Reuben, D. B., & Solomon, D. H. (1997). A report card on geriatrics fellowship training programs. *Journal of the American Geriatrics Society, 45,* 112–113.

Reuben, D. B., Zwanziger, J., Bradley, T. B., Fink, A., Hirsch, S. H., Williams, A. P., et al. (1993). Is geriatrics a primary care or subspecialty discipline? *Journal of the American Geriatrics Society, 41,* 444–453.

Sackett, D. L., Straus, S. E., Richardson, W. S., Rosenberg, W., & Haynes, R. B. (2000). *Evidence based medicine: How to practice and teach EBM* (2nd ed.). Edinburgh: Churchill Livingstone.

Scherger, J. E. (2004). Communicating with your patients online. *Family Practice Management, 11*(3), 93–94.

Solomon, D., Brown, A. S., Brummel-Smith, K., Burgess, L., D'Agostino, R. B., Goldschmidt, J. M., Halter, J. B., Hazzard, W. R., Jahnigen, D. W., Phelps, C., Raskind, M., Schrier, R. W., Sox, H. C., Williams, S. V., Wykle, M. (1988). National Institutes of Health Consensus Development Conference Statement: Geriatric assessment methods for clinical decision-making. *Journal of the American Geriatrics Society, 36,* 342–347.

Soumerai, S. B., & Avorn, J. (1990). Principles of educational outreach ("academic detailing") to improve clinical decision making. *Journal of the American Medical Association, 263*(4), 549–556.

Tolle, S. W., Tilden, V. P. (2002). Changing end-of-life planning: the Oregon experience. *Journal of Palliative Medicine, 5,* 311–7.

von Sternberg, T., Hepburn, K., Cibuzar, P., Convery, L., Dokken, B., Haefemeyer, et al. (1997). Post-hospital sub-acute care: An example of a managed care model. *Journal of the American Geriatrics Society, 45*(1), 87–91.

Wagner, E. H., Austin, B. T., & Von Korff, M. (1996). Organizing care for patients with chronic illness *Milbank Q, 74,* 511–544.

Warshaw, G. A., Bragg, E. J., Shaull, R. W. (2002). Geriatric medicine training and practice in the United States at the beginning of the 21st century: The Association of Directors of Geriatric Academic Medicine Programs (ADGAP) Longitudinal Study of Training and Practice in Geriatric Medicine, New York.

Wenger, N. S., & Shekelle, P. G. (2001). Assessing care of vulnerable elders: ACOVE project overview. *Annals of Internal Medicine, 135,* 642–646.

Whelan, T. B., Levine, M., Willan, A., Gafnia, A., Sanders, I., Mirsky, D., Chambers, S., O'Brien, M. A., Reid, S. & Dubois, S. (2004). Effect of a computer-based decision aid on knowledge, perceptions, and intentions about genetic testing for breast cancer susceptibility: A randomized controlled trial. *Journal of the American Medical Association, 292,* 435–441.

Williams, M. E. (1999). The approach to managing the elderly patient. In W. R. Hazzard, J. P. Blass, W. H. Elttinger, Jr., J. B. Halter, J. G. Ouslander (Eds.) In *Principles of Geriatric Medicine and Geronotology,* New York, McGraw-Hill, pp. 249–253.

Wingo, P. A., Ries, L. A., Rosenberg, H. M., Miller, D. S., & Edwards, B. K. (1998). Cancer incidence and mortality, 1973–1995: A report card for the U.S. *Cancer, 82*(6), 1197–1207.

Winkelman, W. J., & Leonard, K. J. (2004). Overcoming structural constraints to patient utilization of electronic medical records: A critical review and proposal for an evaluation framework. *Journal of the American Medical Information Association, 11,* 151–161.

Woolhandler, S., Himmelstein, D. U., Angell, M., & Young, Q. D. (2003). Physicians' working group for single-payer national health insurance. *Journal of the American Medical Association, 290,* 798–805.

CHAPTER 4

The Analytic Template in the Psychology of Aging

Manfred Diehl and Alissa Dark-Freudeman

THE POTENTIALS AND LIMITATIONS OF PSYCHOLOGICAL AGING

The last 5 decades have seen major developments in the psychology of aging. These developments include an increasingly faster proliferation of knowledge (Birren & Schaie, 2001) and a more detailed understanding of the potentials and limitations of psychological aging in different behavioral domains (Baltes & Baltes, 1990; Craik & Salthouse, 2000; Rowe & Kahn, 1998). Although most psychological aging research in the 1950s and 1960s was influenced by biologically oriented models of decline, findings from longitudinal studies published in the 1970s (Eisdorfer & Lawton, 1973; Palmore, 1970, 1974; Schaie & Labouvie-Vief, 1974; Thomae, 1976) and the increasing acceptance of the life span developmental perspective (Baltes, Lindenberger, & Staudinger, 1998) gave rise to a more optimistic view of psychological aging. Schaie (1973) alluded to such a paradigmatic shift when he pointed out that psychological aging tends to be highly diverse across individuals rather than uniform, and that many different paradigms are required to account for this diversity. Thus, supported by the increasing evidence from longitudinal studies of adult development and aging (Schaie, 1983) and from intervention studies that started in the mid-1970s (Baltes & Lindenberger, 1988; Baltes & Willis, 1982), the overall zeitgeist changed in the 1980s and 1990s and resulted in the acceptance of a differential perspective of psychological aging

(Baltes & Mayer, 1999; Lehr & Thomae, 1987; Rowe & Kahn, 1998; Schaie 1996).

A differential approach distinguishes among three major forms of psychological aging: pathological, normal, and successful aging (Rowe & Kahn, 1998). It also focuses on the description, explanation, and optimization of individual development across adulthood and into old age (Baltes & Baltes, 1990; Baltes & Labouvie-Vief, 1973). In doing so, this approach acknowledges potentials and limitations resulting from person-specific factors (e.g., genetic factors, health, lifestyle, intelligence, personality), contextual influences (e.g., social class membership, historical and cultural influences), and the dynamic interaction of person-specific and contextual influences. Inherent to this approach is also the focus on the behavioral plasticity (Lerner, 1984) and the multidirectionality of processes of aging within and across domains of functioning, as well as the acknowledgment that psychological aging is characterized by vast interindividual differences in intradindividual change (Baltes, 1987, 1997).

This emphasis on the plasticity, multidirectionality, and interindividual variability of age-related changes in adulthood and old age is consistent with the broader view of individuals as producers of their own development (Brandtstädter, 1984, 1999; Lerner & Walls, 1999; Riegel, 1975). For example, Brandtstädter (1999) pointed out that, although earlier approaches to human development acknowledged complex transactions between individual and environment as a driving force of ontogenesis, they have largely disregarded a basic aspect of human development. This basic aspect refers to "the fact that the individual, and the adult in particular, takes an active and creative stance toward his or her personal development" (Brandtstädter, 1999, p. 37). Thus recent developments in psychological aging research have increasingly taken an action-theoretical approach (Brandtstädter & Lerner, 1999) and have emphasized the proactive as well as the reactive nature of human development across the entire life span. In discussing the enduring questions and changing perspectives in select areas of psychological aging, we will adopt this broader theoretical framework because we find it useful in illuminating the continuity between past, present, and future.

Because a discussion of all facets and nuances of psychological aging (Birren & Schaie, 2001) exceeds the scope of this chapter, we will discuss enduring questions and changing perspectives by focusing on three sample cases of psychological aging. The three sample cases are the domains of cognitive, personality, and socioemotional aging. In proceeding in this way, our main objective is to illustrate the enduring questions in the psychology of aging by (1) drawing on important research from the past, (2) discussing current empirical findings, and (3) outlining future directions. For each domain, we limit our discussion to those issues we perceive as being indeed enduring and for which exemplary work exists.

THE SAMPLE CASE OF COGNITIVE AGING: ENDURING QUESTIONS

Cognitive functioning is central for psychological well-being and quality of life throughout the life span. Cognitive aging research has identified age-related changes for a number of cognitive functions, not all of which can be discussed in this chapter. Thus we will focus on three major cognitive functions that have been studied in the laboratory, namely, attention, psychomotor speed, and memory. Next, we will discuss longitudinal research on the development of intellectual abilities. Finally, we will focus on research on cognitive interventions and everyday cognition.

Age-Comparative Findings on Major Cognitive Functions

Attention

Attention is important for individuals of all ages because it determines their orientation to the external world. Whether listening to a conversation, driving a car, or crossing the street, individuals need to be able to select and attend to necessary information. Attention is a multidimensional construct that includes many processes, such as selection of relevant and inhibition of irrelevant information, divided attention, and switching between sources of information (McDowd & Shaw, 2000; Rogers & Fisk, 2001). Current findings regarding attention and aging are mixed. In laboratory settings, older adults often perform worse than younger adults on a variety of attention tasks, and age-related performance differences tend to increase with the complexity of specific tasks. However, these age differences are often reduced when sensory deficits or normal age-related reductions in processing speed and capacity are taken into account. When task complexity and familiarity are considered, older adults perform as well as younger adults on attention tasks, including selection, divided attention, sustained attention, and shifting tasks (McDowd & Shaw, 2000; Stine-Morrow & Soederberg Miller, 1999). These results indicate that ability to attend to relevant information remains mostly intact with age, but it is ultimately compromised by the aging of other processes like vision, working memory, speed of information processing, and very likely neural changes in the aging brain (Raz, 2000; Woodruff-Pak, 1997). Moreover, older adults often develop an awareness of when and where their attention may be slipping and adjust their behavior accordingly so that they stay out of harm's way. One aspect of cognitive aging that is closely related to attention is psychomotor speed and how quickly older adults react to certain stimuli in their environment.

Psychomotor Speed

Research on psychomotor speed and performance has one of the longest traditions in cognitive aging research (Welford, 1959). It is well established that aging is associated with a general slowing, impacting such activities as driving, walking, talking, and thinking. Laboratory research has confirmed that older adults are slower than younger adults both physically and cognitively (Salthouse, 1985). In fact, reaction time (RT) increases linearly with age, starting in young adulthood (Elias, Elias, & Elias, 1977). Although research has reliably shown that slowing occurs with age, the underlying causes are still not well understood, and as a result many questions remain. Some of the main questions that Welford (1959) addressed over 45 years ago are still of interest today. For example, cognitive aging researchers still debate whether observable slowing in psychomotor and perceptual performance may be due to the age-related changes in the overall central nervous system or whether they are primarily due to age-related changes in component processes, including age-related changes in memory and/or sensory systems (Madden, 2001). A recent review concluded that research from the two major approaches to studying psychomotor speed has demonstrated that there is general age-related slowing that is shared across a variety of cognitive tasks, and that it is important to account for this general component before specific cognitive processes are implicated (Madden, 2001). Moreover, there also has been increasingly more research showing that adults' performance on measures of psychomotor speed has high validity for predicting functional outcomes, including mortality. For example, Smits, Deeg, Kriegsman, and Schmand (1999) demonstrated that after self-reported health was statistically controlled, general learning ability and cognitive functioning failed to predict mortality, whereas speed of information processing remained a significant predictor. Thus these findings suggest that psychomotor and perceptual speed of information processing may be reliable indicators of central nervous system functioning and may serve as important predictors of functional status and outcomes such as mortality (Madden, 2001). Recent research using advanced neuroimaging techniques (e.g., functional magnetic resonance imaging) has started to address the extent to which neural changes in the brain may be responsible for age-related changes in psychomotor and perceptual speed (Raz, 2000).

Memory

Research has consistently shown that older adults do not perform as well as younger adults on most laboratory-type memory tasks (Bäckman, Small, & Wahlin, 2001; Zacks, Hasher, & Li, 2000). Although the broad term *memory* includes many types of memory abilities, the majority of the abilities required to process and learn novel information appear to decline slowly and continuously from early to late adulthood. When talking about memory, we can differentiate processes from systems (Craik & Jennings, 1992). Processes include the activities involved in learning, remembering, and accessing information. These processes are generally referred to as encoding, storing, and retrieving. Research on memory has shown that older adults are not as efficient as younger adults at encoding and retrieving newly acquired information—at least, they fail to use spontaneously specific encoding and retrieving strategies (Zacks et al., 2000). Nonetheless, older adults can successfully acquire and apply strategies for the encoding and retrieval of new information, if taught to do so.

Systems include types of memory such as working memory, short-term memory, and long-term memory. Age-related deficits have been documented for many systems, including episodic memory, working memory, prospective memory, source memory, and complex procedural memory tasks (Bäckman et al., 2001). However, there are also some exceptions to this rule, including iconic memory, memory for frequently accessed information, semantic memory, and memory for remote historical and personal events (Poon, 1985; Zacks et al., 2000). An extensive body of research examining older adults' performance with regard to memory for text also has shown that age differences in text memory tend to be small or nonexistent (Hultsch & Dixon, 1990). These findings are consistent with other research showing that when information is meaningful, it is more likely to be remembered by older and younger adults alike (Hultsch & Dixon, 1990). This suggests that memory researchers also need to take into account motivational processes that may impact adults' memory performance.

Future Directions

Future work in cognitive aging research would benefit from three major developments. First, Salthouse (1988) stated that the field of cognitive aging lacks a coherent theoretical framework. Additionally, the field suffers from vague definitions of theoretical constructs, compounded by fairly unspecific interpretations of experimental results. McDowd and Shaw (2000) have voiced the same sentiments and echoed the need for more precise theories in the area of attention research. The theories described above highlight this need. Although several theories attempt to account for changes in attention, psychomotor speed, and memory, at this point none of the accounts provide a comprehensive explanation for current findings. Moreover, explanations are often circular. For example, limitations in working memory capacity are often offered as an explanation for slowing in information processing (Salthouse, 1985), and slowing is often offered as an explanation for decreases in working memory capacity (Poon, 1985). Such circular explanations create the impression that cognitive aging research has been chasing its own tail.

Second, although the focus has shifted from specific to more general factors, researchers need to identify what these general factors are and how they create cognitive changes that tend to increase with age. Is speed of processing the main culprit? Does slowing merely limit expression of an individual's ability, or is speed an important component of ability (Salthouse, 1991)? Does the whole chain of events slow, or are specific links between input and output primarily responsible for slowing (Elias et al., 1977; Salthouse, 1985)? Recent research has suggested that a neurological aging process occurs centrally in the brain, and the aging of this epicenter subsequently affects all other peripheral processes including vision, hearing, balance, speed, and cognition in very complex ways (Baltes & Lindenberger, 1997; Lindenberger & Baltes, 1994; Marsiske, Klumb, & Baltes, 1997). This interesting alternative deserves additional investigation.

Third, neuroscience may provide cognitive aging researchers with new tools and avenues to explore these enduring questions. Neuroimaging research is beginning to identify different patterns or levels of activation required for different types of memory and attention tasks (McDowd & Shaw, 2000; Reuter-Lorenz, Stanczak, & Miller, 1999; Rogers & Fisk, 2001). For example, Madden and colleagues (1999) measured cerebral blood flow in younger and older adults during recognition memory tasks. The results showed that cerebral blood flow during encoding and retrieval was greater for older adults than for younger adults. Thus it appears that memory tasks do require additional neurological resources in older adults (Rogers & Fisk, 2001). This new avenue of research may help define attention, psychomotor speed, and memory more concretely by identifying the mechanisms responsible for success on laboratory tasks. Once mechanisms are identified, researchers can explore how these processes interact with one another and how they change with age.

In addition to these three factors, findings in cognitive aging research have been of limited utility because of an overwhelming reliance on cross-sectional, age-comparative research designs. Rather than relying predominantly on cross-sectional comparisons of older adults with college students, longitudinal follow-up studies in the areas of attention, psychomotor speed, and memory would permit the examination of intraindividual changes that occur with age and would ultimately provide a more complete picture of the cognitive aging process. Studies on the development of intelligence in adulthood have already successfully used longitudinal and cohort-sequential research designs (Schaie, 1983, 1994). These studies can serve as exemplars for cognitive aging researchers. In addition, recent studies using intensive repeated measurement designs to examine short-term intraindividual variability in different domains of cognitive functioning have opened a new window through which basic processes of cognitive aging can be studied effectively (Hultsch & MacDonald, 2000; Hultsch, MacDonald, & Dixon, 2002).

THE DEVELOPMENT OF ADULT INTELLIGENCE

Description of developmental processes in adulthood and aging requires that individuals be observed over time. That is, the same individuals need to be studied over the time period of interest. Thus cross-sectional designs traditionally used in cognitive aging research are inherently limited with regard to the extent to which their data can inform us about aging-related changes. Longitudinal or cohort-sequential designs are needed if statements about intraindividual change and interindividual differences in intraindividual change are the objective (Schaie, 1965, 2000). Thus far, research on development of intelligence is one of the few areas in which such designs have been used (Schaie, 1994).

The Seattle Longitudinal Study (SLS) is the most comprehensive and best known study of adult intelligence. Spanning over 40 years, and having followed over 5,000 participants, the SLS has greatly informed our understanding of intellectual development across the adult years. Through the SLS a general pattern of intellectual development has been identified. In general, gains in intellectual abilities occur until the late 30s or early 40s. This period of gain is followed by a period of stability through the mid 50s or early 60s. After this period of stability, decline begins to occur in the 60s; however, this normative decline tends to be modest and does not affect older adults' daily functioning in any major way. Substantial decline in intellectual functioning does not begin until the mid 70s or early 80s (Schaie, 1996). Although this pattern holds overall, Schaie (1996) has also documented that different intellectual abilities (i.e., the primary mental abilities; Thurstone), change in different ways over time, defying a pattern of uniformity.

As can be seen in Figure 5.1, for most of the abilities measured by Schaie (1994), reliable declines appeared only after age 60. The exception was word

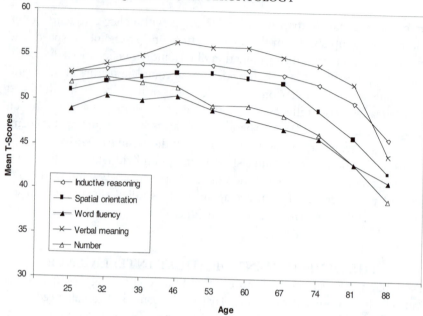

FIGURE 5.1 Longitudinal estimates of mean T scores for single markers of primary mental abilities (from 7-year within-subject data). From Schaie, K. W. (1994). The course of adult intellectual development. *American Psychologist, 49,* p. 306. Copyright 1994 by the American Psychological Association. Reprinted with permission.

fluency, which began to decline at age 53. Examining the pattern of decline more closely revealed a slightly different picture of cognitive aging than laboratory findings would have suggested. For example, the observed decline was not steep and linear, but rather occurred in a gradual, steplike fashion (Schaie, 1994). In general, fluid mental abilities, which tend to be involved in abstract reasoning and complex information processing, declined earlier than crystallized intelligence, which is composed of abilities acquired during the process of education and reflect our everyday knowledge (e.g., vocabulary, numerical ability). However, when crystallized abilities start to decline, their decline tends to be steeper than the decline for fluid abilities.

Using a cohort-sequential design, Schaie (1994, 1996) has also been able to examine whether intellectual development in adulthood differs across different generations or cohorts. Indeed, he found considerable cohort differences in intellectual aging. For example, each subsequent cohort has performed better than the previous one on verbal memory, inductive reasoning, and spatial orientation tasks. In contrast, more recent cohorts have performed more poorly than earlier cohorts on numerical and word fluency tasks (Schaie, 1994). These cohort differences are very likely due to different environmental conditions, such as changes in educational curricula and teaching methods, or technological advances, such as the introduction and dissemination of pocket calculators and personal computers. Such changes in the environment have redefined the cognitive demands that individuals have to respond to on a day-to-day basis and seem to have reshifted the emphasis on certain intellectual abilities (see also Kohn & Schooler, 1978; Schooler, 1984).

Another advantage of Schaie's (1994, 1996) cohort-sequential design is that he has been able to identify long-term correlates of intellectual performance across the adult life span. In addition to cohort differences, person-specific variables affect the development of intellectual abilities. Several factors appear to contribute to individual differences in intellectual abilities, including factors such as physical health (specifically the presence or absence of chronic disease), socioeconomic factors (education, career, income, family structure), social cognitive factors (motivation, self-efficacy), personality factors (flexibility, satisfaction with life), and general cognitive factors (continued involvement in challenging intellectual activities and higher perceptual speed; Schaie, 1994, 1996). It will be essential for cognitive aging research to continue investigating the role these factors play in the maintenance of intellectual abilities in later life, and whether their importance changes for different cohorts of individuals.

Future Directions

Several questions remain to be answered. Although decline has been identified in intellectual abilities after the age of 60, we still know only little about what mechanisms are responsible for the observed declines. We know that biological and environmental factors play a roll in development throughout the life span, but how do these factors interact and affect the aging brain? What are the mechanisms and causes of decline (Schaie, 1996; Schaie & Hofer, 2001)? Are declines in speed of processing the main reason for observed declines in other abilities (Schaie & Hofer, 2001), or is another general factor responsible (Baltes & Lindenberger, 1997)? Do minority groups experience the same patterns of decline (Schaie, 1996)? What do cross-cultural comparisons reveal (Schaie, 1996), and how can environmental conditions, such as the complexity of a person's work environment (Kohn & Schooler, 1978; Schooler, 1984) or involvement in leisure activities (Schooler & Mulatu, 2001), affect the developmental trajectory of his or her intellectual abilities?

Schaie and Hofer (2001) have identified the need for collaboration among investigators and pooling of longitudinal data archives. Longitudinal research is both time-consuming and expensive. Combining efforts across different laboratories and countries will allow cognitive aging researchers to compare results across different populations, and to work with larger populations than might otherwise be possible. To facilitate collaboration, researchers must identify and use standardized and similar measures of intelligence to facilitate the comparison of their findings (Schaie & Hofer, 2001).

Although longitudinal research has shown that declines in cognitive abilities are more gradual and modest than was initially believed, declines still occur and seem to be inevitable in very late life. Thus researchers must continue to examine how and why these declines occur. Are all declines age-related, or are some of the declines due to disuse? Can decline be mitigated or reversed, and if so, to what extent and for what abilities? Cognitive training research has started to address these questions.

FINDINGS FROM COGNITIVE TRAINING RESEARCH

Since the mid 1970s, a number of studies have examined the modifiability of older adults' cognitive functioning. Specifically, since the beginnings of the Adult Development and Enrichment Project (Baltes & Willis, 1982), there has been a substantial body of research showing that older adults can improve their scores on intelligence tests not only through deliberate training, but also through self-instruction and simple practice (Baltes & Lindenberger, 1988; Willis, 1989). Similarly, studies on teaching more effective ways of encoding and retrieving information have also shown that older adults can acquire mnemonic strategies and improve their memory functioning (Neely & Bäckman, 1993; West, 1989; Yesavage, Lapp & Sheikh, 1989). However, one major problem with these intervention studies has been that the obtained improvements tend to be fairly narrow in scope. That is, the training-induced improvements tend to be limited to the trained ability and do not generalize to other cognitive abilities. With regard to memory training, one of the main challenges for researchers has been that older adults fail to use the mnemonic strategies that they learned in the laboratory in their everyday lives (West, 1989). Thus, although a good amount of research has shown that older adults' cognitive functioning can be improved through training, critics have questioned whether such interventions have long-lasting effects and whether they also affect older adults' everyday functioning and quality of life.

To assess whether cognitive training has an effect on older adults' everyday functioning, a large clinical trial, the Advanced Cognitive Training for Independent and Vital Elderly (ACTIVE) study, was conducted, drawing on a large sample of elderly adults from six metropolitan areas (Ball et al., 2002). Results from ACTIVE showed that cognitive abilities improved with training and that training effects were of a magnitude equivalent to the amount of decline expected in healthy elderly persons over 7- to 14-year intervals. However, the cognitive training effects did not transfer to the elderly adults' everyday functioning (Ball et al., 2002). Although this latter finding was somewhat disappointing, the researchers conducting this study argued that longer follow-up may be required to see possible transfer effects, because over the 2-year interval only minimal decline in functional status was observed.

Thus, although the effects of cognitive training may be fairly limited and may not necessarily generalize to older adults' daily lives, it is valuable to understand the range of plasticity in cognitive functioning in late life. Moreover, it is also valuable to know whether reliable decline in cognitive functioning may, in principle, be reversible. Schaie and Willis (1986) addressed this question using data from the SLS. Specifically, they identified study participants who had reliably declined in two intellectual abilities (i.e., spatial orientation and inductive reasoning) over a 14-year period. These participants received five 1-hour training sessions focusing on reasoning and spatial orientation activities and were then assessed again. Significant training effects were achieved for both spatial orientation and inductive reasoning. Most important, however, was that 62% of the participants who had previously declined in their performance were remediated to their predecline level. Interestingly, in both training groups women benefited more from the training than men. In conclusion, this study showed that cognitive training helped to reverse the intellectual decline in a substantial number of older adults who had been studied over an extended time period.

Future Directions in Cognitive Training Research

Willis (2001) pointed out several avenues for future training research. First, training research must remain grounded in experimental design and committed to the advancement of cognitive aging theory and knowledge. Intervention research must not focus solely on cognitive gains, but must also contribute to our understanding of cognitive aging processes by helping to identify the basic mechanisms and processes involved in cognitive decline and cognitive rehabilitation.

In addition to cognitive components, social cognitive factors need to be explored more thoroughly. Willis (2001) mentioned motivation and efficacy as starting points. Social cognitive factors like motivation and feelings of efficacy or beliefs about aging and cognitive functioning in general may affect whether someone chooses to engage in an intervention program. Further, once involved, such factors may also affect whether an individual will put forth the effort required to make an intervention successful; that is, motivational factors may be mostly responsible for the successful transfer of strategies taught in the laboratory into older adults' everyday lives.

Last, researchers must explore ways to maintain training effects by focusing on what older adults can and will employ in their daily lives. The basic goal of cognitive training research is to improve cognitive functioning and ultimately quality of life. If the strategies being taught to older adults do not translate into their daily lives, the entire exercise may become futile. The improvements participants make will be short-lived and consequently, quality of life will not be improved in the long run. Further, intervention research has generally had narrow effects, improving upon the abilities practiced and nothing more. Thus even successful training has not resulted in generalized improvement of cognitive abilities or enhanced daily functional performance. Although ACTIVE and other intervention studies currently seek to identify how training effects can be generalized to older adults' daily lives and everyday functioning, this research has not succeeded yet.

FROM THE LABORATORY TO THE REAL WORLD: EVERYDAY COGNITION

Although experimental research has documented declines in a multitude of cognitive abilities, the majority of community-dwelling older adults appear to function quite well on a daily basis (Salthouse, 1990). This apparent discrepancy has led to a shift in focus from traditional laboratory performance to performance in real-world settings (Park, 1992). What types of activities are important to older adults in their everyday lives? What abilities are necessary to successfully complete these activities? How do we measure these activities and abilities?

Research on older adults' everyday functioning started in the 1960s and 1970s (Kuriansky & Gurland, 1976; Lawton & Brody, 1969). However, it has only been in the past decade or so that researchers have started to examine the cognitive foundation of older adults' everyday competence (Diehl, 1998; Park, 1992; Willis, 1991). Drawing on an extensive literature on assessment of older adults' functional status, Wolinsky and Johnson (1991) reconfirmed that activities of daily living (ADLs) and instrumental activities of daily living (IADLs) are basic building blocks for assessing elderly adults' everyday competence. ADLs include basic tasks related to self-care, such as bathing, feeding, and grooming, whereas IADLs include more complex tasks related to maintaining a household (e.g., balancing a checkbook, food preparation, shopping, and taking medications). In addition to these traditional tasks of daily living, cognitive researchers have increasingly studied older adults' driving competence (Willis, 2000) and their ability to learn using new technologies, such as personal computers (Jay & Willis, 1992) and other devices aiding in performance of home tasks (Czaja, 1997).

The study of older adults' successful performance of everyday tasks has made it clear that researchers need to consider the multidimensional and interactive nature of these tasks and that they must focus on the contribution of a combination of cognitive abilities (Diehl, Willis, & Schaie, 1995). Thus Willis (1996) emphasized that both cognitive and noncognitive factors influence older adults' performance on tasks of daily living. Cognitive factors generally include various measures of fluid and crystallized intelligence and problem solving (Diehl et al., 1995). Noncognitive factors are composed of personal and environmental factors. Personal factors include physical and personal characteristics like health, mobility, personality, and self-efficacy, whereas environmental factors are comprised of an individual's surroundings, including home environment, access to social support, and possibly formal service agencies. At the present time, cognitive factors and health have received the most attention. For example, a number of studies have shown that fluid (e.g., reasoning, fluency of information processing) and crystallized abilities (e.g., verbal comprehension, numerical ability) are not only related to but also predictive of future performance of everyday tasks (Willis, 1996). In addition to cognition, research on health and everyday competence indicates that performance is positively related to general physical health and sensory functioning, specifically cardiovascular health, vision, and hearing (Diehl & Willis, 2003).

Future Directions

Applied research is a new and exciting subdiscipline of cognitive aging research (Park, 1992), and findings from this area will certainly have lasting impact on future generations of aging individuals (Fisk & Rogers, 1997). In a review of the literature on everyday competence and everyday problem solving in older adults, Diehl and Willis (2003) offered several suggestions for how research on everyday cognition should proceed, including the need to consider the impact of technological advances on older adults' lives. Recent decades have seen the rapid introduction and acceptance of new technologies that have affected the lives of many people, young and old alike. Not only has the rate at which such technologies enter the consumer market increased, but each new generation of technology tends to be more complex and requires a more advanced set of skills. If older adults are to take advantage of such technologies, they need to keep up their skills or need to learn new skills that will allow them to perform IADLs and other, more complex tasks of daily living with the assistance of the newly emerging technologies (e.g., online banking). Given this context of rapid technological change, researchers in the field of applied cognitive aging research need to address a number of fundamental questions. For example, how do we define technological competence at different points of the life span, including the later years of life? How do advances in technology impact older adults? How can devices and systems be improved to benefit older adults and to take into account the normative sensory and cognitive changes that take place over the adult life span? Clearly, given the current trends in technological innovation, more attention must be given to technology and its impact on older adults (Diehl & Willis, 2003).

From the perspective of basic research, Allaire and Marsiske (2002) have pointed out the need for multidimensional measures of everyday cognition to fully capture everyday life and the skills necessary to maintain independent living. Combining traditional cognitive measures with well-defined laboratory simulations of everyday tasks and more ill-defined tasks that reflect real-world problem solving holds the promise to greatly contribute to our understanding of how older adults actually use their abilities in their everyday lives (Allaire & Marsiske, 2002; West, 1992).

In summary, cognitive aging research has greatly furthered our understanding of the processes and systems that change during the aging process. Findings from well-designed training studies have clearly documented that older adults' cognitive functioning is modifiable and that even long-term decline may be reversible. Furthermore, research in the area of applied cognition holds the promise of further insights that may lead to improvements in older adults' quality of life.

THE SAMPLE CASE OF PERSONALITY AGING

Unlike research in the domain of cognitive aging, research on personality aging was initiated later in the history of psychological gerontology (Riegel, 1977), but subsequently developed into a major area of inquiry (Neugarten, 1977; Ryff, Kwan, & Singer, 2001). The somewhat delayed start may have been due to the influence of theorists who emphasized the importance of childhood or early learning experiences and proposed that personality was set rather early in life. An additional factor may have been that for a long time only a small number of longitudinal studies were available, which had followed study participants into adulthood and had included measures of personality. Furthermore, the trait approach dominated the field of adult personality research for quite some time, primarily because it provided psychometrically sound measures of personality, and because it amassed substantial evidence in support of personality stability (Costa & McCrae, 1980; McCrae & Costa, 2003). Thus for a long time the major discussion focused on the general question of whether adult personality is stable or whether it can change across adulthood (Heatherton & Weinberger, 1994; Hooker & McAdams, 2003).

Fortunately, recent developments have abandoned this narrow focus and have addressed personality development and aging in a more differentiated way (Caspi & Roberts, 2001; Helson & Kwan, 2000; Hooker & McAdams, 2003; Ryff et al., 2001). As Helson and Kwan (2000) pointed out, recent research and theorizing have given way "to a conception in which personality is relatively enduring but is also expected to change" (p. 78). Moreover, changes in personality are not only anticipated to occur in early and middle adulthood, but are also seen as being possible in old age (Field & Millsap, 1991). As a consequence of this changing view, researchers from different venues are showing a renewed interest in the contributions of personality toward different forms of aging, in general, and toward successful aging, in particular (Hooker & McAdams, 2003; Ryff et al., 2001).

Although definitions of personality abound (Hall, Lindzey, & Campbell, 1998; McAdams, 2001), it is important to define the term *personality* for the purposes of this chapter. Consistent with theories that attempt to bridge the schism between trait theories and more developmentally oriented theories (Hooker & McAdams, 2003; McAdams, 1995), we define personality as the relatively enduring organization of a number of human characteristics, such as traits and states, motives and goals, emotions and coping strategies, and beliefs and self-evaluative processes (Helson & Kwan, 2000; McAdams, 2001; Ryff et al., 2001). Characteristics subsumed under the term *personality* help describe and explain individual differences in behavior and are related to individuals' ways of adapting to challenges over the life span. Moreover, personality characteristics are viewed as major correlates, if not determinants, of psychological well-being and successful aging. Thus it comes as no surprise that Hooker and McAdams (2003) have argued that personality is "the driving force behind all antecedents of successful aging" (p. 296).

Changing Answers to Enduring Questions

Researchers who study personality from a life span perspective have identified several major questions that are enduring in the literature and relevant for evaluating current empirical evidence (Caspi & Roberts, 2001). Of these questions, the following ones are particularly important for aging researchers: (1) When is personality fully developed? (2) How much and what types of continuity can be observed across the adult life span? (3) What factors moderate the amount of continuity or change observed in personality? (4) How is continuity in personality achieved? and (5) How does change in personality come about?

We already mentioned that early theorists postulated that human personality is established fairly early in life. More recently, Costa and Mc-Crae (1994) asserted that personality is fully developed by age 30, which is roughly the age when individuals can be considered adults (Arnett, 2000). These assertions are consistent with the aging stability hypothesis forwarded by Glenn (1980), who argued that as individuals get older, their attitudes, values, and beliefs tend to stabilize and are less likely to change. Although Glenn did not claim that people could not change later in life, his hypothesis has often been interpreted in this way, and only recent theorizing has helped to focus this perspective (Baltes, 1997). Specifically, based on the assumption that processes of development can occur at all stages of the life span, Baltes (1997) has argued that adult behavior, including personality, becomes more consistent yet also retains the potential for change—albeit within a diminished range.

Such a perspective is consistent with a considerable body of empirical research. Roberts and DelVecchio (2000) showed in a comprehensive meta-analysis of 151 longitudinal studies that with age individuals tend to become more consistent, but that change still occurs in midlife and even in old age. For example, based on data from the Berkeley Older Generation Study, Field and Millsap (1991) found that more than one third of the participants increased significantly over time in agreeableness, and both the old-old and oldest-old participants declined in extroversion. Other studies that support the potential for change in adults' personality have been reported by Jones and Meredith (1996), Helson and Kwan (2000), and others (Caspi & Roberts, 2001; Ryff et al., 2001). There is considerable evidence to refute the notion that personality is "set like plaster" by age 30 (Costa & McCrae, 1994). Rather, available evidence suggests personality grows increasingly consistent with age and that this consistency reaches a plateau later in life than originally thought (i.e., around age 50). Moreover, Caspi and Roberts (2001) have pointed out that "life experiences appear to be related to individual differences in personality change well into the 4th decade of life" (p. 51).

Given this more balanced view of adult personality development, researchers have increasingly started to differentiate between different types of continuity. Caspi and Roberts (2001), for example, distinguish among differential, absolute, structural, and ipsative continuity and provide evidence that different conclusions emerge when these different types of continuity are compared with each other. For example, most of the research in the trait tradition has focused on differential continuity, that is, whether individuals retain their ranking within a group over time. This is also often referred to as rank-order stability and is indexed by a test–retest correlation coefficient (i.e., stability coefficient). Indeed, studies have shown high levels of differential continuity of personality traits over time based on self-reports, clinician ratings, and spouse ratings (Caspi & Roberts, 2001; McCrae & Costa, 2003). In addition, some authors have pointed out that several factors moderate the strengths of the stability coefficients (e.g., age of initial assessment; interval of assessment; see Ardelt, 2000), and that the test–retest correlations tend to account for only 35% to 50% of the variance in personality measures (Labouvie-Vief & Diehl, 1998).

Moreover, the focus on rank-order stability has been criticized because it does not take into account changes that may happen with regard to a person's absolute values on a personality dimension. For example, if over the course of a 10-year period the scores of most adults on a scale measuring self-esteem tend to increase by about 10 points, than this change is only insufficiently captured by a correlation coefficient, because the rank order is mostly preserved despite the fact that most individuals changed with regard to their absolute scores. This criticism has led researchers to focus on absolute continuity, or the constancy in the quantity or amount of an attribute over time (i.e., mean-level continuity). Not surprisingly, a number of studies have shown significant mean-level changes in personality characteristics such as conscientiousness, emotional stability, openness to new experiences, self-control, and dominance across the adult life span (Helson & Kwan, 2000). These changes have been documented for several samples, different assessment instruments, and with different statistical methods, including growth curve analysis, and even for individuals in old age (Field & Millsap, 1991; Jones & Meredith, 1996; Mroczek & Spiro, 2003). There is sufficient evidence to infer that for some individuals, personality development continues until late in life and that it may be particularly important for later life resilience (Ryff et al., 2001).

Researchers have not only adopted a more differentiated view when examining the empirical evidence regarding personality development in adulthood, but they have also started to pay greater attention to factors that moderate how much continuity or change can be observed (Ardelt, 2000; Caspi & Roberts, 2001; Labouvie-Vief & Diehl, 1998). Ardelt (2000) and Roberts and DelVecchio (2000) have pointed out that the amount of continuity or change that is observed in longitudinal studies is a function of (1) the age of the participants at the outset, (2) the time span over which participants are observed, and (3) the methods of assessment employed. For example, stability coefficients tend to increase as the age of the participants at entry into the study increases. In contrast, stability coefficients tend to decrease as the time interval between measurements increases and vice versa (Ardelt, 2000). Roberts and DelVecchio (2000) reported that the average retest interval for the 151 studies included in their meta-analysis was 6.8 years. Furthermore, instruments that measure relatively enduring personality traits, such as the big five personality factors (i.e., neuroticism, extroversion, openness to experience, conscientiousness, and agreeableness) tend to produce higher stability coefficients than instruments that are specifically designed to assess change (Ardelt, 2000; Helson & Kwan, 2000).

Besides these methodological and design-related aspects, investigators have increasingly acknowledged that research on adult personality development needs to be more sensitive to the biosocial transitions of adulthood and to historical factors that may impact personality development across the life span (Caspi & Roberts, 2001; Hooker & McAdams, 2003). In this sense, researchers have started to pay closer attention to Neugarten's (1977) advice that "age itself is an empty variable, for it is not merely the passage of time, but the various biological and social events that occur with the passage of time that have relevance for personality change" (p. 633). Underlying this argument is the assumption that changes in personality are most likely to occur at times when an established person–environment fit is challenged either due to biological (e.g., menopause, deteriorating health) or social changes (e.g., transition to retirement). For example, it has been shown that the absolute scores of individuals' self-conceptions changed during important life course transitions (e.g., transition to retirement), whereas the rank order remained fairly stable during these transitions (Caspi & Roberts, 2001).

Similarly, historical factors, such as cohort membership and the experience of specific historical events, may influence personality factors such as norm adherence, behavioral flexibility, and social responsibility in predictable ways (Helson & Kwan, 2000; Schaie & Willis, 1991). For example, Roberts and Helson (1997) showed that the women in the Mills Longitudinal Study changed with regard to Gough's (1991) secular trends index, an index that captures changes in cultural climate in the United States between 1950 and 1985, in a similar way as cross-sectional samples of young adults had changed. Specifically, over the course of their adult years, these women manifested increases in narcissism and individualism and decreases in social responsibility, reflecting the ways in which the overall U.S. culture had changed over the same period.

Given that the empirical findings support a perspective on adult personality that emphasizes both continuity/stability and change (Helson & Kwan, 2000; Ryff et al., 2001), researchers have increasingly asked questions that address mechanisms by which continuity and change are achieved (Caspi & Roberts, 2001). With regard to questions of how continuity in personality is achieved, Caspi and Roberts (2001) offered several possibilities. First, based on findings from behavioral genetics, these authors argued that a good deal of continuity appears to be due to genetic factors. Second, a rival explanation has been that people's personality stays stable because the environment in which they live remains stable. However, because people's genetic makeup does not exist in a vacuum, it is important to acknowledge that continuity is more likely the result of transactional processes between genes and environmental factors. Thus personality characteristics may show continuity not only because of people having a specific set of genes or because they live in stable environments, but because they engage in specific person–environment transactions that promote continuity.

Caspi and Roberts (2001) identified three types of person–environment transactions that contribute to continuity in personality. They refer to these types of transactions as reactive, evocative, and proactive person–environment transactions. Reactive person–environment transactions reflect that individuals extract a subjective psychological life space from the objective surroundings and that they react to the events that take place in that life space. Thus individuals react to their environment by selectively attending to information that confirms their values, beliefs, traits, and behavior, and this process results in personality continuity. In contrast, evocative person–environment transactions contribute to continuity because individuals "evoke distinctive reactions from others on the basis of their unique personality characteristics" (Caspi & Roberts, 2001, p. 58). The more others respond to an individual in a consistent way, the more these others contribute to personality continuity. Finally, individuals are not only reactive or evocative, but also proactive. That is, individuals choose environments deliberately, and they do so based on preferences and similarities. Such proactive transactions are particularly apparent in friendship formation and mate selection (Asendorpf & Wilpers,

1998). For example, it is well known that partners tend to be similar in physical characteristics, cognitive abilities, values, attitudes, and personality traits (Caspi & Herbener, 1990; Epstein & Guttman, 1984). Such assortative mating results in the creation of social networks that further reinforce certain values, attitudes, and behaviors, thus promoting continuity in personality.

Despite these mechanisms promoting continuity, individuals are also capable of changing their behavior. Caspi and Roberts (2001) alluded to several mechanisms that can explain how change in personality comes about. Specifically, they discussed individuals' responding to contingencies, the ability to observe one's own behavior, and listening to and watching others. Although responding to reinforcers and punishers is a simplistic form of behavior change, it is nevertheless powerful and can shape complex behavior, such as socially withdrawn or impulsive behavior. However, besides simply responding to contingencies, people also can observe their own actions, reflect on them, and gradually adopt new behaviors that may be more effective and gratifying. This mechanism may be of particular importance in late life, because age-related losses and impairments often confront older adults with situations that require a reevaluation of personal goals and readjustments of the means by which the goals can be achieved. Finally, watching the behavior of others or listening to the feedback from others can promote change in one's own behavior (Bandura, 1986).

In summary, a growing body of literature suggests that an important part of personality development in adulthood consists of finding the right balance between continuity and change and of developing behavioral repertoires that meet the inherent challenges of the physical, social, and psychological aging process. Theorists like Hooker and McAdams (2003) have been sensitive to these challenges and have proposed a model that integrates personality structures (i.e., factors that promote stability) and personality processes (i.e., factors that facilitate change) into a newly emerging model of human personality.

Future Directions: Putting the "Person" Back into Personality Research

One important development in the area of personality and aging has been the emergence of theoretical models that put the "person" back into personality research (Carlson, 1971). Specifically, the model of Hooker and McAdams (2003) represents an attempt to bridge the long-standing schism between structure-oriented and process-oriented theories of personality and builds on the broader notion that a comprehensive understanding of personality requires studying behavior at multiple levels (McAdams, 1995). These authors postulate three broad levels of personality and specify at each level structures and corresponding processes. For example, at the most general level the structures are traits that account for a person's behavioral signature and consistency over time. The corresponding process construct is that of states, referring to within-person processes that are less stable and more subject to intraindividual fluctuation. At the second level, the structural components are personal action constructs that include goals, personal strivings, and life tasks. The corresponding processes are related to self-regulation in the context of goals, strivings, and life tasks, and include self-efficacy beliefs and outcome expectancies. The third level includes as structure a person's life story, that is, a person's narrative understanding of his or her life, and as corresponding processes forms of self-narration (e.g., remembering, reminiscence, and storytelling).

Although empirical studies can hardly address all of these levels and constructs simultaneously, Hooker and McAdams's (2003) model is important for several reasons. First, it provides a common language and framework to address issues of personality and aging that have often been dealt with in a fragmented way. Second, it helps to address the stability versus change dichotomy and brings a fresh look at some central issues of personality development, including the observation that individuals tend to become more diverse as they age. Third, the proposed model also renews the call for methodological diversity in the study of the aging personality, including the call for intensive repeated observations of individuals with the goal of understanding how within-person variability contributes to between-person differences over time (Nesselroade & Ford, 1985). Finally, this model opens the way for the integration of concepts that traditionally have not been part of adult personality research, such as self-representations and autobiographical memory.

Some of the exciting future directions in this area of psychological aging will see the revisiting of selected key issues within a new theoretical framework, with greater conceptual clarity and more sophisticated statistical methods. One example in support of this argument is the recent focus on adults' self-concept as a psychological resource in the aging process (Brandtstädter & Greve, 1994; Freund & Smith, 1999), and related empirical findings that show the importance of coherent self-representations for psychological well-being in old age (Diehl, Hastings, & Stanton, 2001). Focusing on adults' self-representations as a psychological resource opens the view for cognitive processes that individuals activate in negotiating both continuity and change, showing how individuals tend to construct and reconstruct their self-concept in response to or anticipation of specific developmental tasks and age-related challenges (Brandtstädter, 1999; Markus & Herzog, 1991).

Another promising future direction in studying personality aging is the increased use of multiple assessment procedures and more sophisticated statistical methodology, especially as part of longitudinal investigations. For example, although most of the current personality research is based on self-report data, there is an increasing emphasis on proxy reports (e.g., spouse, family member), observational and behavioral data, and also on new technologies, such as methods of neuroimaging (Craik et al., 1999; Ochsner & Lieberman, 2001). In particular, the use of neuroimaging holds promise that greater insight into the neurological substrates of personality aging can be gained. Similarly, use of new statistical methods, such as multilevel modeling of individual growth curves (Mroczek & Spiro, 2003), and use of latent growth curve modeling (Small, Hertzog, Hultsch, & Dixon, 2003) have introduced new levels of sophistication. Use of these methods promises valuable future contributions to understanding complex person–context interactions and crucial questions related to personality, health, and psychological well-being (Ryff et al., 2001).

THE SAMPLE CASE OF SOCIOEMOTIONAL AGING

Both cognitive and personality aging have often been investigated without major concern for the social context in which they take place. Research on the social relationships of older adults and different dimensions of socioemotional aging, however, have a long and interesting history in psychological aging research (Cumming & Henry, 1961; Havighurst & Albrecht, 1953). Accordingly, we have chosen this area as our third sample case.

Enduring Questions and Changing Perspectives on Socioemotional Aging

The bulk of research in the area of socioemotional aging has addressed the following enduring questions: Is it more adaptive for individuals to reduce their social relationships as they age, or is it better to maintain as many social relationships as possible? How do adults' social relationships change as they age? How and to what extent do social relationships contribute to psychological well-being in adulthood and old age?

Two major theories, disengagement theory and activity theory, focused primarily on the first question. Cumming and Henry's (1961) much debated disengagement theory of aging stated that disengagement from social roles and relationships was a normative, adaptive, and universal process motivated by individuals' preparation for death. Although Cumming and Henry emphasized that optimal disengagement is a mutual process between individual and society, they were also aware that in reality it often occurs in a unilateral way. That is, either society releases an individual from a role (e.g., work) before he or she is ready to be released, or an individual disengages from a role before society is ready to let him or her go. In instances where unilateral disengagement occurs, complications may arise and may result in lowered life satisfaction for the individual.

Although Cumming and Henry (1961) presented a theory that combined individual-psychological variables with social-structural variables, some of the nuances of their theory were often insufficiently assessed in empirical research. Disengagement theory was roundly criticized as being overly negative and restrictive (Hochschild, 1975). However, when researchers paid attention to the more detailed statements of the theory, they found support for the notion that disengagement is not an either-or scenario, but often happens in gradual and selective ways. Moreover, if the person is able to exert control over the timing of the disengagement and can plan for the situation afterwards, then the negative effects of giving up a role or a relationship tend to be diminished or disappear completely, as has been documented in research on retirement (Kim & Moen, 2001). From a historical perspective, disengagement theory represents an important step toward more refined theories of socioemotional aging, and some elements of the theory are still preserved in more recent theories (Carstensen, Isaacowitz, & Charles, 1999).

The second theory that addressed the adaptive nature of social relationships in old age was activity theory (Cavan, Burgess, Havighurst, & Goldhamer, 1949; Havighurst & Albrecht, 1953). Contrary to disengagement theory, activity theory argued that the more socially active older adults are, the greater their satisfaction with life will be. Specifically, proponents of activity theory drew on self-concept and role theory when they argued that individuals' self-conceptions are greatly influenced by the social roles they hold and by the feedback they receive in their relationships with others (i.e., the "looking glass self"; Cooley, 1902). Because the process of aging often brings a loss of roles (e.g., end of active parenting, retirement) and relationships (e.g., loss of spouse and friends), it is essential for maintaining a positive sense of self that older adults stay socially active as much as possible and substitute lost roles and relationships with new ones.

Although there is a good deal of empirical evidence in support of activity theory (Hansson & Carpenter, 1994), there are also reasons why the original version of activity theory has been of limited utility. First, many investigators assumed that all older persons need and desire high levels of social activity and hence neglected that particular social activities and relationships tend to have specific meanings for older adults. Lemon, Bengtson, and Peterson (1972), for example, found that the relationship between well-being and social activity in old age depended strongly on the type of the social role activity. Second, and perhaps most importantly, activity theorists focused primarily on the quantity of social activities rather than the quality. However, a substantial body of research exists showing that the quality of relationships tends to be more important for psychological well-being than the quantity of contact (Lang, 2001).

In summary, although disengagement and activity theory have been important in setting the stage for later theorizing and research, they have been criticized for focusing too narrowly on old age rather than looking at social relationships across the entire life span. Advocates of a life span view have argued that changes in social relationships need to be explained across the whole adult life span rather than just for the period of old age. Two theories that take a life span approach on social relationships are the social convoy theory (Antonucci, 2001; Kahn & Antonucci, 1980) and socioemotional selectivity theory (Carstensen, 1993; Carstensen et al., 1999). In the following sections, we will focus on socioemotional selectivity theory to illustrate how research on adults' social relationships has progressed in recent years, and how it has addressed the role of emotion as part of social relationships.

A Life Span View of Social Relationships: Socioemotional Selectivity Theory

Socioemotional selectivity theory (Carstensen, 1993) contends that social relationships across the life span are motivated by two broad social goals: the acquisition of knowledge and the regulation of emotion. As Figure 5.2 illustrates, which of these goals predominates is related to individuals' perception of personal lifetime (Carstensen et al., 1999). That is, if people have a perception of time as being unlimited, their social relationships will primarily be motivated by the goal of knowledge acquisition. For example, in young adulthood a great deal of social behavior is related to acquiring the skills for being successful in the workplace and in one's chosen profession. Similarly, in middle adulthood social relations often emerge out of instrumental tasks associated with child rearing and with launching one's children beyond the world of the nuclear family. In both of these instances, social relations tend to be primarily motivated by the acquisition and exchange of information. In contrast, in later adulthood or under circumstances in which an individual's personal lifetime is limited (e.g., when diagnosed with a life-threatening illness), the regulation of emotion is of primary importance, whereas the ac-

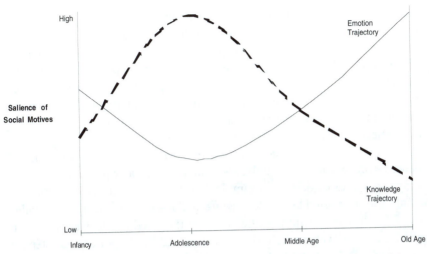

FIGURE 5.2 Idealized model of socioemotional selectivity theory's conception of the salience of two classes of social motives across the life span. From Carstensen, L.L. Gross, J., & Fung, H. (1997). The social context of emotion. *Annual Review of Geriatrics and Gerontology, 17,* p. 331. Copyright 1997 by Springer Publishing Company, Inc. Reprinted with permission.

quisition of new information is less important. When emotion regulation is the primary motivation for individuals' social behavior, they tend to become more selective in their choice of social partners, almost always preferring partners who are familiar to them. By limiting their interactions to familiar partners, people optimize positive emotions, because the behavior of those partners tends to be fairly predictable.

A considerable amount of empirical research from cross-sectional and longitudinal studies supports the main tenets of socioemotional selectivity theory. For example, using longitudinal data from the Child Guidance Study, Carstensen (1992) found that across adulthood frequency of interaction with acquaintances declined, whereas interaction with emotionally close partners was maintained or increased. Similarly, Lang (2000) showed for a sample of older adults that although network size decreased over a 4-year period, relationships with emotionally close partners were maintained. Moreover, the decreases in network size were significantly associated with older adults' subjective perceptions of nearness of death (Lang, 2000).

The contention that it is not a person's age, but his or her perception of personal lifetime that determines the preference for certain social partners has been supported in several studies (for a summary, see Carstensen et al., 1999). Carstensen and Fredrickson (1998) found that in a sample of middle-aged men who differed by human immunodeficiency virus (HIV) status, the men who where HIV-positive and actively experiencing symptoms showed the same pattern of social preferences as older adults. In contrast, HIV-negative and HIV-positive but asymptomatic men had social preferences characteristic of individuals their age. Moreover, studies in which adults' perceptions of personal lifetime were experimentally manipulated have shown that the preferences for social partners changed as predicted by socioemotional selectivity theory (Carstensen et al., 1999).

Finally, there is evidence that the selection of social relationships is a proactive process and tends to be associated with greater psychological well-being. Longitudinal data, for example, have documented that reductions in social relations started long before age-related losses (e.g., decreased mobility, frailty) could have been the cause, and that these reductions were limited to individuals who were perceived as less close and less important (Carstensen, 1992; Lang, 2000; Lang & Carstensen, 1994). However, there is solid support for the hypothesis that the presence of emotionally close social partners is associated with greater well-being, as indicated by lower levels of loneliness and greater social satisfaction (Lang, 2000).

In summary, socioemotional selectivity theory has qualified some of the main statements of disengagement and activity theory and has directed researchers' attention to (1) the broader motivations that underlie social behavior, (2) the central role of personal lifetime awareness, and (3) the proactive nature of selecting social partners. In this sense, socioemotional selectivity theory has helped formulate questions for future research and has contributed to setting the stage on which this future work can take place.

Future Directions in Socioemotional Aging

The future of research on socioemotional aging looks promising because this behavioral domain provides an ideal arena for studying the confluence of a number of influences and for illuminating some positive age-related changes. In the following section we will sketch out what we believe are some likely and promising future directions.

One future direction will likely extend the new emphasis on the role of personal lifetime awareness as a causal factor in socioemotional aging (Carstensen et al., 1999). Specifically, work in this area is likely to examine in more detail how individuals' awareness of developmental stages, transitions, and deadlines (Heckhausen, Wrosch, & Fleeson, 2001) is embedded into the larger context of personal lifetime awareness and how this awareness influences the choices of social roles and relationships across the life span. An additional extension of this work will probably focus on the connection between lifetime awareness and how personal life stories and self-conceptions are subjectively revisited and cognitively reconstructed to promote successful aging (Bluck & Habermas, 2001; Brandtstädter & Greve, 1994).

A second extension of current research will focus more intensively on the exact mechanisms by which social relationships are used to regulate emotions. Although some theorists have suggested older adults may be better in anticipating social situations that meet their emotional needs (i.e., antecedent-focused regulation; Carstensen, Gross, & Fung, 1997), others have pointed out that this phenomenon may not necessarily indicate greater efficiency, but may reflect a fairly simple form of cognitive processing in the service of affect optimization (Labouvie-Vief & Medler, 2002). The increased amount of research on emotional development and aging (Magai & McFadden, 1996) can inform this research and can, in turn, be enriched by contributions from the area of socioemotional aging. Especially, studying the working together of cognitive, personality-related, and emotional factors as they influence adults' social relationships in old age has the potential for providing new insights into the role of social relationships in achieving a good person–environment fit throughout the aging process (Lang, 2001).

Third, although a great deal of research has demonstrated the positive effects of social relationships (Antonucci, 2001; Ryff & Singer, 2001), longitudinal data that describe individuals' social relationships over major portions of the adult life span are still fairly scarce. Future research would benefit from such longitudinal studies and from extensions into very late life (Lang, 2001). Studying adults in very late life can provide a unique window through which we can view how normative cognitive and sensory declines may affect the quality of social relationships during the latter part of the life span.

Finally, although most of the research on social relations in adulthood and old age has focused on their beneficial effects, researchers have increasingly recognized that social relationships can be a mixed blessing (Rook, 1998; Stephens, Kinney, Norris, & Ritchie, 1987). Negative interactions, for example, can take the form of criticizing, demanding, misunderstanding, or overprotecting and can undermine a person's sense of mastery and autonomy. Moreover, negative social relationships may add a burden to older adults' lives by letting them know that their social support resources may not be available when bad things happen (Ingersoll-Dayton, Morgan, & Antonucci, 1997). Future research needs to gain a better understanding of the nature and effects of negative social relations, and how adults may "prune off" burdensome relationships in the process of growing older—very likely another aspect of socioemotional selectivity.

CONCLUSION AND GENERAL OUTLOOK

The purpose of this chapter was to give an overview of some of the enduring questions that psychologists specializing in different areas of human behavior and aging have addressed over the past several decades, and the future directions that may be pursued on the background of the currently available knowledge in these areas. Without a doubt, this overview suggests that the psychology of aging is alive and well and that major insights have been gained with regard to cognitive functioning in adulthood and old age, the role of personality and the role of social relationships in the aging process. Moreover, researchers in all of these areas have increasingly put their findings, which were often obtained under carefully controlled conditions in the laboratory, to the "road test" and have made the step out of the laboratory into the real world in which older adults live. This chapter has also tried to show how bridges can be built between basic and applied research and how such bridge building can be used to optimize the aging process and to improve older adults' quality of life. In terms of general outlook for the field of psychology of aging, we suggest that the most exciting research will result from initiatives that continue to take a multidisciplinary approach and try to translate theoretical questions into real-world applications. Recent initiatives of funding agencies such as the National Institute on Aging and private foundations (e.g., the Retirement Foundation) bear witness to this trend.

REFERENCES

Allaire, J. C., & Marsiske, M. (2002). Well- and ill-defined measures of everyday cognition: Relationship to older adults' intellectual ability and functional status. *Psychology and Aging, 17,* 101–115.

Antonucci, T. C. (2001). Social relations: An examination of social networks, social support, and sense of control. In J. E. Birren & K. W. Schaie (Eds.), *Handbook of the psychology of aging* (5th ed., pp. 427–453). San Diego, CA: Academic Press.

Ardelt, M. (2000). Still stable after all these years? Personality stability theory revisited. *Social Psychology Quarterly, 63,* 392–405.

Arnett, J. J. (2000). Emerging adulthood: A theory of development from the late teens through the twenties. *American Psychologist, 55,* 469–480.

Asendorpf, J. B., & Wilpers, S. (1998). Personality effects on social relationships. *Journal of Personality and Social Psychology, 74,* 1531–1544.

Bäckman, L., Small, B. J., & Wahlin, A. (2001). Aging and memory: cognitive and biological perspectives. In J. E. Birren & K. W. Schaie (Eds.), *Handbook of the psychology of aging* (5th ed., pp. 349–377). San Diego, CA: Academic Press.

Ball, K., Berch, D. B., Helmers, K. F., Jobe, J. B., Leveck, M. D., Marsiske, M., et al. J. N., (2002). Effects of cognitive training interventions with older adults: A randomized controlled trial. *Journal of the American Medical Association, 288*, 2271–2281.

Baltes, P. B. (1987). Theoretical propositions of life-span developmental psychology: On the dynamics between growth and decline. *Developmental Psychology, 23*, 611–626.

Baltes, P. B. (1997). On the incomplete architecture of human ontogeny: Selection, optimization, and compensation as foundation of developmental theory. *American Psychologist, 52*, 366–380.

Baltes, P. B., & Baltes, M. M. (1990). Psychological perspectives on successful aging: The model of selective optimization with compensation. In P. B. Baltes & M. M. Baltes (Eds.), *Successful aging: Perspectives from the behavioral sciences* (pp. 1–34). New York: Cambridge University Press.

Baltes, P. B., & Labouvie-Vief, G. (1973). Adult development of intellectual performance: Description, explanation, and modification. In Eisdorfer, C., & Lawton, M. P. (Eds.), *The psychology of adult development and aging* (pp. 157–219). Washington, DC: American Psychological Association.

Baltes, P. B., & Lindenberger, U. (1988). On the range of cognitive plasticity in old age as a function of experience: 15 years of intervention research. *Behavior Therapy, 19*, 283–300.

Baltes, P. B., & Lindenberger, U. (1997). Emergence of a powerful connection between sensory and cognitive functions across the adult life span: A new window to the study of cognitive aging? *Psychology and Aging, 12*, 12–21.

Baltes, P. B., Lindenberger, U., & Staudinger, U.M. (1998). Life-span theory in developmental psychology. In W. Damon (Series Ed.) & R. M. Lerner (Vol. Ed.), *Handbook of child psychology: Theoretical models of human development* (Vol. 1, pp. 1029–1143). New York: Wiley.

Baltes, P. B., & Mayer, K. U. (Eds.). (1999). *The Berlin Aging Study: Aging from 70 to 100*. New York: Cambridge University Press.

Baltes, P. B., & Willis, S. L. (1982). Enhancement (plasticity) of intellectual functioning in old age: Penn State's Adult Development and Enrichment Project (ADEPT). In F. I. M. Craik & S. E. Trehub (Eds.), *Aging and cognitive processes* (pp. 353–389). New York: Plenum.

Bandura, A. (1986). *Social foundations of thought and action*. Englewood Cliffs, NJ: Prentice-Hall.

Birren, J. E., & Schaie, K. W. (Eds.). (2001). *Handbook of the psychology of aging* (5th ed.). San Diego, CA: Academic Press.

Bluck, S., & Habermas, T. (2001). Extending the study of autobiographical memory: Thinking back about life across the lifespan. *Review of General Psychology, 5*, 135–147.

Brandtstädter, J. (1984). Personal and social control over development: Some implications of an action perspective in life-span developmental psychology. In P. B. Baltes & O. G. Brim, Jr. (Eds.), *Life-span development and behavior* (Vol. 6, pp. 1–32). New York: Academic Press.

Brandtstädter, J. (1999). The self in action and development: Cultural, biosocial, and ontogenetic bases of intentional self-development. In J. Brandtstädter & R. M. Lerner (Eds.), *Action and self-development: Theory and research through the life span* (pp. 37–65). Thousand Oaks, CA: Sage.

Brandtstädter, J., & Greve, W. (1994). The aging self: Stabilizing and protective processes. *Developmental Review, 14,* 52–80.

Brandtstädter, J., & Lerner, R. M. (Eds.). (1999). *Action and self-development: Theory and research through the life span.* Thousand Oaks, CA: Sage.

Carlson, R. (1971). Where is the person in personality research? *Psychological Bulletin, 75,* 203–219.

Carstensen, L. L. (1992). Social and emotional patterns in adulthood: Support for socioemotional selectivity theory. *Psychology and Aging, 7,* 331–338.

Carstensen, L. L. (1993). Motivation for social contact across the life span: A theory of socioemotional selectivity. In J. E. Jacobs (Ed.), *Nebraska Symposium on Motivation 1992: Developmental perspectives on motivation* (Vol. 40, pp. 209–254). Lincoln: University of Nebraska Press.

Carstensen, L. L., & Fredrickson, B. F. (1998). Socioemotional selectivity in healthy older people and younger people living with the human immunodeficiency virus: The centrality of emotion when the future is constrained. *Health Psychology, 17,* 1–10.

Carstensen, L. L., Gross, J. J., & Fung, H. H. (1997). The social context of emotion. In M. P. Lawton & K. W. Schaie (Eds.), *Annual review of gerontology and geriatrics* (Vol. 17, pp. 325–352). New York: Springer.

Carstensen, L. L., Isaacowitz, D. M., & Charles, S. T. (1999). Taking time seriously: A theory of socioemotional selectivity. *American Psychologist, 54,* 165–181.

Caspi, A., & Herbener, E. S. (1990). Continuity and change: Assortative mating and the consistency of personality in adulthood. *Journal of Personality and Social Psychology, 58,* 250–258.

Caspi, A., & Roberts, B. W. (2001). Personality development across the life course: The argument for change and continuity. *Psychological Inquiry, 12,* 49–66.

Cavan, R. S., Burgess, E. W., Havighurst, R. J., & Goldhamer, H. (1949). *Personal adjustment in old age.* Chicago: Science Research Associates.

Cooley, C. H. (1902). *Human nature and the social order.* New York: Scribner.

Costa, P. T., Jr., & McCrae, R. R. (1980). Still stable after all these years: Personality as a key to some issues in adulthood and old age. In P. B. Baltes & O. G. Brim, Jr. (Eds.), *Life-span development and behavior* (Vol. 3, pp. 65–102). New York: Academic Press.

Costa, P. T., Jr., & McCrae, R. R. (1994). "Set like plaster"?: Evidence for the stability of adult personality. In T. F. Heatherton & J. L. Weinberger (Eds.), *Can personality change?* (pp. 21–40). Washington, DC: American Psychological Association.

Craik, F. I. M., & Jennings, J. M. (1992). Human memory. In F. I. M. Craik & T. A. Salthouse (Eds.), *The handbook of aging and cognition* (pp. 51–110). Hillsdale, NJ: Erlbaum.

Craik, F. I. M., Moroz, T. M., Moscovitch, M., Stuss, D. T., Winocur, G., Tulving, E., et al. (1999). In search of the self: A positron emission tomography study. *Psychological Science, 10,* 26–34.

Craik, F. I. M., & Salthouse, T. A. (Eds.). (2000). *The handbook of aging and cognition* (2nd ed.). Mahwah, NJ: Erlbaum.

Cumming, E., & Henry, W. E. (1961). *Growing old: The process of disengagement.* New York: Basic Books.

Czaja, S. J. (1997). Using technologies to aid the performance of home tasks. In A. D. Fisk & W. A. Rogers (Eds.), *Handbook of human factors and the older adult* (pp. 311–334). San Diego, CA: Academic Press.

Diehl, M. (1998). Everyday competence in later life: Current status and future directions. *The Gerontologist, 38,* 422–433.

Diehl, M., Hastings, C. T., & Stanton, J. M. (2001). Self-concept differentiation across the adult life span. *Psychology and Aging, 16,* 643–654.

Diehl, M., & Willis, S. L. (2003). Everyday competence and everyday problem solving in aging adults: The role of physical and social context. In H.-W. Wahl, R. J. Scheidt, & P. G. Windley (Eds.) *Annual review of gerontology and geriatrics* (Vol. 23, pp. 130–166). New York: Springer.

Diehl, M., Willis, S. L., & Schaie, K. W. (1995). Everyday problem solving in older adults: Observational assessment and cognitive correlates. *Psychology and Aging, 10,* 478–491.

Eisdorfer, C., & Lawton, M. P. (Eds.). (1973). *The psychology of adult development and aging.* Washington, DC: American Psychological Association.

Elias, M. F., Elias, P. K., & Elias, J. W. (1977). *Basic processes in adult developmental psychology.* Saint Louis, MO: C. V. Mosby.

Epstein, E., & Guttman, R. (1984). Mate selection in man: Evidence, theory, and outcome. *Social Biology, 31,* 243–278.

Field, D., & Millsap, R. E. (1991). Personality in advanced old age: Continuity or change? *Journal of Gerontology: Psychological Sciences, 46,* P299–P208.

Fisk, A. D., & Rogers, W. A. (Eds.). (1997). *Handbook of human factors and the older adult.* San Diego, CA: Academic Press.

Freund, A. M., & Smith, J. (1999). Content and function of the self-definition in old and very old age. *Journal of Gerontology: Psychological Sciences, 54B,* P55–P67.

Glenn, N. D. (1980). Values, attitudes, and beliefs. In O. G. Brim, Jr., & J. Kagan (Eds.), *Constancy and change in human development* (pp. 596–640). Cambridge, MA: Harvard University Press.

Gough, H. (1991, August). *Scales and combinations of scales: What do they tell us, what do they mean?* Invited address presented at the Division of Evaluation and Measurement, annual scientific meeting of the American Psychological Association, San Francisco.

Hall, C. S., Lindzey, G., & Campbell, J. B. (1998). *Theories of personality.* New York: Wiley.

Hansson, R. O., & Carpenter, B. N. (1994). *Relationships in old age.* New York: Guilford.

Havighurst, R. J., & Albrecht, R. (1953). *Older people*. New York: Longmans, Green.

Heatherton, T. F., & Weinberger, J. L. (Eds.). (1994). *Can personality change?* Washington, DC: American Psychological Association.

Heckhausen, J., Wrosch, C., & Fleeson, W. (2001). Developmental regulation before and after a developmental deadline: The sample case of "biological clock" for childbearing. *Psychology and Aging, 16,* 400–413.

Helson, R., & Kwan, V. S. Y. (2000). Personality development in adulthood: The broad picture and processes in one longitudinal sample. In S. E. Hampson (Ed.), *Advances in personality psychology* (Vol. 1, pp. 77–106). Hove, UK: Psychology Press.

Hochschild, A. (1975). Disengagement theory: A critique and proposal. *American Sociological Review, 40,* 553–569.

Hooker, K., & McAdams, D. P. (2003). Personality reconsidered: A new agenda for aging research. *Journal of Gerontology: Psychological Sciences, 58B,* P296–P304.

Hultsch, D. F., & Dixon, R. A. (1990). Learning and memory in aging. In J. E. Birren & K. W. Schaie (Eds.), *Handbook of the psychology of aging* (3rd ed., pp. 258–274). San Diego, CA: Academic Press.

Hultsch, D. F., & MacDonald, S. W. S. (2004). Intraindividual variability in performance as a theoretical window onto cognitive aging. In R. A. Dixon, L. Bäckman, & L. G. Nilsson (Eds.), *New frontiers in cognitive aging* (pp. 65–88). New York: Oxford University Press.

Hultsch, D. F., MacDonald, S. W. S., & Dixon, R. A. (2002). Variability in reaction time performance of younger and older adults. *Journal of Gerontology: Psychological Sciences, 57B,* 101–115.

Ingersoll-Dayton, B., Morgan, D., & Antonucci, T. C. (1997). The effects of positive and negative social exchanges on aging adults. *Journal of Gerontology: Social Sciences, 52B,* S190–S199.

Jay, G. M., & Willis, S. L. (1992). Influence of direct computer experience on older adults' attitudes toward computers. *Journal of Gerontology: Psychological Sciences, 47,* P250–P257.

Jones, C., & Meredith, W. (1996). Patterns of personality change across the life span. *Psychology and Aging, 11,* 57–65.

Kahn, R. L., & Antonucci, T. C. (1980). Convoys over the life course: Attachment, roles, and social support. In P. B. Baltes & O. G. Brim, Jr. (Eds.), *Life-span development and behavior* (Vol. 3, pp. 253–286). New York: Academic Press.

Kim, J. E., & Moen, P. (2001). Moving into retirement: Preparation and transitions in late midlife. In M. E. Lachman (Ed.), *Handbook of midlife development* (pp. 487–527). New York: Wiley.

Kohn, M. L., & Schooler, C. (1978). The reciprocal effects of the substantive complexity of work and intellectual flexibility: A longitudinal assessment. *American Journal of Sociology, 84,* 24–52.

Kuriansky, J., & Gurland, B. (1976). The Performance Test of Activities of Daily Living. *International Journal of Aging and Human Development, 16,* 181–201.

Labouvie-Vief, G., & Diehl, M. (1998). Life-span developmental theories. In A. S. Bellak & M. Hersen (Series Eds.) & C. E. Walker (Vol. Ed.), *Comprehensive clinical psychology: Foundations* (Vol. 1, pp. 261–296). Oxford: Pergamon.

Labouvie-Vief, G., & Medler, M. (2002). Affect optimization and affect complexity: Modes and styles of regulation in adulthood. *Psychology and Aging, 17*, 571–587.

Lang, F. R. (2000). Endings and continuity of social relationships: Maximizing intrinsic benefits within personal networks when feeling near to death? *Journal of Social and Personal Relationships, 17*, 157–184.

Lang, F. R. (2001). Regulation of social relationships in later adulthood. *Journal of Gerontology: Psychological Sciences, 56B*, P321–P326.

Lang, F. R., & Carstensen, L. L. (1994). Close emotional relationships in late life: Further support for proactive aging in the social domain. *Psychology and Aging, 9*, 315–324.

Lawton, M. P., & Brody, E. M. (1969). Assessment of older people: Self-maintaining and instrumental activities of daily living. *The Gerontologist, 9*, 179–185.

Lehr, U., & Thomae, H. (Eds.). (1987). *Formen seelischen Alterns: Ergebnisse der Bonner Gerontologischen Längsschnittstudie—BOLSA* [Patterns of psychological aging: Findings from the Bonn Longitudinal Study of Aging]. Stuttgart, Germany: Enke.

Lemon, B. W., Bengtson, V. L., & Peterson, J. A. (1972). An exploration of the activity theory of aging: Activity types and life satisfaction among in-movers to a retirement community. *Journal of Gerontology, 27*, 511–523.

Lerner, R. M. (1984). *On the nature of human plasticity.* New York: Cambridge University Press.

Lerner, R. M., & Walls, T. (1999). Revisiting individuals as producers of their development: From dynamic interactionism to developmental systems. In J. Brandtstädter & R. M. Lerner (Eds.), *Action and self-development: Theory and research through the life span* (pp. 3–36). Thousand Oaks, CA: Sage.

Lindenberger, U., & Baltes, P. B. (1994). Sensory functioning and intelligence in old age: A strong connection. *Psychology and Aging, 9*, 339–355.

Madden, D. J. (2001). Speed and timing of behavioral processes. In J. E. Birren & K. W. Schaie (Eds.), *Handbook of the psychology of aging* (5th ed., pp. 288–312). San Diego, CA: Academic Press.

Madden, D. J., Turkington, T. G., Provenzale, J. M., Denny, L. L., Hawk, T. C., Gottlaub, L. R., & Coleman, R. E. (1999). Adult age differences in the functional neuroanatomy of verbal recognition memory. *Human Brain Mapping, 7*, 115–135.

Magai, C., & McFadden, S. H. (Eds.). (1996). *Handbook of emotion, adult development, and aging.* San Diego, CA: Academic Press.

Markus, H. R., & Herzog, R. A. (1991). The role of the self-concept in aging. In K. W. Schaie (Ed.), *Annual review of gerontology and geriatrics* (Vol. 11, pp. 110–143). New York: Springer.

Marsiske, M., Klumb, P., & Baltes, M. M. (1997). Everyday activity patterns and sensory functioning in old age. *Psychology and Aging, 12*, 444–457.

McAdams, D. P. (1995). What do we know when we know a person? *Journal of Personality, 63,* 365–396.

McAdams, D. P. (2001). *The person: An integrated introduction to personality psychology* (3rd ed.). Fort Worth, TX: Harcourt.

McCrae, R. R., & Costa, P. T., Jr. (2003). *Personality in adulthood: A five-factor theory perspective* (2nd ed.). New York: Guilford.

McDowd, J. M. & Shaw, R. J. (2000). Attention and aging: A functional perspective. In F. I. M. Craik & T. A. Salthouse (Eds.), *The handbook of aging and cognition* (2nd ed., pp. 221–292). Mahwah, NJ: Erlbaum.

Mroczek, D. K., & Spiro, A., III. (2003). Modeling intraindividual change in personality traits: Findings from the Normative Aging Study. *Journal of Gerontology: Psychological Sciences, 58B,* P153–P165.

Neely, A. S., & Bäckman, L. (1993). Long-term maintenance of gains from memory training in older adults: Two 3½-year follow-up studies. *Journal of Gerontology: Psychological Sciences, 48,* P233–P237.

Nesselroade, J. R., & Ford, D. H. (1985). P-technique comes of age: Multivariate, replicated, single-subject designs for research on older adults. *Research on Aging, 7,* 46–80.

Neugarten, B. L. (1977). Personality and aging. In J. E. Birren & K. W. Schaie (Eds.), *Handbook of the psychology of aging* (pp. 626–649). New York: Van Nostrand Reinhold.

Ochsner, K. N., & Lieberman, M. D. (2001). The emergence of social cognitive neuroscience. *American Psychologist, 56,* 717–734.

Palmore, E. (Ed.). (1970). *Normal aging.* Durham, NC: Duke University Press.

Palmore, E. (Ed.). (1974). *Normal aging II.* Durham, NC: Duke University Press.

Park, D. C. (1992). Applied cognitive aging research. In F. I. M. Craik & T. A. Salthouse (Eds.), *The handbook of aging and cognition* (pp. 449–493). Hillsdale, NJ: Erlbaum.

Poon, L. W. (1985). Differences in human memory with aging: Nature, causes, and clinical implications. In J. E. Birren & K. W. Schaie (Eds.), *Handbook of the psychology of aging* (2nd ed., pp. 427–462). New York: Van Nostrand Reinhold.

Raz, N. (2000). Aging of the brain and its impact on cognitive performance: Integration of structural and functional findings. In F. I. M. Craik & T. A. Salthouse (Eds.), *The handbook of aging and cognition* (2nd ed., pp. 1–90). Mahwah, NJ: Erlbaum.

Reuter-Lorenz, P. A., Stanczak, L., & Miller, A. C. (1999). Neural recruitment and cognitive aging: Two hemispheres are better than one, especially as you age. *Psychological Science, 10,* 494–500.

Riegel, K. F. (1975). Toward a dialectical theory of development. *Human Development, 18,* 50–64.

Riegel, K. F. (1977). History of psychological gerontology. In J. E. Birren & K. W. Schaie (Eds.), *Handbook of the psychology of aging* (pp. 70–102). New York: Van Nostrand Reinhold.

Roberts, B. W., & DelVecchio, W. F. (2000). The rank-order consistency of personality from childhood to old age: A quantitative review of longitudinal studies. *Psychological Bulletin, 126,* 3–25.

Roberts, B. W., & Helson, R. (1997). Changes in culture, changes in personality: The influence of individualism in a longitudinal study of women. *Journal of Personality and Social Psychology, 72,* 641–651.

Rogers, W. A., & Fisk, A. D. (2001). Understanding the role of attention in cognitive aging research. In J. E. Birren & K. W. Schaie (Eds.), *Handbook of the psychology of aging* (5th ed., pp. 267–287). San Diego, CA: Academic Press.

Rook, K. (1998). Investigating the positive and negative sides of personal relationships: Through a lens darkly. In B. H. Spitzberg & W. R. Cupach (Eds.), *The dark side of close relationships* (pp. 369–393). Mahwah, NJ: Erlbaum.

Rowe, J. W., & Kahn, R. L. (1998). *Successful aging: The MacArthur Foundation Study.* New York: Pantheon Books.

Ryff, C. D., Kwan, C. M. L., & Singer, B. H. (2001). Personality and aging: Flourishing agendas and future challenges. In J. E. Birren & K. W. Schaie (Eds.), *Handbook of the psychology of aging* (5th ed., pp. 477–499). San Diego, CA: Academic Press.

Ryff, C. D., & Singer, B. (2001). *Emotion, social relationships, and health.* New York: Oxford University Press.

Salthouse, T. A. (1985). Speed of behavior and its implications for cognition. In J. E. Birren & K. W. Schaie (Eds.), *Handbook of the psychology of aging* (2nd ed., pp. 400–426). New York: Van Nostrand Reinhold.

Salthouse, T. A. (1988). Initiating the formalization of theories of cognitive aging. *Psychology and Aging, 3,* 3–16.

Salthouse, T. A. (1990). Cognitive competence and expertise in aging. In J. E. Birren & K. W. Schaie (Eds.), *Handbook of the psychology of aging* (3rd ed., pp. 310–319). San Diego, CA: Academic Press.

Salthouse, T. A. (1991). *Theoretical perspectives on cognitive aging.* Hillsdale, NJ: Erlbaum.

Schaie, K. W. (1965). A general model for the study of developmental problems. *Psychological Bulletin, 64,* 91–107.

Schaie, K. W. (1973). Developmental processes and aging. In C. Eisdorfer & M. P. Lawton (Eds.), *The psychology of adult development and aging* (pp. 151–156). Washington, DC: American Psychological Association.

Schaie, K. W. (Ed.). (1983). *Longitudinal studies of adult psychological development.* New York: Guilford.

Schaie, K. W. (1994). The course of adult intellectual development. *American Psychologist, 49,* 304–313.

Schaie, K. W. (1996). *Intellectual development in adulthood: The Seattle Longitudinal Study.* New York: Cambridge University Press.

Schaie, K. W. (2000). The impact of longitudinal studies on understanding development from young adulthood to old age. *International Journal of Behavioral Development, 24,* 257–266.

Schaie, K. W. & Hofer, S. M. (2001). Longitudinal studies in aging research. In J. E. Birren & K. W. Schaie (Eds.), *Handbook of the psychology of aging* (5th ed., pp. 53–77). San Diego, CA: Academic Press.

Schaie, K. W., & Labouvie-Vief, G. (1974). Generational versus ontogenetic components of change in adult cognitive behavior: A fourteen-year cross-sequential study. *Developmental Psychology, 10,* 305–320.

Schaie K. W., & Willis, S. L. (1986). Can decline in adult intellectual functioning be reversed? *Developmental Psychology 22,* 223–232.

Schaie, K. W., & Willis, S. L. (1991). Adult personality and psychomotor performance: Cross-sectional and longitudinal analyses. *Journal of Gerontology: Psychological Sciences, 46,* P275–P284.

Schooler, C. (1984). Psychological effects of complex environments during the life span: A review and theory. *Intelligence, 8,* 259–281.

Schooler, C., & Mulatu, M. S. (2001). The reciprocal effects of leisure time activities and intellectual functioning in older people: A longitudinal analysis. *Psychology and Aging, 16,* 466–482.

Small, B. J., Hertzog, C., Hultsch, D. F., & Dixon, R. A. (2003). Stability and change in adult personality over 6 years: Findings from the Victoria Longitudinal Study. *Journal of Gerontology: Psychological Sciences, 58B,* P166–P176.

Smits, C. H. M., Deeg, D. J. H., Kriegsman, D. M. W., & Schmand, B. (1999). Cognitive functioning and health as determinants of mortality in an older population. *American Journal of Epidemiology, 150,* 978–986.

Stephens, M. A. P., Kinney, J., Norris, V., & Ritchie, S. W. (1987). Social networks as assets and liabilities in recovery from stroke by geriatric patients. *Psychology and Aging, 2,* 125–129.

Stine-Morrow, E. A. & Soederberg Miller, L. M. (1999). Basic cognitive processes. In J. C. Cavanaugh & S. K. Whitbourne (Eds.), *Gerontology: An interdisciplinary perspective* (pp. 186–212). New York: Oxford University Press.

Thomae, H. (Ed.). (1976). *Patterns of aging.* Basel, Switzerland: Karger.

Thurstone, L. L. (1938). *The primary mental abilities.* Chicago: University of Chicago Press.

Welford, A. T. (1959). Psychomotor performance. In J. E. Birren (Ed.), *Handbook of aging and the individual* (pp. 562–613). Chicago: The University of Chicago Press.

West, R. L. (1989). Planning practical memory training for the aged. In L. W. Poon, D. C. Rubin, & B. A. Wilson (Eds.), *Everyday cognition in adulthood and late life* (pp. 573–597). New York: Cambridge University Press.

West, R. L. (1992). Everyday memory and aging: A diversity of tests, tasks, and paradigms. In R. L. West & J. D. Sinnott (Eds.), *Everyday memory and aging: Current research and methodology* (pp. 3–21). New York: Springer-Verlag.

Willis, S. L. (1989). Improvement with cognitive training: Which old dogs learn what tricks? In L. W. Poon, D. C. Rubin, & B. A. Wilson (Eds.), *Everyday cognition in adulthood and late life* (pp. 545–569). New York: Cambridge University Press.

Willis, S. L. (1991). Cognition and everyday competence. In K. W. Schaie & M. P. Lawton (Eds.), *Annual review of gerontology and geriatrics* (Vol. 11, pp. 80–109). New York: Springer.

Willis, S. L. (1996). Everyday problem solving. In J. E. Birren & K. W. Schaie (Eds.), *Handbook of the psychology of aging* (4th ed., pp. 287–307). San Diego, CA: Academic Press.

Willis, S. L. (2000). Driving competence: The person x environment fit. In K. W. Schaie & M. Pietrucha (Eds.), *Mobility and aging* (pp. 269–277). New York: Springer.

Willis, S. L. (2001). Methodological issues in behavioral intervention research with the elderly. In J. E. Birren & K. W. Schaie (Eds.), *Handbook of the psychology of aging* (5th ed., pp. 78–108). San Diego, CA: Academic Press.

Wolinksy, F. D., & Johnson, R. J. (1991). The use of health services by older adults. *Journal of Gerontology: Social Sciences, 46*, S345–S357.

Woodruff-Pak, D. S. (1997). *The neuropsychology of aging.* Malden, MA: Blackwell.

Yesavage, J. A., Lapp, D., & Sheikh, J. I. (1989). Mnemonics as modified for use by the elderly. In L. W. Poon, D. C. Rubin, & B. A. Wilson (Eds.), *Everyday cognition in adulthood and late life* (pp. 598–611). New York: Cambridge University Press.

Zacks, R. T., Hasher, L., & Li, K. Z. H. (2000). Human memory. In F. I. M. Craik & T. A. Salthouse (Eds.), *The handbook of aging and cognition* (2nd ed., pp. 293–358). Mahwah, NJ: Erlbaum.

CHAPTER 5

The Dynamic Nature of Societal Aging in a Global Perspective

Chris Phillipson

The purpose of this chapter is to assess the scope of sociological work within the field of gerontology, exploring changes in key research areas over the past 50 years and likely developments for the future. The time period is itself providential. In 1954, the *American Journal of Sociology* published a special issue on aging, with contributions from researchers such as Clark Tibbitts, Robert Havighurst, Ernest Burgess, and David Reisman. The range of topics covered included participation in the labor force, the emergence of retirement, social roles in later life, leisure activities, and the development of retirement communities. This collection of subject areas was to reappear 6 years later, together with what would become staple themes relating to the family, health, and income, in influential books edited by Tibbitts (*The Handbook of Social Gerontology,* 1960) and Burgess (*Aging in Western Societies,* 1960).

By the mid 1970s, Bell's *Contemporary Social Gerontology* (1976), subtitled *Significant Developments in the Field of Aging,* retained many of these areas but had some notable additions, including an extensive discussion on theories of aging, a section on minority aging, and a review of research strategies in social gerontology. This broad list of topics continued through successive editions of what were to become established handbooks, such as *Handbook of Aging and the Social Sciences* (Binstock & George, 2001), but with the contribution of a broader range of interests and disciplines now in evidence. At the same time, subdivisions within social gerontology were opening up new ways of classifying and analyzing the discipline (Katz, 1996). Collections by

Minkler and Estes (1991, 1999) and Cole, Achenbaum, Jakobi, and Kastenbaum (1993) represented different ways of understanding the influence of economy and society on older people, but they were in broad agreement on the need to challenge the prevailing orthodoxy within gerontology.

As the above might indicate, social gerontology has evolved in a variety of ways since that initial review in 1954. This is especially the case regarding the contribution made by sociologists to the study of aging, where it is possible to discern a potent mix of uncertainty in direction but with considerable variety of subject matter and styles of discourse about the experience of growing old. The former almost certainly reflects instabilities within gerontology as a whole, with the questioning of whether it ever can really be a discipline in its own right (Achenbaum, 1995; Katz, 2003). The latter reflects the breakdown of a theoretical consensus in the 1980s and 1990s, with an array of perspectives coming forward, from the development of neo-Marxist political economy at one end (Estes, Biggs, & Philipson, 2003) to narrative and ethnographic accounts at the other (Gubrium & Holstein, 2003).

Given the above context, this chapter will reflect upon the likely development of the sociology of aging over the next decade. The issues will be presented in four main ways: First, the distinctive contribution made by sociology to the study of old age will be briefly stated; second, changes affecting the context for gerontological research will be reviewed; third, emerging themes and questions in key areas of the sociology of aging will be examined; finally, prospects for the future of sociological perspectives in aging will be assessed.

SOCIOLOGICAL PERSPECTIVES ON AGING

This section begins by asking: What is the distinctive contribution of a sociological perspective to the study of aging and later life? What do sociologists bring to the study of growing old that is different from other disciplines? One answer to such questions was provided by Matilda White Riley in her 1986 Presidential Address to the American Sociological Association, entitled "On the Significance of Age in Sociology" (1987). In her presentation, Riley provided a review of her personal odyssey as a sociologist—starting in the 1930s—exploring how her increasing interest in the nature of aging stemmed naturally from wider sociological concerns with the impact of social and cultural change. In this essay the author explores her preoccupation with individual aging on the one side, and social change on the other. Riley (1987) comments:

In studying age, we not only bring people (women as well as men) . . . back into society, but recognize that *both* people and society undergo process and change. The aim is to understand each of the two dynamisms: (1) the *aging of people* in successive cohorts who grow up, grow old, die, and are replaced by other people; and (2) the *changes in society* as people of different ages pass through the social institutions that are organized by age. The key to this understanding lies in the interdependence of aging and social change, as each transforms the other. (p. 2)

Together with the above emphasis must be added core sociological concerns relating to inequality and difference, along with the mechanisms through which social variations are produced and maintained in later life. This is an explicit concern of approaches focusing on the impact of cumulative advantage and disadvantage over the life course, as well as issues relating to the impact of social and cultural diversity. Biggs and Daatland (2004) express this point as follows:

That there are more older adults around than at any time in history is now well known. It is less well understood that, as the population ages, it becomes more diverse. In part, this is because individuals have had time to develop a more integrated and particular sense of self, in other words, who they believe themselves to be. Additionally, we are exposed to many more cultural pathways than preceding generations, making life appear richer and with substantially more options than has traditionally been the case. Diversity is also a consequence, however, of cumulative inequalities that have been accrued across a lifetime and now accentuate difference in later life. Each of these trends contributes to a widening variety of experiences of aging in contemporary societies—for good or bad. (p. 1)

Another aspect of sociological work (along with allied research in the humanities) has been a questioning of many of the "taken for granted" categories around which growing old is constructed. The work of Gubrium (1993; see also Gubrium & Wallace, 1990) has been especially influential in this regard, for example, in highlighting the "ordinary theorizing" engaged in by individuals about the process of growing old and the way this might be given equal (complementary) status to that of professionals in the field. This approach focuses on the idea of age as a phenomenon negotiated by older people both through personal relationships and through social institutions. Rather than determined by given structural processes—whether biological or social or in combination—age emerges as a social construction in this approach, descriptively organized through "prevailing stocks of knowledge" (Lynott & Lynott, 1996, p. 754).

Despite the clear role and justification for a sociological perspective, it has nonetheless struggled for position alongside other disciplines within the discipline of gerontology. The reasons for this are probably threefold. First, Biggs, Hendricks, and Lowenstein (2003, p. 3) make the point that gerontology was itself "part of the great push for social improvement" characteristic of the 1950s and 1960s, becoming in the process closely allied with public concerns about the impact of demographic change. The dominance of social policy perspectives on aging was especially true of European countries such as Britain, particularly in those contexts where there was a strong welfare state (Phillipson & Biggs, 1998). Second, for much of the last half of the 20th century the study of social aspects of aging was squeezed between the natural sciences on the one side and biomedicine on the other (Achenbaum, 1995). Both areas were to undergo dramatic expansion in funding over the postwar period, with support for sociological research falling steadily behind in Europe as well as North America. Finally, the sociology of aging appears to have suffered most from the dominance of theoretical perspectives such as structural functionalism and modernization theory in sociology over the 1950s and 1960s (Hendricks & Achenbaum, 1999). The discipline of social gerontology emerged when functionalist views of the family and related institutions were at their most influential. This may partly explain why this perspective became so strongly embedded within the discipline, and the consequential "longevity" of debates relating, for example, to the relative merits of disengagement over activity theory (Biggs et al., 2003, p. 3).

Despite these problems, by the 1990s sociological perspectives on aging had begun to embrace a variety of approaches, with important contributions from feminism, economics, life history perspectives, and developmental psychology. In some cases, as Katz (2003, p.16) observes, social gerontology began to draw upon areas that were losing ground in the rest of the social sciences (the influence of Marxism in critical gerontology being one such example). In other instances, researchers drew upon new approaches within the discipline (the application of cultural studies to the field of aging representing a case in point).

At the same time, the underlying question for all sociological models concerned with aging remained that of clarifying the basis of social integration in later life, with competing points of emphasis around questions of self and identity, the influence of economic relationships, and the impact of social differences through the life course. Awareness of the impact of globalization brought new challenges to the idea of social integration, an area usually examined in national as opposed to global settings. Traditional sociological interests remained, for example, around the role of the family and patterns of social inequality in old age. Increasingly, however, such topics were addressed in global and transnational contexts, reflecting the movement of populations and the impact of international agencies and corporations on the quality of daily living. In short, although the enduring question remains that of understanding the nature of integration in old age, the answers are to be found in an increasingly diverse range of institutions and relationships. It is to an examination of these that we now turn.

SOCIAL GERONTOLOGY IN CONTEXT

By the end of the 1990s, it was clear that a new type of social gerontology was emerging alongside a transformed sociology of aging. Before reviewing some of the key elements and the way these are likely to develop, the wider context will first be assessed. Three main developments can be highlighted that have influenced the application of sociology to the study of old age: (1) changes to the theoretical context; (2) changes to the welfare state; (3) changes in the broader social context.

Changing Theory

In terms of social theory, a traditional concern has been with the "data rich but theory poor" nature of the application of sociology to gerontology (Birren & Bengston, 1988, p. ix). In one sense, this last statement seems much less accurate now than at the time it was made. The broad range of theories discussed in collections such as those edited by Andersson (2002), Biggs et al. (2003), or Binstock and George (2001) illustrates the diversity of approaches now characteristic of social theory within gerontology. Approaches such as critical gerontology are certainly strong but in no way hegemonic, with important subdivisions—Foucaldian, Marxist, and humanistic—even within this single area (Estes et al., 2003). Or to take another instance, perspectives on the family in old age retain some elements of functionalism, but many other approaches—symbolic interactionist, network theory, feminist arguments, life course perspectives—offer competing models (Bengston & Lowenstein, 2003; Estes, 2004; Phillipson & Allan, 2003).

The variety of social theories contrasts strongly with the early phase of social gerontology and must be regarded as a positive development. Paradoxically, however, one side effect is that theory, given its diversity, can too often be ignored in the development of research. This point was highlighted by Bengston, Rice, and Johnson (1999), as follows:

[M]any journal editors and reviewers seem to have little concern for theory or its development. The disenchantment with "general theories" of aging, and the push for practical solutions to problems of the aged, have led to a devaluation of theory, particularly among gerontological practitioners and policy-makers. We [suggest] that applications of knowledge in gerontology—whether in medicine, practice or policy—demand good theory, since it is on the basis of *explanation* about problems that interventions should be made; if not they seem doomed to failure. (p. 16)

Nonetheless, interest in the nature of theorizing about old age seems an important part of the landscape of gerontology at the present time, with increased support for the view that "[w]ithout theorizing and theoretical development social gerontology will stall out with piecemeal empiricism but relatively few insights" (Biggs et al., 2003, p. 10). At the same time, it will be essential to link theoretical developments with the practice of gerontology as a discipline, and methodological advances at an empirical level. Reflecting this is the need to develop concepts that can integrate advances in theories applied to aging with models that can drive the collection of data on the ground. Areas within the sociology of aging where this is beginning to emerge include research relating to understanding the range of influences on quality of life in old age (Walker, 2005; Walker & Hennessy, 2004), work on the impact of cumulative advantage/disadvantage over the life course (Crystal & O'Shea, 2002; Dannefer, 2003), and studies of self and identity in a context of social change and life span development (Giarrusso, Mabry, & Bengston, 2001).

Changing Welfare

The importance of connecting theory to wider social change is illustrated by the second major contextual development, namely, changes to the welfare state. For much of the past 50 years, the lives of older people were shaped by aspirations to develop welfare states, expressed with contrasting structures and value orientations in the different states of Europe and North America (Esping-Andersen, 1990; Pierson & Castles, 2000). Such arrangements were to develop, from the late 1940s onward, as a crucial source of support for older people. Indeed, as John Myles (1984) and others have argued, much of welfare state provisions have traditionally been built around the needs and aspirations of older people.

At the same time, the dominance of the welfare state was to restrict discussions about aging to concerns about a limited range of health and social services with little underlying debate or critique about the way in which such services had evolved. This changed radically beginning in the 1970s, for two main reasons. The first concerned the impact of economic recession on the welfare state and the subsequent questioning of its aims and values by neoliberal governments in Britain, the United States, and elsewhere (Estes & Phillipson, 2002). Second, within gerontology there was the rise of a political economy perspective that, although supportive of state provisions, also raised issues about its role in the development of what Peter Townsend (1981) defined as "structured dependency." These developments were to pull the direction of social theory away from its traditional preoccupation with explaining individual lifestyles and patterns of adjustment in later life (Estes, 1979). Instead, the focus moved to exploring causal linkages between aging on the one side and characteristics of the social, economic, and political structure on the other.

From a sociological perspective, subsequent moves toward what has been termed "the privatization of social policy" (O'Rand, 2000) raise additional issues for the study of old age. On the one hand, growing older seems to have become more secure in certain respects, with longer life expectancy, rising levels of economic well-being (Disney & Whitehouse, 2002), and enhanced lifestyles in old age. Set against this, the pressures associated with the achievement of security are themselves generating fresh anxieties and divisions among older people as well as younger cohorts. Risks once carried by social institutions have now been displaced onto the shoulders of individuals and/or their families (Bauman, 2000; O'Rand, 2000). Dannefer (2000, p. 270) summarizes this process in the following way: "[C]orporate and state uncertainties are transferred to citizens—protecting large institutions while exposing individuals to possible catastrophe in the domains of health care and personal finances, justified to the public by the claim that the pensioner can do better on his or her own, and that Social Security can do better diversified into equity markets." More generally, Stiglitz (2003) argues that risk has been turned into "a way of life" through a combination of changes in the labor market (with the erosion of jobs for life) and reliance on private pension arrangements—these subject to the volatility of the global stock market (Blackburn, 2002; Minns, 2001).

Changing Society

Changes in the organization of welfare have been further reinforced by a third dimension affecting the sociology of old age, notably the impact of various aspects of globalization on the lives of older people and the communities in which they live. By the end of the 1990s, the need to extend work in gerontology beyond the nation-state had become apparent. Pressures on welfare states were increasingly global rather than national in scope (Estes & Phillipson, 2002). The globalization of capital itself had a destabilizing effect in many spheres, most notably on the organization of work and welfare. Beck (2000) has analyzed the link between globalization and the development of deregulated labor markets, accompanied by greater levels of insecurity in the workplace in advanced capitalist economies. Globalization has also been a crucial influence in shaping debates around the future of welfare policy, with International Governmental Organizations (IGOs) feeding into what Estes (1991) identifies as the "crisis construction and crisis management" of state policies for older people (see further below).

Anthony Giddens (1999) describes two views on globalization: those of the "skeptics," who view globalization as a myth, not altogether different from earlier transformational changes in society; and those of the "radicals," who view globalization as real, and with consequences that are largely indifferent to national borders. Giddens himself takes the view of the "radicals," noting that globalization is revolutionary on multiple economic, political, cultural, and societal levels. He argues that globalization is characterized by a complex set of forces, embodied by contradictory, oppositional processes that pull away power and influence from the local and nation-state level while also creating new pressures for local autonomy and cultural identity.

The new challenge for gerontology is linking aging issues to global as well as national contexts. Urry's (2000) analysis of the "new mobilities" affecting the 21st century and Castells' (1996, 2004) focus on the role of networks, rather than countries, providing the architecture for the global economy come to similar conclusions in highlighting the various pressures facing nation-states. Increasingly, national sovereignty is influenced, to a greater or lesser degree, by transnational organizations and communities of different kinds. Older people themselves experience a range of global, national, regional, and local forces influencing the construction of later life, leading to considerable diversity of lifestyles and experiences. From a theoretical perspective, this has introduced significant discontinuities into the lives of older people, notably in terms of widening the pathways and options that might be followed through the life course (Daatland & Biggs, 2004).

Changes at the level of theory, the welfare state, and global society have transformed the context within which social gerontology operates. To illustrate this in more detail, a number of major societal transitions and issues arising from these developments will be assessed. The areas to be examined are: the sociology of the life course, family life and personal communities, the sociology of inequality, and modernization and globalization.

These may be seen to represent major strands in research in social gerontology over the past 50 years but which are now undergoing significant
change, given the above social and economic contexts. The implications for
a reconfigured sociology of old age will be addressed in the final section of
this chapter.

RECONSTRUCTING THE LIFE COURSE

For much of its brief history, social gerontology has been influenced
by a particular view about the shape of the life course. In general terms,
the period from 1945 to the mid 1970s was dominated by the idea of a
"standardized" life course built around what Best (1980) termed as the "three
boxes" of education, work, and leisure. In the case of western industrial
societies (and especially so for men rather than women), this phase is associated with the creation of retirement as a major social institution, with the
growth of entitlements to leisure and the gradual acceptance of an extended
period of leisure following the ending of full-time work (Phillipson, 1998).
Kohli and Rein (1991) summarize this development as follows. By the
1960s, retirement for men had become a normal feature of the life course, a
taken-for-granted part of one's biography. The tripartition of the life course
into a period of preparation, one of "active work," and one of retirement
had become firmly established. Old age had become synonymous with the
period of retirement: a life phase set apart from "active" work life and with a
relatively uniform beginning defined by the retirement age limit as set by the
public old age pension system. With the increasing labor force participation
of women, they too have increasingly been incorporated in this life course
regime.

What has been termed by Mayer and Muller (1986) as "the institutionalization of the life course" lasted a short span of time viewed from a historical perspective, with the period 1945 to 1975 defining its outer limits.
After the mid 1970s, a number of changes can be discerned arising from
the development of more flexible patterns of work, along with the impact
of globalization on patterns of employment. These produced what may be
termed the reconstruction of middle and old age, with the identification of a
"third age" between the period of work and employment (the "second age")
and that of a period of mental and physical decline (the "fourth age"). A
characteristic feature of this new period of life is the ambiguity and flexibility of its boundaries, at both the lower and upper ends (Moen, 2003).
Both these boundaries are seen to involve complex periods of transition,
with greater ambiguity associated with the move away from employment,

and with the blurring of dependence and independence with physical and mental deterioration.

The above changes will set a comprehensive research agenda for gerontology over the next decade. The sociological dimension concerns the extent to which "age integration" or "age segregation" is likely to characterize the individual's journey through the life course. The argument for the former is advanced by those advocating the likelihood of a "blurring" in age divisions and the tendency for adulthood to be interspersed with periods of education and leisure rather than wholly devoted to the sphere of work (Neugarten & Neugarten, 1986; Riley & Riley, 1994). This relaxation of age divisions may be accelerated through the significance of consumption in middle and later life, with the development of lifestyles that cross traditional generational boundaries (Gilleard & Higgs, 2002). Polivka (2000) sees these developments as reflecting the "improvisational" nature of the life course, with people increasingly cultivating the capacity to adjust to discontinuity in key areas of their life.

Against this, evidence for continuing age segregation has been advanced in a number of empirical and theoretical studies. Uhlenberg and De Jong Gerveld (2004, p. 22), drawing on survey research from the Netherlands, found evidence indicating "a deficit of young adults in the networks of older people." Their data, supported by other studies in the United States and Britain, confirmed the extent of age homogeneity in social networks, with younger network members being drawn overwhelmingly from kin. These researchers note demographic factors that may increase the extent of age segregation: (1) aging populations that will further decrease the relative supply of younger adults as potential network members; (2) the continued decline in the average number of adult children, these forming a highly significant group in social networks in middle and later life.

From a different perspective, Ekerdt (2004) suggests that the divisions between working life and retirement may actually increase as emphasis is placed on lifelong planning and preparation for leaving work. Retirement is no longer a concern solely for the second half of life. Rather, the idea that we will someday retire is increasingly present to all adults, and it is even urged on adolescents. The earliest reaches of adulthood are being colonized by frequent reminders that it takes individual effort to achieve retirement. The changing nature of pensions, the identification of retirement saving with financial markets, the aging baby boom generation, and the interests of a powerful industry and of government are daily compelling people's attention to retirement as a lifelong goal.

How far life course divisions will dissolve or be retained remains open to conjecture. Moen (2003) identifies an emerging life stage between the years of career building and old age, a period stretching roughly from age 50 to age 75. She sees this new phase as creating a mixture of uncertainties and opportunities: the former reflected in pressures and insecurities in the workplace (with downsizing and forced early retirement), the latter developed through a broadening in the range of productive activities (with combinations of work, caring, and leisure activities). Arising from what Moen refers to as a yet "unscripted life stage" are what she sees as a number of challenges for social research over the coming decades. In particular, research will need to assess: (1) the range of pathways to and through the midcourse years and beyond (2) those patterns most conducive to productive engagement and social integration (3) Inequalities in terms of the distribution of advantage and disadvantage across subgroups of people moving into, through, and out of the midcourse years (4) The institutional arrangements that can be invented, recombined, or reinvented to foster the life chances and life quality in the later years of adulthood (Moen, 2003, p. 93).

The above issues represent a significant research agenda and emergent set of concerns around transformations in the shape of the life course. Changing relationships at work are one vital element in these developments. Of equal importance, however, are the relationships and experiences that flow from the social ties maintained by older people, notably those linked to family and friends. These have produced a range of enduring issues and questions for researchers in aging, and it is to a consideration of these that we now turn.

THE NEW SOCIOLOGY OF FAMILY LIFE

The study of family ties has been a major concern for work in the sociology of old age. Research on this topic in Britain by Townsend in the 1950s and Shanas in the United States in the 1960s and 1970s became highly influential in setting a research agenda exploring patterns of care of support in a context of geographical and social mobility (Litwak, 1960). This work examined the social world of older people as dominated by families, first of all; friends and neighbors, second; and voluntary and bureaucratic organizations, a distant third (to roughly paraphrase the formulation expressed in the 1970s by Ethel Shanas, 1979). By the 1990s, the extent of social change, with "reconstituted families," the rise of childlessness, and the trend toward living alone or "going solo," was raising major new questions for the sociology of family life in old age. A crucial element here, as the foregoing suggests, was the range of experiences now contained within the institution of the family.

Bernades (cited in Allan & Crow, 2001) asks the question Do we really know what "the family'" is? The answer is almost certainly more uncertain than it was when Parsons (1943) was developing his model of the "nuclear family" in the 1930s and 1940s. Yet, in some ways, gerontology seems uneasy with the idea that family practices have become much less predictable and certainly more diverse. Shanas's (1979) "family first" model has become embedded to a substantial degree within the core assumptions of the discipline, mirrored in part by neoliberal social policies focusing on family support as the first line of defense in the provision of care for older people.

The issue of diversity has also been sidelined by the main theoretical tradition used to explain family relationships. Social exchange theory, along with the related concept of reciprocity, has been employed in numerous studies of the family life of older people. Lowenstein (1999) summarizes this approach as follows:

In the study of intergenerational relations, there is an increased emphasis on the interdependence of generations, that is, the mutual exchange of resources between elderly parents and their adult children, based on social exchange theory. Social exchange theory deals with the balance between dependence and power as an important determinant of the satisfaction which two persons experience in their relationship. (p. 400)

As broad principles underpinning social relationships, ideas about exchange and reciprocity continue to exert considerable force. They have been especially important in the debate about intergenerational equity and have been used to explain a number of findings from research in the area of family sociology (Arber & Attias-Donfut, 2000; Katz et al., 2003). At the same time, this approach may need some modification, given a context of greater fluidity and instability in personal relationships. Reciprocity, in the "risk society" as advanced by Beck (1999) and Giddens (1998), may have a different quality when compared with the "environment of kin" (Frankenberg, 1966) into which older people's lives have traditionally been absorbed. Gouldner's (1960) view about the universality of reciprocity may still apply, but the associated mechanisms—given accelerated geographical and social mobility—is likely to produce different outcomes for kin as well as nonkin relations.

The possibility of open or porous kinship boundaries has been a long-established theme in the research literature. Stack's (1974) study of an African American urban community in the United States demonstrated how standard definitions of nuclear or extended families often failed to capture the complex way in which people lived their lives. Added to this is the importance of demographic changes such as later age of marriage, delayed childbirth, and cohabitation, all of which underline the significance of the view that there can be "little doubt that the network of potentially significant relationships is becoming enlarged" (Riley & Riley, 1993, p. 187; see also Allan & Crow, 2001).

A key point is the level of analysis to consider when exploring changes in relationships. Generational perspectives are vital when tracing developments at the macroeconomic and macrosocial levels, as the debate around intergenerational equity and the link between family and welfare generations demonstrate (Hills, 1996). But this must be complemented by approaches better able to explore microsocial developments, especially in respect to the process and dynamics of family and community change. Here, the concept of "personal communities" (i.e., the world of friends, neighbors, leisure associates, and kin) has some merit when attempting to capture the interplay of different kinds of social ties in old age. Wellman and Wortley (1990, p. 560) define a "personal community network" as a person's set of active community ties, [which] is usually socially diverse, spatially dispersed, and sparsely knit . . . its ties vary in characteristics and in the kinds of support they provide.

Until now, community (and kinship) analysts have concentrated on documenting the persistence, composition, and structure of these networks in order to show that community has not been lost in contemporary societies. They have paid less attention to evaluating how characteristics of community ties and networks affect access to the supportive resources that flow through them.

Placing people within the context of personal communities also bears upon an important sociological issue, namely, what may be characterized as the development of a more "voluntaristic" element in personal relations. Instead of people locked into family groups, they may be more accurately perceived as "managing" a broad spread (or "convoy," to use Kahn and Antonucci's, 1980, term) of relationships, with friends, kin, neighbors, and other supporters, exchanging and receiving help at different points of the life course (Pahl, 2000). Viewing people as managers of a network of relationships offers a different approach to that usually adopted within gerontology. Here, the traditional focus (as noted earlier) has been upon a preordained sequence starting with the family first, and leading outward toward other sets of relationships. However, an alternative approach is to view older people as active network participants, adopting a range of strategies in maintaining social ties.

The changes described amount to a research agenda for gerontologists to develop in the new century. Demographic changes will almost certainly lead, as Bengston (2001) suggests, to the increased salience of multigenerational ties, with bonds of friendship complementing these but also in some cases substituting for kin-based support. However, it is also the case that a broad range of social ties will be needed to cope with the pressures and conflicts affecting family relationships. Global changes associated with migration and increased mobility (see further below) represent one major element. Of additional importance is the tension between work relations on the one hand, and family support on the other. Sennett (1999), for example, has argued that the new flexibility and mobility associated with paid work may have a corrosive effect on long-term ties to friends and family. His analysis suggests that family relationships may be compromised by the insecurities and anxieties affecting people in employment. This raises the important question of the extent to which the social environment appropriate for an aging society may conflict with the economic goals associated with advanced capitalism. Family groups and personal communities, as argued in this chapter, are traditionally associated with high levels of support to older people. However, this may be disrupted through work ties that encourage short-term forms of association rather than the long-term connections characteristic of family ties.

This last comment suggests the possibility of new forms of social division and inequality in later life. This has traditionally been a major concern for sociological research applied to old age, and the next section of this chapter reviews some of the key developments that are likely to emerge over the next decade.

SOCIAL INEQUALITY AND SOCIAL DIVISIONS IN LATER LIFE: CURRENT AND FUTURE TRENDS

Hendricks (2003, p. 63) suggests that a key task for social gerontology has been to "redress previous assumptions of homogeneity among older actors." He goes on to make the important point that "[p]eople do not become more alike with age; in fact the opposite may well be the case. . . . Their heterogeneity is entrenched in disparate master status characteristics, including membership groups and socio-economic circumstances, race and ethnicity, gender, subcultural, or structural conditions on the one hand, and personal attributes on the other."

Attention to social class has been a major issue for those taking a political economy approach within gerontology, with the view taken that older people are as deeply divided along class and other structural lines as younger and middle-aged adults (Minkler & Estes, 1999). Sociological research has begun to clarify the range of processes likely to maintain social divisions in later life. From a life course perspective, the role of education appears highly influential. O'Rand (2002) concludes from a summary of U.S. longitudinal data that the enduring effect of educational attainments confirms the force of selection effects early in the life course on later life outcomes. Farkas (2002) argues that education may play a crucial role in improving access to stocks of social and cultural capital, thus increasing psychological resources, healthy lifestyles, and general well-being. O'Rand (2002) further suggests that education may be seen as the anchor point of several cumulative pathways, these formed around three types of life course capital: human capital that influences employment and income; social capital, which links to social integration and support; and personal capital that relates to the individual's sense of efficacy and personal control. She concludes that

> origins and destinations in the life course are linked by patterns of appreciation, depreciation and compensation of life course capital that are highly complex and interdependent with age. Early socio-economic resources benefit from a process of appreciation over time, although adverse life events can reorient early pathways. Similarly, early economic hardship can be mediated or compensated for by the intervening accumulation of resources, especially education. (O'Rand, 2002, p. 27)

An additional approach to understanding social divisions concerns the multidimensional way in which inequality and deprivation might be experienced in old age. In this context, the concept of "social exclusion" has been helpful in pointing to the range of factors that might limit involvement in mainstream social institutions (Hills, Le Grand, & Piachaud, 2002; Scharf & Smith, 2004). Room (1995) argues that the idea of social exclusion is intended to recognize

> not only the material deprivation of those in poverty but also the broader process of isolation, detachment and low participation in social, cultural and political life which accompany it. . . . As a concept, it does not seek to diminish the importance of distributional issue of material resources but serves to focus upon relational issues—of inadequate social participation, lack of social integration and lack of power. (p. 85)

Research in Britain by Scharf, Phillipson, Smith, and Kingston (2002) demonstrates the extent to which older people living in areas of acute social deprivation may face multiple forms of exclusion, with clear links operating between different domains of exclusion. In particular, there appeared a strong relationship between exclusion from social relations and exclusion from material resources, confirming the way in which poverty and deprivation can combine to restrict participation in a range of informal social relationships. This kind of research raises issues about the role of social institutions in supporting older people's participation in daily life and, conversely, their potential to contribute to "'disengagement," where financial and social resources drop below certain levels.

A central question for the sociology of old age concerns future trends in social inequality through the life course. The likelihood is for a continuation of patterns of cumulative advantage/disadvantage, these constructed around gender, cohort, class, and ethnic divides. Gender is likely to remain a crucial component of inequality, with women especially affected by changes to the organization of welfare and social security (Arber, Davidson, & Ginn, 2003). Casey and Yamada (2004) highlight the problems facing women in Organization for Economic Cooperation and Development (OECD) countries, with those living alone especially likely to fall into those groups with the lowest income. Price and Ginn (2003, p. 145), analyzing British data, find that divorced and separated people are at a particularly high risk of poverty in later life: "For divorced/separated women this matches the individual poverty and lack of independent pension building of married women—a situation from which they find it difficult to recover if they are caring for young children and in the part-time labor force."

Recognition of growing diversity and inequality within cohorts will be another major theme in the sociology of aging (Dannefer & Uhlenberg, 1999). Here, studies of the baby-boom generation are likely to show wide variations in future income and consumption prospects, reflecting educational, occupational, gender, class, and other social factors (American Association of Retired Persons [AARP], 2003). Johnson and Crystal (2002) find from their study drawing upon U.S. longitudinal data that there is the prospect for "high income inequalities among [American] baby boomers during their retirement years." They report that

> [i]n comparing levels of income inequality across cohorts, we found that income inequality at ages 40–45 was quite similar for boomers as for the immediate preceding (1923–1937) cohorts. However, consistent with other research on cohorts born in the early part of the twentieth century . . . we also found that the 1923–37 cohorts demonstrated a marked increase in within cohort inequality beginning at age 50 and continuing into retirement years. If the experience of the baby boom cohorts is similar—which appears likely—they will experience a high level of economic inequality in their retirement years. (p. 266)

This may be compounded by changes in employment conditions across the class divide, with improvements in the remuneration of professional and white-collar workers on the one hand, but with reduced support for blue-collar workers on the other. The driving factors here will include the growth of flexible employment (associated with a decline in company benefits), changes to pensions with the move from defined benefit to defined contribution schemes, and the further deterioration in manufacturing employment in developed economies (Beck, 2000; Sennett, 1999; Wilson, 1997). More generally, inequalities associated with the rise of globalization will be an additional factor for sociologists to address. A review of some of the main issues affecting older people in this area will now be addressed.

GLOBALIZATION AND THE SOCIOLOGY OF AGING

Debates around the theme of globalization were highly influential in many areas of the social sciences during the 1990s, notably in sociology and political science (Held, McGrew, Goldblatt, & Perraton, 1999). Subsequently, this work was to broaden out with extensive discussions in social policy (George & Wilding, 2002; Mishra, 1999; Yeates, 2001) and more recently within social gerontology (Estes & Phillipson, 2002; Vincent, 2003; Walker & Deacon, 2003). However, it might be argued that much work remains to be done exploring the full impact of globalizing processes both on older people and on the social institutions through which they are supported.

In general terms, globalization has produced a distinctive stage in the history of aging, with tensions between nation-state-based policies concerning demographic change and those formulated by global actors and institutions. Social aging can no longer be viewed solely as a national problem or issue but one that affects individuals, groups, and communities across the globe. Local and national interpretations of aging had substance where nation-states (at least in the developed world) claimed some control over the construction of welfare policies. They also carried force where social policies were being designed with the aim or aspiration of leveling inequalities, and where citizenship was still predominantly a national issue. The changes affecting all of these areas, largely set in motion by different aspects of globalization, is generating significant implications for work in the field of gerontology (O'Rand, 2000).

Viewing aging from a global perspective will have at least three major implications for work in the sociology of aging. In the first place, a global perspective raises issues about the construction of the life course as typically understood within social gerontology (see above). Dannefer (2003) makes the point:

> [q]uite different patterns are found in the "Majority World"—the poorer and less developed countries where most of the people inhabiting the earth

live. . . . If the life course area is to encompass the full range of human diversity and human possibility, these diverse patterns cannot be ignored. Many "alternative" life course configurations are also strongly institutionalized. Such established patterns can be observed in spite of the high population turnover of countries that have not undergone the demographic transition—witnessing powerfully to the fact that the life course is indeed a social institution that transcends, and yet encases, the biographies of individuals. In some cases, such patterns are well entrenched, and are clearly older than the "three boxes" of the "modern" life course which the term institutionalization has often been equated. (p. 649)

The challenge for studies in aging lies in acknowledging the way in which the life course may, as a result of the above processes, assume a "nonlinear" shape, with features of so-called normal aging occurring earlier or later in life, depending on a particular sequence of biographical events (Hoerder, 2001). By extension, an additional issue concerns greater variability in respect of images and definitions of aging. In the context of accelerated movement of populations, interlaced with powerful global networks, ideas about the meaning of old age, when old age begins, and normative behaviors for later life will demonstrate greater variation within any one society than has historically been the case (Phillipson & Ahmed, 2004).

The second issue brought out from research on globalization concerns the degree of restlessness and uncertainty expressed about the meaning of home. Gardner (2002, p. 209), in her research on older Bangladeshi migrants, expresses this in terms of the "perpetual re-assessment of in which place it is best to be, the sense that wherever one goes, one has always left part of oneself behind in the 'other' place." For gerontology, this raises new research questions about how uncertainty and insecurity about the meaning of home are managed in old age. Traditionally, we have tended to see a secure attachment to a domestic space called "home" as a vital anchor, the loss of which may cause illness and even premature mortality (arising, e.g., from relocation to a residential home). But the complex life histories of some migrants reminds us of other possibilities: that with large-scale global movements, people arrive in old age with unresolved issues about where one's true home is located and the space that it is best to be to live out one's old age. The implications of this for understanding issues relating to identity and transition in old age are worthy of further investigation in gerontology.

Third, globalization, both through the spread of worldwide communications and via the power of global organizations, has elevated aging to an issue that transcends individual societies or states. Gerontology, for much of the 20th century, was preoccupied with issues affecting older people in advanced capitalist societies (Dannefer, 2003). Indeed, theories such as disengagement and modernization theory took the view that the Western model of aging would ultimately be diffused across all cultures of the world (Fennell, Phillipson, & Evers, 1988). Globalization has provided a fundamental challenge to vestiges of this approach. Global interests may indeed continue to be subject to U.S. hegemony and/or Western imperialism in various guises, but globalization also illustrates the emergence of new social and political forms at international, national, regional, and local levels (Held & McGrew, 2000). Cerny and Evans (2004) make this point in the following way:

> The central paradox of globalization, the displacement of a crucial range of economic, social and political activities from the national arena to a cross-cutting global/transnational/domestic structured field of action, is that rather than creating one economy or one polity, it also divides, fragments and polarizes. Convergence and divergence are two sides of the same process. Globalization remains a discourse of contestation that reflects national and regional antagonisms and struggles. (p. 63)

But the globalization of communications has introduced a further dimension into the understanding of demographic change. Thompson (2000) explored the processes involved in the appropriation of globalized media products as follows:

> I want to suggest that the appropriation of globalized symbolic materials involves what I shall describe as the *accentuation of symbolic distancing from the spatial-temporal contexts of everyday life* [author's emphasis]. The appropriation of symbolic materials enables individuals to take some distance from the conditions of their day-to-day lives—not literally but symbolically, imaginatively, vicariously. Individuals are able to gain some conception, however partial, of ways of life and life conditions that differ significantly from their own. They are able to gain some conception of regions of the world which are far removed from their own locales. (p. 212)

The process Thompson describes is transforming aging in a variety of ways. Global communications sharpened awareness in the 1990s of the suffering of older people in zones of conflict, notably in the former Eastern bloc countries and in sub-Saharan Africa (Lloyd-Sherlock, 2004). But from another perspective it also generated ideas about the new lifestyles that might be possible to develop in middle and older age. Older people in developed countries became aware of the possibilities of travel and migration and the potential benefits of global tourism. Bauman (1998, p. 78) observes that "spiritually at least we are all travelers." During the past 10 years this been put into practice by a minority of wealthier retirees, even though many of their contemporaries remained tied to localities experiencing the costs associated with global change (Phillipson & Scharf, 2004).

Such examples confirm the way in which globalization has been radical in its transformation of aging, with, to paraphrase Beck (1999), few social groups or societies immune to its effects. Further work in this area will certainly be a key dimension to social gerontological research over the next decade.

CONCLUSION

This chapter has explored a number of key questions and concerns arising from sociological research in the field of gerontology. To conclude this assessment, a number of lessons will be drawn from the literature, along with some questions that might be raised for future research. Four issues will be considered: first, the relationship between population aging and other types of social change; second, changes to the life course; third, changes in personal ties; and fourth, issues relating to inequality and difference.

First, an important development at a macrolevel arises from the interplay between demographic change (notably longer life expectancy) and the trends associated with political and cultural globalization. Awareness of living in an interconnected world brings to the fore questions of cultural diversity, different understandings about what it means to grow old, and the issue of who we take to be an older person. The tendency in gerontology has been to use Western models of development to define old age, these taking age 60–65 as the boundary set by conventional retirement and pension systems. But on some continents (notably sub-Saharan Africa) old age may be more meaningfully defined as starting at age 50 (or even earlier). Access to pension systems to mark the onset of old age is itself a culturally specific process. Relevant to Western contexts (though changing even here with privatization), it has little resonance in countries such as China, where out of 90 million people age 65 plus, just one quarter have entitlement to a pension (Lloyd-Sherlock, 2004). In a number of senses the traditional formulation of "aging societies" is unhelpful, given global inequalities. Global society contains numerous demographic realities: aging Europe certainly, as compared with increasingly youthful United States, and plummeting life expectancy in Russia and sub-Saharan Africa. Such contrasts create significant variations in the construction of growing old—national, transnational, subcultural—producing as a result new questions and perspectives for research in gerontology.

Second, research into the changing life course will remain an important concern within the field of social gerontology. An enduring question here concerns the tension between the retention of boundaries between different life stages and opposing trends toward more flexible lifestyles. Social gerontology as a discipline was itself founded on the notion of people occupying roles specific to certain periods of life. Managing the transition from one role to another was viewed as crucial in successful adjustment to aging. This may continue as an important theme in some instances (the study of widowhood being one such example). In other instances the idea of clear transitions between different roles may break down as individuals combine work, leisure, caring, and personal roles well into advanced old age. This will pose questions about the development of new forms of social engagement in later life, and the different opportunities available to individuals according to class, gender, and ethnic origin.

A third area concerns changes in personal ties and the shifting balance between family and friends. The significance of family ties will almost certainly remain an enduring issue for gerontology, as reflected in studies of informal care and the various exchanges of support and help across generations. But a key development for the future must be to recognize the salience of other types of relationships, notably those linked to long-standing friendships. These may play a key role in the provision of support for gay and lesbian older people as well as for people living alone. More widely—as social relations of choice—ties of friendship may be seen to represent a major contribution to sustaining quality of life in old age. Indeed, deprivation of the means to sustain friendships may come to be ranked of equal importance to that associated with the loss of family, both contributing in equal albeit different ways to the maintenance of identity in old age.

Finally, issues of inequality will continue to provide enduring questions for research in gerontology. For a significant group in the developed world, growing old will continue to develop as a time of freedom and extended choice. For a majority, however, and especially those in the global south, a secure old age seems scarcely possible. On the one hand, baby boomers in the United States and Europe will be rewriting traditional scripts about what it means to grow old. On the other, millions will continue to experience aging as a time of exclusion from access to those resources that make for a decent and meaningful life. The enduring question for gerontology will be how to embrace the diversity of lives that will comprise aging populations in the 21st century. A gerontology that brings together a range of disciplines to the study of human aging will remain crucial to addressing this fundamental task.

REFERENCES

Achenbaum, W. A. (1995). *Crossing frontiers: Gerontology emerges as a science.* New York: Cambridge University Press.

Allan, G., & Crow, G. (2001). *Families, households and society.* London: Palgrave

American Association of Retired Persons (AARP). (2003). *Boomers at midlife (Wave 2, 2003).* Washington: Author.

Andersson, L. (Ed.). (2002). *Cultural gerontology.* Westport, CT: Auburn House.

Arber, S., & Attias-Donfut, C. (2000). *The myth of generational conflict: The family and state in generational conflict.* London: Routledge.

Arber, S., Davidson, K. & Ginn, J. (Eds.). (2003). *Gender and ageing.* Buckingham, UK: Open University Press.

Bauman, Z. (1998). *Globalization.* Oxford: Polity Press.

Bauman, Z. (2000). *Liquid modernity.* Oxford: Polity Press.

Beck, U. (1999). *World risk society.* Cambridge: Polity Press.

Beck, U. (2000). *The brave new world of work.* Cambridge: Polity Press.

Bell, B. (Ed.). (1976). *Contemporary social gerontology.* Springfield, IL: Charles C Thomas.

Bengston, V. L. (2001). Beyond the nuclear family: The increasing importance of multigenerational bonds, *Journal of Marriage and the Family, 63,* 1–16.

Bengston, V. L., & Lowenstein, A. (Eds.). (2003). *Global aging and challenges to families.* New York: Aldine de Gruyter.

Bengtson, V. L., & Schaie, K.W. (Eds.). (1999). *Handbook of theories of aging.* New York: Springer.

Bengston, V. L., Rice, C. J., & Johnson, M. (1999). Are theories of aging important? Models and explanations in gerontology at the turn of the century. In V. L. Bengtson & K. W. Schaie (Eds), *Handbook of theories of aging* (pp. 3–20). New York: Springer.

Best, F. (1980). *Flexible life scheduling.* New York: Praeger.

Biggs, S., & Daatland, S. (2004). Ageing and diversity: A critical introduction. In S. Biggs & S. Daatland (Eds.), *Ageing and diversity: Multiple pathways and cultural migrations* (pp. 1–12). Bristol, UK: Policy Press.

Biggs, S., Hendricks, J., & Lowenstein, A. (2003). The need for theory in gerontology. In S. Biggs, A. Lowenstein, & J. Hendricks (Eds.), *The need for theory: Critical approaches to social gerontology* (pp. 1–14). Amityville, NY: Baywood Publishers.

Binstock, R., & George, L. (Eds.). (2001). *Handbook of aging and the social sciences* (5th ed.). New York: Academic Press.

Birren, J., & Bengtson, V. L. (Eds.). (1988). *Emergent theories of aging.* New York: Springer.

Blackburn, R. (2002). *Banking on death.* London: Verso Books.

Burgess, E. W. (Ed.). (1960). *Aging in western societies: A survey of social gerontology.* Chicago: The University of Chicago Press.

Casey, B., & Yamada, A. (2004). The public-private mix of retirement income in nine OECD countries: Some evidence from micro data and an exploration of its implications. In M. Rein & W. Schmähl (Eds.), *Rethinking the welfare state: The political economy of pension reform* (pp. 395–411). Cheltenham, UK: Edward Elgar.

Castells, M. (1996). *The rise of the network society* (Vol. 1). Oxford: Blackwell Publishers.

Castells, M. (2004). *The power of identity* (2nd ed.). Oxford: Blackwell.

Cerny, P. G., & Evans, M. (2004). Globalization and public policy under new labour. *Policy Studies, 25*(1), 51–65.

Cole, T. R., Achenbaum, W. A., Jakobi, P. L., & Kastenbaum, R. (Eds.). (1993). *Voices and visions of aging: Toward a critical gerontology.* New York: Springer.

Crystal, S., & O'Shea, D. (Eds.). (2002). Economic outcomes in later life. *Public Policy, Health and Cumulative Advantage. Annual Review of Gerontology and Geriatrics, 22.* New York: Springer, 293.

Dannefer, D. (2002). Whose life course is it anyway? Diversity and "linked lives" in global perspective. In R. Settersten (Ed.), *Invitation to the life course* (pp. 259–268). Amityville, NY: Baywood.

Dannefer, D. (2003). Cumulative advantage/disadvantage and the life course: Cross-fertilizing age and social science theory. *Journal of Gerontology, 58B*(6), S327–S337.

Dannefer, D., & Uhlenberg, P. (1999). Paths of the life course: A typology. In V. L. Bengtson & K. W. Schaie (Eds.), *Handbook of theories of aging* (pp. 306–326). New York: Springer.

Daatland, S. O., & Biggs, S. (Eds.). (2004). *Ageing and diversity.* Bristol, UK: Policy Press.

Disney, R., & Whitehouse, E. (2002). The economic well-being of older people in international perspective: A critical review. In S. Crystal & D. Shea (Eds.), *Economic outcomes in later life: Public policy, health and cumulative advantage* (pp. 59–94). *Annual Review of Gerontology and Geriatrics,* Vol. 22. New York: Springer.

Ekerdt, D. (2004). Born to retire: The foreshortened life course. *The Gerontologist, 44*(1), 3–9.

Esping-Andersen, G. (1990). *The three worlds of welfare capitalism.* Cambridge: Polity Press.

Estes, C. (1991). The Reagan legacy: Privatization, the welfare state, and aging in the 1990s. In J. Myles & J. Quadagno (Eds.), *States, labour markets and the future of old age policy,* (pp. 58–83). Philadelphia: Temple University Press.

Estes, C. L. (2004). Social Security privatization and older women: A feminist political economy perspective. *Journal of Aging Studies, 18*(1), 9–26.

Estes, C., Biggs, S., & Phillipson, C. (2003). *Social theory, social policy and ageing: A critical introduction.* Maidenhead, UK: Open University Press.

Estes, C., & Phillipson, C. (2002). The globalization of capital, the welfare state and old age policy. *International Journal of Health Services, 32*(2), 279–297.

Farkas, G. (2002). Human capital and the long-term effects of education in later-life inequality. *Annual Review of Gerontology and Geriatrics, 20.* New York: Springer, 138–154.

Fennell, G., Phillipson, C., & Evers, H. (1988). *The sociology of old age*. Milton Keynes, UK: Open University Press.

Finch, J., & Mason, J. (1993). *Negotiating family responsibilities*. London: Routledge.

Frankenberg, R. (1966). *Communities in Britain*. London: Penguin Books.

Gardner, K. (2002). *Age, narrative and migration*. Oxford: Berg.

George, V., & Wilding, P. (2002). *Globalization and human welfare*. London: Palgrave.

Giddens, A. (1998). *The third way: The renewal of social democracy*. Cambridge: Polity Press

Giarruso, R., Mabry, B., & Bengston, V. L. (2001). The aging self in social contexts. In R. Binstock & L. George (Eds.), *Handbook of aging and the social sciences* (pp. 295–312). New York: Academic Press.

Giddens, A. (1999). Globalization (BBC Reith Lectures, No. 1). Retrieved from www.lse.ac.uk/Giddens/lectures.htm

Gilleard, C., & Higgs, P. (2002). *Cultures of ageing: Self, citizen and the body*. London: Prentice-Hall.

Gouldner, A. (1960). The norm of reciprocity: A preliminary statement. *American Sociological Review, 25*(2), 169–178.

Gubrium, J. F. (1993). Voice and context in a new gerontology. In T. Cole, W. A. Achenbaum, P. Jakobi, & R. Kastenbaum (Eds.), *Voices and visions of aging: Toward a critical gerontology*. New York: Springer, 46–63.

Gubrium, J. F., & Holstein, J.A. (Eds.). (2003). *Ways of aging*. Malden, MA: Blackwell.

Gubrium, J. F., & Wallace, J. B. (1990). Who theorises age? *Ageing and Society, 10*(2), 131–149.

Held, D., McGrew, A., Goldblatt, D., & Perraton, J. (1999). *Global Transformations*. Cambridge: Polity Press.

Hendricks, J. (2003). Structure and identity—Mind the gap: Toward a personal resource model of successful aging. In S. Biggs, A. Lowenstein, & J. Hendricks (Eds.), *The need for theory: Critical approaches to social gerontology* (pp. 63–90). Amityville, NY: Baywood.

Hendricks, J., & Achenbaum, A. (1999). Historical development of theories of aging. In V. L. Bengtson & K. W. Schaie (Eds.), *Handbook of theories of aging* (pp. 21–39). New York: Springer.

Hills, J. (1996). Does Britain have a welfare generation? In A. Walker (Ed.), *The new generational contract* (pp. 56–80). London: UCL Press.

Hills, J., Le Grand, J., & Piachaud, D. (2002). *Understanding social exclusion*. Oxford: Oxford University Press.

Hoerder, D. (2001). Reconstructing life courses: A historical perspective on migrant experiences. In V. Marshall, W. Heinz, H. Kruger, & A. Verma (Eds.), *Reconstructing work and the life course*. Toronto: University of Toronto Press, 525–539.

Johnson, R.W., & Crystal, S. (2002). The economic future of the baby boom generation. In S. Crystal & D. O'Shea (Eds.), *Annual Review of Gerontology and Geriatrics, 22*, 239–268.

Kahn, R., & Antonucci, T. (1980). Convoys over the life course: Attachment, roles and social support. In P. B. Baltes & O. Brim (Eds.), *Life span development and behaviour*. New York: Academic Press, 253–286.

Katz, R., Daatland, S. O., Lowenstein, A., Bazo, M. T., Ancizu, I., Herlofston, K., et al. (2003). Family norms and preferences in intergenerational relations: A comparative perspective. In V. L. Bengston & A. Lowenstein (Eds.), *Global aging and challenges to families* (pp. 305–326). New York: Aldine de Gruyter.

Katz, S. (1996). *Disciplining old age*. Charlottesville: The University Press of Virginia.

Katz, S. (2003). Critical gerontological theory: Intellectual fieldwork and the nomadic life of ideas. In S. Biggs, A. Lowenstein, & J. Hendricks (Eds.), *The need for theory: Critical approaches to social gerontology* (pp. 15–31. Amityville, NY: Baywood.

Kohli, M., & Rein, M. (1991). The changing balance of work and retirement. In M. Kohli, A. Rein, A. M. Guillemard, & H. van Gunsteren (Eds.), *Time for retirement: Comparative studies of early exit from the labor force* (pp. 1–35). Cambridge: Cambridge University Press.

Litwak, E. (1960). Occupational mobility and extended family cohesion. *American Sociological Review, 25,* 9–21.

Lloyd-Sherlock, P. (2004). *Living longer: Ageing, development and social protection*. London: Zed Books.

Lowenstein, A. (1999). Intergenerational family relations and social support. In Hirsh, R. D., Brendebach, C., Wahl, H. W., & Kruse, A. (Eds.) *Key Note Lectures, Fifth European Congress of Gerontology* (pp. 398–407). Darmstadt, Germany: Steinkopff.

Lynott, R. J., & Lynott, P. P. (1996). Tracing the course of theoretical development in the sociology of aging. *The Gerontologist, 36*(6), 749–760.

Mayer, K.-U., & Muller, W. (1986). The state and the structure of the life course. In A. B. Sorensen, F. Weinert, & L. Sherrod (Eds.), *Human development and the life course: Multidisciplinary perspectives* (pp. 217–245). Hillsdale, NJ: Erlbaum.

Minkler, M., & Estes, C. L. (Eds.). (1991). *Critical perspectives on aging: The political and moral economy of growing old*. Amityville, NY: Baywood.

Minkler, M., & Estes, C. L. (Eds.). (1999). *Critical gerontology: Perspectives from political and moral economy*. Amityville, NY: Baywood.

Minns, R. (2001). *The cold war in welfare: Stock markets versus pensions*. London: Verso.

Mishra, R. (1999). *Globalization and the welfare state*. Cheltenham, UK: Edward Elgar.

Moen, P. (2003). Mid course: Reconfiguring careers and community service for a new life stage. *Contemporary Gerontology, 9*(3), 87–94.

Myles, J. (1984). *Old age in the welfare state: The political economy of public pensions*. Lawrence: University of Kansas Press.

Neugarten, B., & Neurgarten, D. (1986). Changing meanings of age in the ageing society. In A. Pifer & L. Bronte (Eds.), *Our ageing society: Paradox and promise* (pp. 33–52). New York: Norton.

O'Rand, A. M. (2000). Risk, rationality, and modernity: social policy and the aging self. In K. W. Schaie (Ed.), *Social structures and aging* (pp. 225–249). New York: Springer.

O'Rand, A. M. (2002). Cumulative advantage theory in life course research. *Annual Review of Gerontology and Geriatrics, 22,* 14–30.

Pahl, R. (2000). *On friendship.* Oxford: Polity Press.

Parsons, T. (1943). The kinship system of the contemporary United States. *American Anthropologist, 45,* 22–38.

Phillipson, C. (1998). *Reconstructing old age.* London: Sage.

Phillipson, C. & Ahmed, N. (2004). Transnational communities, migration and changing identities in later life: A new research agenda. In S. O. Daatland & S. Biggs (Eds.), *Ageing and diversity* (pp. 157–179). Bristol, UK: Policy Press.

Phillipson, C., & Allan G. (2003). Aging and the Life Course. In J. Scott, J., Thea S., and Richards, M. *Blackwell Companion to the Sociology of the Family.* Oxford: Blackwell (126–140).

Phillipson, C., & Biggs, S. (1998). Modernity and identity: Themes and perspectives in the study of older adults. *Journal of Age and Identity, 3*(1), 11–23.

Phillipson, C., & Scharf, T. (2004). The impact of government policy on social exclusion of older people: A review of the literature. London: Stationery Office.

Pierson, C., & Castles, F. (2000). *The welfare state reader.* Cambridge: Polity Press.

Polivka, L. (2000). Postmodern aging and the loss of meaning. *Journal of Aging and Identity, 5*(1), 3–14.

Price, D., & Ginn, J. (2003). Sharing the crust: Gender, partnership, status and inequalities in pension accumulation. In S. Arber, K. Davidson & J. Ginn (Eds.), *Gender and ageing* (127–146). Buckingham, UK: Open University Press.

Riley, M. W. (1987). On the significance of age in sociology. *American Sociological Review, 52,* 1–14.

Riley, M. W., & Riley, J. W. (1993). Connections: Kin and cohort. In V. L.Bengston & W. A. Achenbaum (Eds.), *The changing contract across generations* (pp. 169–190). New York: Aldine de Gruyter.

Riley, M. W., & Riley, J. W. (1994). Structural lag. In M. W. Riley, R. L. Kahn, & A. Foner (Eds.), *Age and structural lag* (pp. 15–36). New York: Wiley.

Room, G. (Ed.). (1995). *Beyond the threshold: The measurement and analysis of social exclusion.* Bristol, UK: Policy Press.

Scharf, T., Phillipson, C., Smith, A. E., & Kingston, P. (2002). *Growing older in socially deprived areas: Social exclusion in later life.* London: Help the Aged.

Scharf, T., & Smith, A. E. (2004). Older people in urban neighborhoods: Addressing the risk of social exclusion in later life. In C. Phillipson, G. Allan, & D. Morgan (Eds.), *Social networks and social exclusion* (pp. 162–179). Aldershot, UK: Ashgate.

Sennett, R. (1999). *The corrosion of character.* London: Norton.

Shanas, E. (1979). The family as a social support system in old age. *The Gerontologist, 19*(2), 169–174.

Stack C. (1974). *All our kin: Strategies for survival in a black community.* New York: Harper.

Stiglitz, J. (2003). *The roaring nineties.* London: Penguin Books.

Thompson, J. B. (2000). The globalization of communication. In D. Held & A. Mc-Grew (Eds.), *The global transformations reader.* Cambridge: Polity Press.

Tibbitts, C. (Ed.). (1960). *The handbook of social gerontology.* Chicago: The University of Chicago Press.

Townsend, P. (1981). The structured dependency of the elderly: The creation of policy in the twentieth century. *Ageing and Society, 1*(1), 5–28.

Uhlenberg, P., & De Jong Gerveld, J. (2004). Age segregation in later life: An examination of personal networks. *Ageing and Society, 24*(1), 5–28.

Urry, J. (2000). *Sociology beyond societies.* London: Routledge.

Vincent, J. (2003). *Old age.* London: Routledge.

Walker, A. (Ed.). (1996). *The new generational contract.* London: UCL Press.

Walker, A. (Ed.). (2005). *Growing older in Europe.* Buckingham, UK: Open University Press.

Walker, A., & Deacon, B. (2003). Economic globalization and policies on aging. *Journal of Societal and Social Policy, 2*(1), 1–18.

Walker, A., & Hennessy, C. (Eds.). (2004). *Growing older: Quality of life in old age.* Maidenhead, UK: Open University Press.

Wellman, B., & Wortley, S. (1990). Different strokes from different folks: Community ties and social support. *American Journal of Sociology, 96,* 558–588.

Wilson, W. J. (1997). *When work disappears: The world of the new urban poor.* Chicago: The University of Chicago Press.

Yeates, N. (2001). *Globalization and social policy.* London: Sage.

CHAPTER 6

Whatever Happened to Culture?

Christine L. Fry

As it is currently used in practice, culture is an idea that grew in a world of economic and political expansion. Peoples of vastly different backgrounds were drawn into long-term interaction and interdependency. Culture is rather hard to miss when people not only look different, dress differently, but have markedly different beliefs, speak dissimilar languages, and behave in alien ways. Culture became the central concept of anthropology and was influential in the development of many of the social sciences. The late 19th–early 20th century was the golden age for the development and elaboration of the phenomena of culture. In the early 21st century, how has this concept endured for research into age and aging? The thesis of this chapter is that we are running the risk of losing contact with the phenomena we study. The reason is straightforward. We increasingly have turned our attention to the familiar cultural worlds of home (Ikels & Beall, 2001). Not only is it increasingly difficult to study alien worlds, but those worlds have become increasingly familiar and homogenized with globalization. Age is doubly familiar, especially when we study it at home, simply because everyone has experience with it either in self or others.

THE NATURE OF CULTURAL THINGS

Culture means a lot of different things, depending on what one is intending to accomplish. The intent of this section is to discuss what we have come to understand as culture as a phenomenon that is researchable. Edward Tylor first defined the idea in 1871. His short definition is "culture or civilization. . . is that complex whole that includes knowledge, belief, art, law, morals, customs, and any other capabilities and habits acquired by man as a member of society." Although Tylor's definition is rather dated, we will take this as our point of departure to look at the ways it is used in contemporary anthropology. This original conception of culture was designed to facilitate the examination of traits among other peoples with the hope of arranging them in an evolutionary progression to discover the "laws of evolution."

About the only component of Tylor's definition that is modern is that in being acquired as a member of society, the implication is that culture is learned. Most anthropologists would agree with this and would argue that, because culture is learned from others, it is also shared to a certain extent. One of the refinements in the definition of culture in the 20th century was that culture is self-organized. Each individual in learning is actually figuring out the world and creating their own models of how the cultural worlds of others work. Likewise, all social groups use their cultures to self-organize in response to an ever-changing world. Also, culture is primarily a cognitive phenomenon anchored in symbols. This symbolic world gives humans the ability to think about the world and devise strategies, and it ultimately shapes behavior and action.

Beyond the notion that culture is learned, shared, self-organized, and symbolic, the idea itself is sufficiently abstract to allow for multiple perspectives and multiple ways of operationalizing the concept. For ecological anthropology, culture becomes a system of knowledge, social structure, and material culture that enables humans to respond to and adapt to an environment. For social anthropologists, culture becomes the institutional basis for social life. For cognitive anthropologists, culture becomes a system of knowledge about the world. For others, culture provides the meaning that makes experience understandable.

The invention of culture has to be among one of the best success stories of all time. Back in the 1870s Tylor was unsure of his new concept of "culture" or "civilization." He later dropped the term *civilization* because it implies the existence of a state and opted for the more generalized term *culture*. It took some 50 years for the term to be widely used in anthropology. One hundred years later, this word has been incorporated into the vocabulary of everyday language. The idea of culture has lost its scientific, restricted, and jargonistic meaning. Nearly every undergraduate entering an introductory anthropology class has a good idea that culture has to do with ethnicity and different designs for living.

THE NATURE OF CULTURE AND ETHNOGRAPHY

How do anthropologists use culture in presenting the lives of alien peoples around the world to audiences at home? The products of anthropological work are presented in a distinctive genre of writing called ethnography. Although anthropological data may be obtained by specific research strategies such as interviews, card sorts, free listing, life histories, or even a census, all are anchored in a holistic understanding of a context. This understanding is rooted in participant observation, which provides the cultural knowledge of life in that context. In its simplest form, ethnography is a representation of another culture. Written forms such as monographs or articles are common, but other media are used as well. Film or video is perhaps the best-known medium other than writing. Regardless of the media, the task of ethnography is to take an alien culture and make it believable to an intended audience.

Ethnographies are far more complicated than a journalistic travelogue. An ethnographer takes multiple perspectives in the construction of ethnography. At a minimum the ethnographer takes into account at least two perspectives. Anthropologists refer to these as the emic (the native point of view, the alien) and the etic (the observer's point of view, the familiar). By interweaving these perspectives, the alien people and their culture are made into an "other." The other is socially distant and appears to be objectified. This gives the ethnographer considerable latitude in the presentation of the other. The ethnographer makes the other into an object of study to be described and analyzed.

AN ETHNOGRAPHY OF AGE: AGE AMONG THE NACIREMA

What would an ethnography of age look like? To accomplish this, we have to turn to what is known about a specific people. We select a little studied but highly significant iconic tribe in North America, the Nacirema. These people are known for their unusual attitudes toward the body. Back in 1956, Horace Miner, then president of the American Anthropological Association, wrote a short article titled "Body Ritual among the Nacirema" (Miner, 1956). In this article Miner describes the preoccupation of the Nacirema with the body and their assumption that it is in the process of decay. He describes rather barbaric and harsh body rituals of this little known tribe, including facial lacerations, baking of heads in small ovens, and intentionally drilling holes in their teeth and filling them with magical substances. Subsequently, a physician, Joel Dimsdale, visited the Nacirema and further documented many of their medical beliefs (Dimsdale, 2001). An edited volume further documents social structure, kinship, economics, law, religion, and values (Spradley & Rynkiewich, 1975). We will further investigate the Nacirema and examine their preoccupation with age, which is just as extreme as their concerns with body decay, presumably because they are related in the eyes of Nacirema natives. In presenting a brief ethnography of age, we will examine the following issues among tribal Nacirema: the birthday complex, the age class system, the body ritual specialists who help old people delay body decay; the diseases associated with older people, especially animism disorder, and what the high priests of aging do to try to help this unfortunate class of people.

The Birthday Complex

In investigating other cultures, anthropologists have noted distinct complexes elaborated by specific cultures. For instance, the Inuit are known for the snow complex, in which over 20 different terms are used to classify unique types of snow. In East Africa, cattle herders have elaborated on cows. There is an extensive vocabulary to describe the color and confirmation of cattle, along with an extensive differentiation of cow body parts. This is viewed as excessive by other peoples of the world but not by those whose cultures are bound up with the well-being of their cattle. The Nacirema are known for their birthday complex. Clearly, age is an obsession among these people. The birth date of each and every individual is recorded on the sacred scrolls. Every infant is issued a certificate to document his or her birth date. Later in life, all members of the tribe carry evidence of their age. Beside a great sacred lake in the western part of the Nacirema range is located a temple devoted to the Book of the Dead, in which the birth date and death date of every known Nacirema are recorded. Death itself is so revered that the Nacirema devote significant portions of their assets to launch their deceased into the next world. A whole culture of preparation has grown up in support of the ritual.

Time among the Nacirema is carefully studied and recorded through the use of a solar calendar, which has remnants of an earlier lunar calendar embedded in it. Although they acknowledge earlier times, the present era is anchored in the birthday of an important god, Susej. Each year is noted, and each individual knows and has a special relationship to the year in which he or she was born. All members acknowledge the day of their birth on an annual basis. Some birthdays are more important than others. The first birthday is very important. Clan members gather to impress on the child the gravity of the day and to celebrate with ceremonial foods. Throughout childhood, ceremonies are held on children's birthdays to impress upon them the importance of knowledge of age. Other important birthdays are the 16th and the 21st. On these days transitions toward adult status are given special recognition. Throughout adulthood, every 10th birthday is a little more special, but some Nacirema also give extra recognition to every 5th birthday. Birthdays call for messages of congratulations, special foods, and fairly elaborate rituals including fire and song.

The Age Class System

Anthropologists make a distinction between age grades and age classes. Every culture recognizes a series of age grades, which are loosely defined, fairly broad divisions of life from birth to death (Radcliffe-Brown, 1929). Age classes, sometimes called age sets, are less common. In the creation of an age class, individuals, usually male, are recruited on the basis of age. Once recruited, a corporate group is formed, with the members passing through life together in opposition to the groups more senior and more junior to them. Usually the basis of group formation is generations (Bernardi, 1985; Eisenstadt, 1956; Spencer, 1996). Nacireman age sets are a little different, reflecting their preoccupation with chronological age. Individuals of both genders are recruited explicitly on the basis of age. Before the onset of puberty, usually after the fifth or sixth birthday, a child is initiated into the first of 10 to 16 age classes. Groups of age peers are formed on an annual basis. At the end of the annual cycle, each group is promoted to replace the group senior to it. As Maybury-Lewis (1974) notes, among the Akwi-Shavanti, age classes are most active for the young. Among the functions of the Nacirema age classes are acculturation and the denial of full adult status to adolescents. Once an individual leaves his or her last narrowly defined age class, the person enters the class of householder, when he or she focuses on productive activities and raising children. Around the 60th or 70th birthday, the individual enters the class of the *Deriter*. The focus of the individual's life turns to leisure and taking care of the decaying body.

Body Ritual Specialists and the Aged

As Miner (1956) noted, the Nacirema are fearful of the body forever falling into a state of decay or disrepair. Unfortunately, with increased age, one also experiences more rapid bodily deterioration. The shamans, or medicine men, struggle with each of their clients to prevent decay. Miner (1956) documented a number of specialized shamans, such as the "Holy Mouth Man" and the "Listener," who remove the products of decomposition or cast out demons. Also, the *latipso* is a specialized temple where most of the curing takes place, with an emphasis on extremely painful rituals. It is interesting to note that, despite the increased need for body ritual specialists among aged Nacirema, very few of these medicine men specialize in advanced states of decay. Obviously, the success rate of curing is marginal, and no shaman wants to risk his or her reputation. There are extensive pharmacopeias devoted to age reversals. These, however, simply mask the decay and do not cure it.

Animism Disorder

In his celebrated study of primitive religion, Edward Tylor (1871) discovered the phenomenon of animism. Animistic spirits, in leaving the body during dreams, also leave the dreamer with a shadowy memory. Tylor argued that in this animistic experience, we find the origin of all religion. Once the spirit leaves the body and does not return, the dreamer experiences death. The Nacirema have a disease that is best described as animism disorder (AD), or the loss of the soul. The soul leaves the body, but the individual does not die. In the early stages of this disease, the soul makes an attempt to return, and the afflicted individual experiences difficulties in interpreting immediate and present stimuli and retreats into past memories. Despite the efforts of the shamans to attract the soul back into the body, eventually the abandoned body succumbs to decay and dies several years later. Given the presumed absence of the soul, the medicine men cease addressing the Nacirema directly but instead address all comments through an intermediary, most often a family member, usually a spouse, who then presumes to speak for the one whose soul has left. No one knows for sure whether the soul stays gone without any brief revisitations or whether the soul returns to roost for brief periods until finally leaving completely, and the body passes to the next stage.

The High Priests of Age

If aging exacerbates the decay the Nacirema abhor, is there anything that can be done? In the village of the paramount chief, they have established a temple to house the priests who search for an antiaging elixir. These priests belong to a collectivity known as the Tsigolotnoreg. This is a multifaceted attack on aging inclusive of experts in the body and body systems, curers, listeners, and those who search for the social origins of well-being. So far the Tsigolotnoreg have not been successful in their search for the fountain of youth, but they have commandeered a sizeable portion of the chief's wealth to finance their efforts. They have also organized themselves into subtribes and often seem to feud with one another rather than tend to their missions.

One might ask what kind of society is the Nacirema. They are located in North America just south of the Cree of Canada, north of the Tarhumara of Mexico, and north of the Carib of the Caribbean basin. They are noted for their advanced economy organized by the marketplace. The Nacirema are quick to distance themselves from other tribal peoples who have rituals they do not immediately understand but are wont to admit that their own may strike others as just as strange. Among the Nacirema the value of paper seems to become the measure of people and an indicator of who is most deserving of what the culture has to offer. Though they represent a tribal society, Nacirema easily identify internal differences and seem to adjudicate among petitioners for cultural benefits on the basis of their accumulation of paper and other indicators of wealth. They are also noted for writing backward, including the name by which they refer to themselves. If one were to hold a mirror up to the culture of the Nacirema, one would quickly discover they are Americans.

HAVE WE LOST CULTURE IN OUR EXPLORATIONS OF AGE?

The intent of our etic ethnography of age among the Nacirema is to demonstrate the importance of social distance in ethnographic reporting. In writing about another culture, it is far easier to describe a cultural world that is alien and can be made into an object of study. It is far more difficult to ethnographically write about the familiar. Both the writer and the reader are likely to respond, "So what? I already knew that." Have we lost culture in our explorations of age as we have increasingly turned our attention to the familiar and to the alien that has become more familiar as peoples of different cultures have entered a globalized world? In this section we explore the difference in the detail and the way the data are reported in research at home and abroad. My intent here is not to indicate we have lost culture, but that we are at risk of not being as distant and objective with our cultural models.

Much of what we do in gerontology, at least in sociocultural gerontology, is based on the survey. Survey data are useful for associational or statistical modeling. We use mathematical techniques and technology to search for patterns in the data that enable us to make generalizations about the world. These models, however, are very abstract and tend to reify the statistical mean as typical of actual human beings. There is very little or no information about context. There is no ethnography to be found in these models. There is not much that is human about them other than the humans who provided the data. Although the models are cultural, there is very little about culture that is reported.

Ethnography brings humans and context back into our accounts and back to our efforts to understand the nature of experience and the creation of meaning. Participant observation familiarizes a researcher with the context, daily routine, environment, cast of characters, social structure, and issues shaping life. Doing ethnography abroad is difficult in that it takes time, and as one enters an alien cultural world, one's own cultural world is set on end. It is also increasingly difficult to do foreign research because of national restrictions placed on foreign researchers in the third world. In addition, with globalization many of the alien worlds are no longer alien through universal education and participation in the global economy. Yet the exotic in the alien worlds catches our attention and make us think. Death-hastening behavior is shocking regardless if it involves abandonment or actual killing. Widow inheritance or arranged marriages is not something that is ordinary at home. Placing men in age classes after an initiation that may involve scarification or circumcision is impressive. Filial piety sounds wonderful, but it is not practiced by Americans.

Ethnography at home is a little easier on the researcher in certain practical respects but far more difficult in terms of setting aside preconceptions. Usually linguistic barriers are minimized, and the amount the ethnographer has to learn is reduced because of prior cultural knowledge. Because of the scale of the home social field, ethnographers try to restrict the boundaries or even define the boundaries of the context. The real difficulty is that we are describing the familiar. It is hard to make the familiar as interesting as the alien. Ethnographers try to find the not so obvious or the counterintuitive to avoid sounding like chamber of commerce members. Another strategy is to take a concept developed in another context and apply it to the familiar. For instance, liminality is an excellent way of describing the endless transition in a nursing home (Shield, 1988). In our Nacirema ethnography, we described age through concepts developed in smaller scaled societies to create the illusion of social distance. Nevertheless, we are increasingly focused on the familiar. Do we learn more about age in America by writing about it as if we are describing the alien Nacirema? Do some of the explanations and rituals sound somewhat off-kilter when put in the context of the unfamiliar?

What has happened to culture? Are we running the danger of missing it or losing it because we are researching contexts that are familiar? The real problem is not that we are describing culture in which both the researcher and the audience already share many cultural assumptions. The real problem is that in any scientific account, our data must be objectified. Data have to be operationalized into objective categories. If our data are not socially distant, we run the danger of weakening our hold on culture. Early anthropologists actually increased the distance and objectivity with tribal peoples around the world. Not only were they geographically distant, but they also thought these people were archaeological fossils. They represented a different time (Fabian, 1983). Thus cultural facts and the "other" were objectified in time and space. Of course, there are times when one does not want to objectify culture. This is a more humanitarian use of culture, such as in literature or philosophy, where one intends to extend the experience or broaden the horizon of our audience. Have we lost culture, or is it simply changing?

REDISCOVERING CULTURE AND AGE

Anthropology awoke to age about the same time as other disciplines in the post –World War II era. It was 1945 when Leo Simmons published *The Role of the Aged in Primitive Society*. This volume is a landmark in gerontological research not only because it introduced culture and cross-cultural analysis to research on aging, but because it is the cornerstone of more recent anthropological inquiry into aging. Simmons used the then new Human Relations Area Files (HRAF), a topically organized file of existing published ethnographic work. The book is a combination of two very large tables of traits for 71 different cultures, along with ethnographic descriptions, including Simmons' own work among the Hopi. Simmons' work was the primary contribution of anthropology to gerontology until the 1960s. Following directly in Simmons' footsteps, a number of researchers have used a research strategy known as holocultural, which is a more sophisticated use of the HRAF. Questions explored relate to decrepitude and death-hastening behavior toward older people (Glascock, 1982, 1997; Glascock & Feinman, 1981), the motive for gerontocide (Maxwell, Silverman, & Maxwell, 1982), information and power for older people (Silverman & Maxwell, 1987), respect and deference toward older people (Maxwell, 1986; Silverman & Maxwell 1978), and contempt for older people (Maxwell & Maxwell, 1980).

Cross-cultural research has remained a steady and important contribution to aging research from anthropology. Some of the questions introduced by Simmons have continued to be explored using primary data rather than the secondary data to be found in the HRAF. Status of the aged has been linked to resource control using a regional sample (Press & McKool, 1972). Aging and modernization theory, introduced by Cowgill and Holmes (1972; Cowgill, 1986), explicitly formulates a hypothesis that links modernization to the declining status of older people. This hypothesis, in its simplicity, triggered one of the most productive debates in gerontology. The net result is a much more sophisticated and complex view of the implications of the cultural transformations that resulted in contemporary capitalistic societies for old people. Cross-cultural research can also have an integrated theory and methods. One such project is Project AGE, reported by Keith et al. (1994). Very different communities with differing economies and of dissimilar scale were ethnographically studied in Botswana, Ireland, Hong Kong, and the United

States. This project examined the features of seven different communities in shaping pathways to well-being in old age; the effects of different family organization; and the meaning of age, the life course, and health and functionality. With globalization, a cross-cultural and cross-national perspective is vital in understanding variations in experiences of aging around the world (Albert & Cattell, 1994). Not only do we need to know what has happened in the recent past, but we also need to use that knowledge to make the future more predictable. That future in all likelihood will involve far more economic integration and expansion of both labor and consumer markets. We will see differential participation in these markets, with an increase in homogeneity for some people and an increase in diversity or creolization for others, especially with the expansion of consumer markets.

The comparative method remains a strong component of the anthropological perspective. Despite the difficulties of foreign research and loss of cultural distinctness because of globalization, anthropologists have studied older people around the world, including Africa (Cattell, 1990, Draper & Harpending, 1994; Stucki, 1992), Asia (Beall & Goldstein, 1986; Cohen, 1998; Elliott & Campbell, 1993; Ikels, 1993; Keifer, 1990), Oceania (Barker, 1997; Counts & Counts, 1985; Dickerson-Putman, 1994; Holmes & Holmes, 1987; vanWilligen, Chadha & Kedia, 1995), Native North America (Amoss, 1981; Hennessy & John, 1995; Schweitzer, 1999), Central America, and South America. Closer to home, research among different ethnic groups is yet another use of the comparative method (Barker, Morrow, & Mitteness, 1998; Becker & Beyene, 1999; Groger & Kunkel, 1995).

In the late 1960s anthropological studies of aging took a major turn. The shift was to bring our research to American and European populations and a shift in perspectives. Margaret Clark (1967) brought medical anthropology to studies of aging. She saw her own work as contributing to furthering investigations of culture and personality. Her major study of mental illness and mental wellness among elderly San Franciscans linked mental problems and adjustment in old age to adherence to American values (Clark & Anderson, 1967). She also examined value orientations and the issue of dependency in later life (Clark, 1972). Margaret Clark went on to found the Medical Anthropology Program at the University of California–San Francisco and trained a whole generation of medical anthropologists specializing in aging.

Anthropologists seemed to thrive once introduced to aging. Sources of meaning in late life were explored (Kaufman, 1986; Luborsky, 1993). Retirement and its meanings were also investigated (Luborsky, 1994, Savishinsky, 2000). Gender has not been overlooked, with studies of older and middle-aged women (Kerns & Brown, 1992) and of older men living alone (Rubinstein, 1986). Comparative studies of menopause raise serious questions about its universality and its medicalization (Du Toit, 1990; Lock, 1993). Issues relevant to later life have proven to be fertile ground for anthropological inquiry.

Once anthropologists shifted their attention from tribal peoples and peasants to urban Americans, locations where older people were found became prime targets for ethnographic research. Age-homogenous or retirement communities were a comparative novelty. They also were viewed as potentially problematic because of the age segregation (Mumford, 1956). Once anthropologists moved in and participated in these newly created communities (Counts & Counts, 2001; Francis, 1984; Fry, 1977; Hochschild, 1973; Keith, 1977, 1979; Myerhoff, 1978), the picture changed completely toward the positive. Older people in quite diverse settings, including the deaf (Becker, 1980), are very much involved in their community's life and in shaping their future. Likewise, nursing homes became another target for ethnographic research, revealing both strengths and weaknesses in these settings (Foner, 1994; Henderson & Vesperi, 1995; Kayser-Jones, 1981; Savishinsky, 1991; Shield, 1988). Even inner-city residents in single-room occupancy (SRO) hotels were found to have created distinctive communities in these blighted areas (Cohen & Sokolovsky, 1989; Eckert, 1980; Sokolovsky & Cohen, 1987). Older people in age-heterogeneous communities also have received anthropological attention. Most notably are the aged in Appalachia (van Willigen, 1989), who face a changing and industrializing world. Women in rural communities also face distinctive challenges (Shenk, 1998).

One of the advantages of doing ethnography and becoming familiar with an alien context is that it is possible to create a holistic model of social life and social structure. Of all the cultural diversity in the world, one of the anthropological problems in social organization that has caught the attention of gerontologists is the discovery of societies that have age classes. In these societies, males are explicitly stratified by age into age-homogenous groups (Baxter & Almagor, 1978; Bernardi, 1985; Spencer, 1990, 1996). A man will pass through life together with his age peers. These age classes take many forms and are multifunctional, but they appear to be political in nature and serve to reduce conflict between father and son. Although the models of these societies are inappropriate for the study of industrialized societies, they stimulated the early theoreticians of the life course in formulating ideas about age norms, age grades, age stratification, and the meaning of cohorts. As the life course became a major paradigmatic framework in gerontology, anthropologists embraced it as a potential cross-cultural unit (Fry & Keith, 1982). On a comparative basis we know that life courses are organized or calibrated differently (Fry, 1999). In nonindustrial, small-scale societies, without the Gregorian calendar, age is relative, and the life course is calibrated by generational differences. Age class societies are a special case in which relative age and generations are formalized. The life course in industrialized societies is very distinctive in that it is staged through age-explicit norms created by the state. Age is chronological, which means it is not relative, but calculated in absolute terms through the use of a calendar. This has produced a tripartite life course organized around work: (1) childhood and adolescence, (2) adulthood, and (3) old age.

ENDURING QUESTIONS FROM ANTHROPOLOGY

Anthropological theory about aging has been transformed over the past 50 years. Anthropologists are no longer are exclusively concerned with relatively simple questions of how older people are faring in other societies. Instead, they look at how specific contexts shape the experience of aging. Researchers consider such things as gender, the meaning of age itself, and the configurations of life courses or a plan for aging. Ethnographers investigate how age has become medicalized and a whole host of questions involving older people and physicians, hospitals, nursing homes, and health and functionality. On a comparative basis, intergenerational relations and expectations of kin incorporating older people into family life are explored. Another issue is to probe the roles that resources and technology play in promoting a good old age.

When anthropology embraced gerontology, many of the anthropologists involved in aging saw it as an opportunity for reciprocal interdisciplinary exchange. Despite efforts to promote the study of aging in the field of anthropology (Kertzer & Keith, 1984), the exchange has been primarily one way, with anthropologists contributing and being welcomed into the field of gerontology. What is the contribution that makes anthropology appreciated in gerontology? What is the anthropological enduring question? It has to be culture in all its complexity and diversity.

I (Fry, 2003) have argued that we in aging research are a little disadvantaged in that we do not have a word that both indicates the phenomena we study and communicates something about cultural dimensions. People who research gender have the term *gender,* which is suggestive of cultural meanings. In contrast, the term *sex* refers to the phenotypic differences between men and women. When we use the term *age,* we seem to think about senescence—the physical phenomena, not culture. In my previous work (2003) I made an attempt to come up with a useful term. I used *age/time.* That earlier chapter was in a volume on the life course and lives unfold in different kinds of time, and the double word made sense. Here, with the emphasis on culture, I would like to argue that *age* is a perfectly good word that encompasses the cultural aspects of the phenomena. Thus my parallel with gender studies is this: Gender is to sex as age is to time. Absolutely everything we do with age has to do with culture. Biologists build models of the temporal process of aging; social scientists build models of caregiving, of family support, of political economies, of age structure, of demography. It is all culture. The physical aspect of aging is time and what happens along many dimensions in time.

The only downside to the use of the term *age* to capture culture is that it has a prior meaning in naturally occurring English. A quick check of a dictionary or thesaurus on the meanings of *age* shows (1) decrepitude and (2) geology. We should think about this dual meaning. Geological eras capture the order of change through time. Decrepitude, in contrast, is random insults and the resulting disorder in a biological organism or a social world. In aging, we study order and structure through time along many dimensions. We study the processes that try to restore order or make the results of chaos tolerable. We do not study chaos simply because it is random with no pattern. There is no way to make sense of chaos. Yet, if we take the commonsense observation that with increasing age, we find increasing disorganization or decrepitude, we fall into a trap. Age will forever be associated with the negative consequences of chaos and things we cannot change. We will never find an antiaging drug, and we will never invent an antiaging medicine (Hayflick, 2004). If we see age as culture and models of order, then age becomes much more positive and interesting. There are things we can do to promote and prolong order and structure once we understand them. Not only is it time that gerontology recaptures culture and recognizes that its endeavor is cultural, it is time for us to recapture the central phenomenon of our discipline, age as culture.

Age as culture is both enduring and revolutionary. It is enduring because anthropologists have emphasized the cultural aspects of age in all of their research. It is revolutionary because it brings culture center stage. Absolutely everything we investigate about age and how we research age is cultural. Science is cultural. The humanities are cultural. Every model we build about age or the experience of aging is cultural. Every path model, regression equation, or ethnographic model about age is cultural. This is not cultural imperialism, but it reminds us that culture is the way we come to understand the world. Because culture is the nexus of that understanding, it is one of the most difficult phenomena to be aware of.

As stated above, the whole idea of culture was born in a context of colonialism and economic and political expansion that brought culturally diverse peoples into long-term contact and interdependency. If the world were completely culturally homogenous, then we would not need to think of culture. But the world did not turn out that way. Culture is necessary to understand and represent the worlds of the people we study. Culture can also be used to advantage in understanding the gerontological enterprise and ourselves. If we are to make major breakthroughs in gerontology, we must move beyond our own nativistic, emic views of age. The prevalent themes of gerontological research such as senescence, antiaging medicine, caregiving, and well-being are rooted in cultural assumptions of age as decrepitude. Decrepitude is not the phenomenon of gerontological inquiry. Time is the phenomenon. Age is a temporal phenomenon. Age as culture is our understanding and interpretations of what happens in time.

Age as culture makes gerontology far more exciting and far more complicated than age as decrepitude. Lots of things happen in time. Further complicating the picture, there are many kinds of time with different clocks. This can range from the time Einstein introduced into physics the models we have of the universe. However, there are different dimensions of time calibrating the life course, such as work, family, health, and leisure. Age as a temporal phenomenon is enduring, not revolutionary. Age as culture in interpreting temporal phenomena is revolutionary. If the Nacireman Tsigolotnoregs embrace this perspective, the door is wide open for new lines of inquiry, and in the next 50 years we will see a very different gerontology.

REFERENCES

Albert, S. M., & Cattell, M. G. (1994). *Old age in global perspective: Cross-cultural and cross-national views.* New York: G. K. Hall.

Amoss, P. (1981). Cultural centrality and prestige for the elderly: The Coast Salish case. In C. Fry (Ed.), *Dimensions: Aging, culture and health* (pp. 47–64). South Hadley, MA: Bergin & Garvey Press.

Barker, J. (1997). Between humans and ghosts: The decrepit elderly in a Polynesian society. In J. Sokolovsky (Ed.), *The cultural context of aging: Worldwide perspectives* (pp.407–424). Westport, CT: Bergin & Garvey Press.

Barker, J., Morrow, J., & Mitteness, L. S. (1998). Gender and informal support networks, and elderly urban African Americans. *Journal of Aging Studies, 12,* 199–222.

Baxter, P. T., & Almagor, U. (Eds.) (1978). *Age, generation and time.* London: Hurst.

Beall, C., & Goldstein M. (1986). Family change, case and the elderly in a rural locale in Nepal. *Journal of Cross-Cultural Gerontology, 1,* 305–316.

Becker, G. (1980). *Growing old in silence.* Berkeley: University of California Press.

Becker, G., & Beyene, Y. (1999). Narratives of age and uprootedness among older Cambodian refugees. *Journal of Aging Studies, 13,* 295–314.

Bernardi, B. (1985). *Age class systems*. London: Cambridge University Press.

Cattell, M. G. (1990). Models of old age among the Samia of Kenya: Family support of the elderly. *Journal of Cross-Cultural Gerontology, 5*, 375–394.

Clark, M. M. (1967). The anthropology of aging: A new area for studies of culture and personality. *Gerontologist, 11*, 55–65.

Clark, M. M. (1972). Cultural values and dependency in later life. In D. O. Cowgill & L. D. Holmes (Eds.), *Aging and modernization* (pp. 263–274). New York: Appleton-Century-Crofts.

Clark, M. M., & Anderson, B. G. (1967). *Culture and aging: An anthropological study of older Americans*. Springfield, IL: Charles C Thomas.

Cohen, C. I., & Sokolovsky, J. (1989). *Old men of the Bowery: Strategies for survival among the homeless*. New York: Guilford.

Cohen, L. (1998). *No aging in India: Alzheimer's, the bad family, and other modern things*. Berkeley: University of California Press.

Counts, D. A., & Counts, D. R. (Eds.). (1985). *Aging and its transformations: Moving toward death in Pacific societies*. New York: University Press of America.

Counts, D. A., & Counts, D. R. (2001). *Over the next hill: An ethnography of RVing seniors in North America*. Peterborough, Ontario: Broadview Press.

Cowgill, D. O. (1986). *Aging around the world*. Belmont, CA: Wadsworth.

Cowgill, D. O., & Holmes, L. D. (Eds.). (1972). *Aging and modernization*. New York: Appleton-Century-Crofts.

Dickerson-Putman, J. (1994). Old women at the top: An exploration of age stratification among Bena Bena women. *Journal of Cross-Cultural Gerontology, 9*, 193–205.

Dimsdale, J. E. (2001). The Nacirema revisited. *Annals of Behavioral Medicine, 23*, 78–79.

Du Toit, B. M. (1990). *Aging and menopause among Indian South African women*. Albany: State University of New York.

Eckert, K. (1980). *The unseen elderly: A study of marginally subsistent hotel dwellers*. San Diego, CA: Campanile Press.

Eisenstadt, S. N. (1956). *From generation to generation*. New York: Free Press.

Elliott, K. S., & Campbell, R. (1993). Changing ideas about family care for the elderly in Japan. *Journal of Cross-Cultural Gerontology, 8*, 119–135.

Fabian, J. (1983). *Time and the other: How anthropology makes its object*. New York: Columbia University Press.

Foner, N. (1994). *The caregiving dilemma: Work in an American nursing home*. Berkeley: University of California Press.

Francis, D. (1984). *Will you still need me, will you still feed me, when I'm 84?* Bloomington: Indiana University Press.

Fry, C. L. (1977). Community as commodity: The age-graded case. *Human Organization, 3*, 115–123.

Fry, C. L. (1999). Anthropological theories of age and aging. In V. L. Bengtson & K. W. Schaie (Eds.), *Handbook of theories of aging* (pp. 271–286). New York: Springer.

Fry, C. L. (2003). The life course as a cultural construct. In R. A. Settersten, Jr. (Ed.), *Invitation to the life course: Toward new understandings of later life* (pp. 269–294). Amityville, NY: Baywood.

Fry, C. L., & Keith, J. (1982). The life course as a cultural unit. In M. Riley, R. Ables, & M. Teitelbaum (Eds.), *Aging from birth to death* (pp. 51–70) Boulder, CO: Westview Press.

Glascock, A. P. (1982). Decrepitude and death-hastening: The nature of old age in third world societies. In J. Sokolovosky (Ed.), *Aging and the aged in the Third World: Part I. Studies in Third World Societies* (pp. 43–66) Williamsburg, VA: College of William and Mary.

Glascock, A. P. (1997). When is killing acceptable?: The moral dilemma surrounding assisted suicide in America and other societies. In J. Sokolovsky (Ed.), *The cultural context of aging: worldwide perspectives* (pp. 56–70). Westport, CT: Bergin & Garvey Press.

Glascock, A. P., & Feinman, S. L. (1981). Social asset or social burden: Treatment of the aged in non-industrial societies. In C. Fry (Ed.), *Dimensions: Aging, culture and health* (pp. 13–12). South Hadley, MA: Bergin & Garvey Press.

Groger, L., & Kunkel, S. (1995). Aging and exchange: Differences between black and white elders. *Journal of Cross-Cultural Gerontology, 10,* 269–287.

Hayflick, L. (2004). From here to immortality. *Public Policy and Aging Report, 14*(1), 3–7.

Henderson, J. N., & Vesperi M. (Eds.). (1995). *The culture of long-term care: Nursing home ethnography.* Westport, CT: Greenwood.

Hennessy, C. H., & John, R. (1995). The interpretation of burden among Pueblo Indian caregivers. *Journal of Aging Studies, 9,* 231–244.

Hochschild, A. R. (1973). *The unexpected community: Portrait of an old age subculture.* Berkeley: University of California Press.

Holmes, L. D., & Holmes, E. (1987). Aging and change in Samoa. In J. Sokolovsky (Ed.), *Growing old in different societies: Cross-cultural perspectives* (pp. 119–129). Acton, MA: Copley.

Ikels, C. (1993). Chinese kinship and the state: Shaping of policy for the elderly. In G. L. Maddox & M. P. Lawton (Eds.), *Annual review of gerontology and geriatrics: Focus on kinship, aging and social change.* New York: Springer. (pp. 123–146).

Ikels, C., & Beall, C. M. (2001). Age, aging and anthropology. In R. H. Binstock & L. K. George (Eds.), *Handbook of aging and the social sciences* (5th ed., pp. 125–140). San Diego, CA: Academic Press.

Kaufman, S. R. (1986). *The ageless self: Sources of meaning in late life.* Madison: University of Wisconsin Press.

Kayser-Jones, J. S. (1981). *Old, alone, and neglected: Care of the aged in Scotland and the United States.* Berkeley: University of California Press.

Keifer, C. (1990). The elderly in modern Japan: Elite, victims or plural players. In J. Sokolovsky (Ed.), *The cultural context of aging: Worldwide perspectives* (pp. 181–196). New York: Bergin & Garvey Press.

Keith, J. (1977). *Old people, new lives: Community creation in a retirement residence.* Chicago: The University of Chicago Press.

Keith, J. (1979). The ethnographics of old age. Special Issue. *Anthropological Quarterly.* 52: 1, 69.

Keith, J., Fry, C. L., Glascock, A. P., Ikels, C., Dickerson-Putman, J., Harpending, H. C., & Draper, P. (1994). *The aging experience: Diversity and commonality across cultures.* Thousand Acres, CA: Sage.

Kerns, V., & Brown, J. K. (1992). *In her prime: New views of middle-aged women.* Urbana: University of Illinois Press.

Kertzer, D., & Keith, J. (Eds.). (1984). *Age and anthropological theory.* Ithaca, NY: Cornell University Press.

Lock, M. (1993). *Encounters with aging: Mythologies of menopause in Japan and North America.* Berkeley: University of California Press.

Luborsky, M. (1993). The romance with personal meaning in gerontology: Cultural aspects of life themes. *The Gerontologist, 33,* 440–454.

Luborsky, M. (1994). The retirement process: Making the person and cultural meanings malleable. *Medical Anthropology Quarterly, 8,* 411–429.

Maxwell, E. (1986). Fading out: Resource control and cross-cultural patterns of deference. *Journal of Cross-Cultural Gerontology, 1,* 73–89.

Maxwell, E., & Maxwell, R. J. (1980). Contempt for the elderly: A cross-cultural analysis. *Current Anthropology, 24,* 569–570.

Maxwell, R. J., Silverman, P., & Maxwell, E. K. (1982). The motive for gerontocide. In J. Sokolovosky (Ed.), *Aging and the aged in the Third World: Part I. Studies in Third World societies* (pp. 67–84). Williamsburg, VA: College of William and Mary.

Maybury-Lewis, D. (1974). *Akwe-Shavante society.* Clarendon UK: Oxford University Press.

Miner, H. (1956). Body ritual among the Nacirema. *American Anthropologist, 58,* 503–507.

Mumford, L. (1956). For older people: Not segregation, but integration. *Architectural Record, 119,* 191–194.

Myerhoff, B. G. (1978). *Number our days.* New York: Dutton.

Press, I., & McKool, M. (1972). Social structure and status of the aged: Toward some valid cross-cultural generalizations. *Aging and Human Development, 3,* 297–306.

Radcliffe-Brown, A. R. (1929). Age organization terminology. *Man, 29,* 21.

Rubinstein, R. L. (1986). *Singular paths: Old men living alone.* New York: Columbia University Press.

Savishinsky, J. (1991). *The ends of time: Live and work in a nursing home.* Westport, CT: Bergin & Garvey Press.

Savishinsky, J. (2000). *Breaking the watch: The meanings of retirement in America.* Ithaca, NY: Cornell University Press.

Schweitzer. M. M. (Ed.). (1999). *American Indian grandmothers: Traditions and transitions.* Albuquerque: University of New Mexico Press.

Shenk, D. (1998). *Someone to lend a helping hand: Women growing old in rural America*. Amsterdam: Gordon & Breach.

Shield, R. R. (1988). *Uneasy endings: Daily life in an American nursing home*. Ithaca, NY: Cornell University Press.

Silverman, P., & Maxwell, R. J. (1978). How do I respect thee? Let me count the ways: Deference toward elderly men and women. *Behavioral Science Research, 13*, 91–108.

Silverman, P., & Maxwell, R. J. (1987). The significance of information and power in the comparative study of the aged. In J. Sokolovsky (Ed.), *Growing old in different societies: Cross-cultural perspectives* (pp. 43–55). Acton, MA: Copley.

Simmons, L. W. (1945). *The role of the aged in primitive society*. New Haven, CT: Yale University Press.

Simmons, L. W. (1960). Aging in preindustrial societies. In C. Tibbits (Ed.), *Handbook of social gerontology: Societal aspects of aging* (pp 62–91). Chicago: The University of Chicago Press.

Sokolovsky, J., & Cohen, C. (1987). Networks as adaptation: The cultural meaning of being a "loner" among the inner city elderly. In J. Sokolovsky (Ed.), *Growing old in different societies: Cross-cultural perspectives* (pp. 189–201). Acton, MA: Copley.

Spencer, P. (1990). *Anthropology and the riddle of the sphinx: Paradoxes of change in the life course*. London: Routledge.

Spencer, P. (1996). Age sets, age grades, and age generation systems. In D. Levinson, and Ember, M. (eds). *The encyclopedia of cultural anthropology*. New York: Henry Holt.

Spradley, J. P., & Rynkiewich (Eds.), (1975). *The Nacirema*. Boston: Little, Brown.

Stucki, B. (1992). The long voyage home: Return migration among aging cocoa farmers of Ghana. *Journal of Cross-Cultural Gerontology, 7*, 363–378.

Tylor, E. B. (1871). *Primitive culture: Researches into the development of mythology, language, art and custom*. London:

van Willigen, J. (1989). *Getting some age on me. Social organization of older people in a rural American community*. Lexington, KY: The University Press of Kentucky.

van Willigen, J., Chadha, N. K., & Kedia, S. (1995). Personal networks and personal texts: Social aging in Delhi, India. *Journal of Cross-Cultural Gerontology, 10*, 175–198.

CHAPTER 7

The Contributions of Philosophy and Ethics in the Study of Age

Martha Holstein and Mark Waymack

When the ripe fruit falls
Its sweetness distills and trickles away into the veins of the earth.
When fulfilled people die
The essential old of their experience enters
The veins of living space, and adds a glisten
To the atom, to the body of immortal chaos.
For space is alive
And it stirs like a swan whose feathers glisten
D. H. Lawrence, "When the Ripe Fruit Falls," 1929, quoted in Cole and
Winkler (1994), p. 76.

In recent decades philosophical interest in aging has focused primarily on applied questions in medicine and long-term care (Holstein & Mitzen, 2002; Kane & Caplan, 1993; Parks, 2003), on specific topics such as ethics and Alzheimer's disease (Binstock, Post, & Whitehouse, 1992; Holstein, 1998; Nelson & Nelson, 1996), and somewhat less often on distributive justice—inquiries about resource allocation and intergenerational justice (are the elderly getting "too much"?) (Binstock & Post, 1991; Callahan, 1987; Homer & Holstein, 1990), advance directives, ageism, and pleas for respecting autonomy. In contrast, only a handful of writers have addressed larger themes about meaning and other normative concerns (Cole, 1985; Cole & Holstein, 1993; Manheimer, 1993; Moody, 1984; Rentsch, 1997). Yet, despite the dilatory attention paid to it, the essential Socratic question "How shall I live?" endures. Reflective people ask that question periodically—and often painfully—during their lives. The answers to deeper and broader questions about aging and meaning—essential philosophical notions about what it means to be old—have societal as well as personal significance, for without having some idea about what old age ought to be about—the core normative questions—we cannot conceptualize the elderly as a group about whom we can frame questions about social policy. Lacking such a notion, for example, how can we decide on the goals of programs such as Social Security or Medicare or support or attack retirement as a social institution? Without an idea of aging, what sense can we make of "antiaging" medicine? Tacit or otherwise, then, we must be operating with some implicit ideas about what it means to be old. Yet what are they? And what do those conceptions mean to those of us who are, or will, live them? Such questions are generally invisible to the dominant scientific mode of gerontology, gradually disappearing during the early modern period, when aging became a problem to be solved rather than a mystery to be lived (Cole, 1992).

What might happen if we allowed a return, however slight, to the mystery of old age? If we could accept that it is more than a problem to be solved and acknowledge that even if we understand the processes of aging at the molecular level, and know what social relationships facilitate a good quality of life, that mystery will always remain. We'll never "get it" all because, as the Italian philosopher Norberto Bobbio (2000) reminded us: "He who praises old age has not stared it in the face." Neither ancient myths nor modern stereotypes capture the challenges or the uncertainties of late life (Cole & Holstein, 1994). We cannot deny old age away by such trite advice as "You are only as old as you feel"; nor would the existential problems of old age disappear if age became irrelevant, something of a mythic dream, in any case. No matter the length of the telomerase at the end of our chromosomes, we are different at 80 than at 40; we are different at 60 even if we can still climb a mountain. Because we don't age only at the cellular level (Hayflick, 1994), our old age will be complicated—a blend of loss and strength, of burning passions but limited ability to act upon them (Maxwell, 1968/1979). If we allow ourselves, we will come to know that the fact of finitude makes our choices about how to live ever more urgent. With his experiences in the Nazi concentration camps as a backdrop, Victor Frankl (1968) observed that there are many things we cannot change, that instead we must adopt an attitude toward them. Even if biomedicine further democratized longevity and gave us the means to live in relative good health until we reached 120, we still would have to decide how to respond to those years and how to use them. Perhaps accepting that old age will always be something of a mystery, not ever fully understood, can inform the attitude we adopt toward old age. Mystery is often writ larger than a single life and suggests that even if we understand all the givens from relevant disciplines, that "the last of life for which the first was made" will still be filled with ambiguities, intricacies, the nearness to death, and a certain ad hoc quality. These realities make the enduring—the "ought"—questions alive and new while guaranteeing that there will be no permanent answers.

FACING ENDURING QUESTIONS

Philosophy and the humanities, more broadly, engage with these "ought" questions. What is a good old age? How will I know how I ought to live as an old person? What will support my self-respect, the sense that I have a real place in the world? What is expected of me? What does society owe to me so that I can live without undue anxiety about my financial security? How do I make my life coherent and purposeful? Who am I? For what purposes have I lived? Did my life matter? How do I hold myself accountable for the life I have lived and am living? To whom am I accountable? What values and belief systems give me the cognitive maps of my life so my experiences are more than a string of unrelated events? What happens when I cannot make sense of what is happening to me? The need to feel confident that we are doing what we "ought" to be doing is probably important to most, if not all, of us. This need escalates when we can no longer depend on our former roles and activities to instruct us and structure our lives. But how do we decide how to live? Are there cultural messages available to help us in wrestling with these questions? We may hear much about our rights, but what about our duties? Without obligations, am I not excluded from the moral community?

These questions may seem hopelessly old-fashioned, an indication that we have missed those seminars on Lyotard (1984) and postmodern aging. However, they may also mean that we tried to re-create ourselves in some radical way but that something still doesn't feel right. Can such questions be made relevant again? Can they survive existentialism, the linguistic "turn," philosophical neglect, postmodernism, applied ethics, "antiaging" medicine and death denial, and the multidisciplinarity of gerontology? We too are skeptical of abstract meta-narratives, such as the once-popular debate about disengagement and activity theory (although it seems that activity theory, in a new guise, is alive and well), yet we are convinced that, rather than being hopelessly old-fashioned, making informed decisions about the good life becomes more important as our life spans increase and our choices expand.

MAKING QUALITATIVE DISTINCTIONS

In his monumental book *Sources of the Self* (1984), philosopher Charles Taylor uses the concept "horizons of meaning" to remind us that we believe, often in- choately, that some ways of living are infinitely better than others. We choose, for example, those actions for which we can give the best reasons (Rachels, 2003) or those that facilitate moral understandings among people (Walker, 1998) or support our strongly held religious values. Different philosophers have approached the "ought" differently. They might, for example, consider the harms or benefits of different choices, or the way choices conform to his- torically honored values (MacIntyre, 1989; Taylor, 1984), or how choices fit the narrative of particular lives. Modern philosophical naturalists (Flanagan, 1991; Moreno, 1995) would further remind us that, although we cannot be held accountable for what is impossible, we are not absolved from acting morally. No matter how hard we try, we cannot scale Mount Everest, but that does not free us from making our bodies move in whatever way works.

We value a variety of approaches to the enduring questions and do not believe that any particular rule or principle will provide all answers; rather, a process of critical thinking that starts with acknowledging the worth of the questions seems essential. We start with culture, because its values and representations of old age are primary sources for our ideals of the good. Though we are free to make choices, to assess possibilities, to alter the status quo, and to adopt an attitude toward events, we are generally limited by some defining community (Taylor, 1984) that "gives us the symbols, images, and rituals upon which we can build meaningful lives within inevitable limits". (Cole & Holstein, 1994). Indeed, these social ways of thinking create the possibility for individuality, for constructing a meaningful life. The problem that we face today, however, is a map without directions, one full of shadows. There are few, if any, criteria, other than seemingly random personal prefer- ence, to inform our choices.

A normative discourse should minimally be able to suggest some grounds for making choices about how to live. They must not be, for example, perceived as oppressive (Holstein & Minkler, 2003; Ruddick, 1999). One of our strongest objections to the successful aging framework is this very limita- tion. To be successful, as Rowe and Kahn (1987) describe it, is probably not within the range of many older people, especially those who have struggled all their lives in low-wage, back-breaking jobs. Nor is it sufficiently rich to give us guidance about what to do if we are so fortunate as to have good health or if we do not.

As we consider the possibilities for criteria that will be neither oppressive nor impossible for many older people, cultural, sociopolitical, socioeconomic, and often gendered constraints are critical variables. These constraints are present and interact with one another in often invisible ways; they set boundaries, though not impermeable ones, around our life choices. Even more subtly, however, our choices are further limited by the way society describes and understands old age. In ordinary language, the descriptive or the ascriptive, the "is" and the normative "ought," are frequently conflated. So, when old age is described in a certain way, that is also the way the old are expected to be. These ideas help create the moral economy (Minkler & Cole, 1999), which identifies the obligations that society has toward its members. More specifically, this moral economy shapes public policy that, in turn, influences how we experience our old age. Social Security and Medicare, for example, came about in part because of certain ideas of the neediness of the old and their deservingness. As these impressions change, taken-for-granted policies may also change (Phillipson, 1998). In turn, these boundaries "furnish the markers by which life's chances are organized and representations of people grounded" (Hendricks, 2004, p. 248). In a never-ending circle, policy shifts, based on modifications of the ascriptive status held by older people, often force a rethinking of one's identify—where once the old were needy and deserving, today they are "geezers" who use too much of our collective resources, or they are considered vigorous enough to work until 70 (even if there are few jobs).

THE LIMINALITY OF OLD AGE

Such cultural confusion, though not unique to old age, is certainly more visible than at any other time. At all other ages, at least the structural outlines of how we ought to live are givens (Fahey & Holstein, 1993). We tend to conform because it is difficult not to. Law mandates that we go to school and punishes us if we do not support the families we create. Even the most rebellious among us generally play by at least most of the rules. At different times in our history, gender or race or ethnicity or class has shaped how we engaged with these institutionalized norms, but we cannot easily evade them—for example, it is not easy to drop out of the workforce at age 44, if we are not independently wealthy. If we were lucky enough and possessed the acceptable characteristics, we had much choice within these boundaries. Those boundaries, in turn, shaped us.

But old age has been different. Although powerfully influenced by the political and moral economy, by culture, and by our health and family status—all interactive with one another—we face no socially normative expectations. We exit one stage and enter another that is devoid of any culturally affirmed philosophical or existential meaning. Until recently, no one expected anything of people who were 70 or 80 or older. "The triumph of mass longevity was not accompanied by culturally rich notions of what old age could or should mean for individuals or society. Instead modern old age loomed as a permanently liminal state, with neither shared ideals or purposes." (Cole & Holstein, 1994). Even now, in professional and popular circles, the prevailing norm for old age is no more than being as we were in middle age. This norm requires accepting the pretense that chronological age is an artifact that should have no influence on how we subjectively experience our old age. But this norm places real pressures on many older people to accept the ever-escalating expectations that to modify our bodies, faces, and hair so as to mitigate the obvious signs of aging. Advertisements show us the penalty of "letting ourselves go," and a visit to a nursing home reminds us that we too can fail (i.e., be in a wheelchair at 82 rather than sailing in the Bahamas) if we do not maintain good health habits all of our lives. If we become disabled, if we are and feel subjectively old, we are then failures, with the singular goal of not entering a nursing home (Cohen, 1988; Minkler, 1990).

As such, American culture is strangely impoverished. It does not ask the enduring philosophical questions about aging and old age. These questions are necessary because, contrary to current ideologies, age is a unique time in human life, one not to be denied away. Because there is a time for every purpose, as both Ecclesiastes and 1960s folk music reminded us, the enduring questions are still worth exploring. If we engage consciously and vigorously with these enduring questions of how to live, we are more likely to find the cognitive maps we need for ourselves; it is also more likely that public policies will reflect deeply held values rather than threaten them.

The absence of such sustained engagement fit well with the impugning of grand narratives, initiated by Lyotard (1984) and other pioneer post-modernists; it is reflected in the relative absence of prevailing philosophical reflections about old age, even among philosophers. For the most part, philosophers who are interested in applied questions focus on the ethical ideal of autonomy and rather narrowly circumscribed ethical problems. Applying the core concept of autonomy, for example, to old age supports ideals of freedom. With a few important exceptions (Callahan, 1996; Mackenzie & Stoljar, 2000; Meyers, 1997), to applied ethicists choice, much like good health to Rowe and Kahn (1987), is what matters. What ought to be done with good health or how to ensure that an array of meaningful choices is available to most, if not all, older people is left unaddressed.

Instead we have "empirical" ideas about how to age well (Rowe & Kahn, 1987) that tend to act as implicit norms; we have a large literature on the self in old age (e.g., Atchley, 1987; Holstein & Gubrium, 2000; Kaufman, 1986) with suggestive normative content, and sociological ideas about what we do and how we live in old age. We see images of "busyness," as reflected in the National Public Radio series produced by Connie Goldman in the 1980s, "I'm Too Busy to Talk Now," and articles critiquing the "busy" ethic in old age (Ekerdt, 1996; Katz, 2000), but without offering a substantive alternative. Measuring our days so that we can face death is answered most often by hospice and not by taking account of finitude in our daily lives. It is only acceptable to think about death when it is immediately upon us and we have little time to prepare. Where would we fit this story from the Midrash: A rabbi tells his companion that one must always prepare for death by atoning for one's sins the day before one dies; the other rabbi is puzzled. "How do I know it is the day before I die?" he asks. The first rabbi then answers, "It is for that reason that we must live everyday as if it were our last."

If for no other reason than to prepare for death, focused normative reflection, whether inductive or deductive, can offer a toolbox of ideals and images for us to think about. This need becomes ever more important as we edge toward the inevitable losses that accompany old age. If old age is not always joyful and positive, as the postmodern ideal would have it, older people may need cultural assistance in making sense of the particular untoward events of later life (Bruner, 1990).

We now turn to some specific ways in which cultures across time have engaged with philosophical issues that aging and old age raise for us as individuals and as social entities. The limits of time and space will make this scan a brief one—a sampling rather than a history of humanistic reflections on aging (Cole & Gadow, 1986; Cole, Kastenbaum, & Ray, 1999). Some of the best sources, to which we cannot give the attention they deserve, are literary—poetry, prose, memoirs, and journals. We hope our brief foray will entice readers to further pursue these sources, as they are not only intellectually enticing but also personally essential.

AGES AND STAGES

Historically, two images—the division of life into ages (or stages) and the metaphor of life as a journey—to represent the wholeness, unity, or meaning of life have dominated Western thinking about aging (Cole & Holstein, 1994). In the image of the stages of life, expectations for each "age of man" were clear: The proverbial stages of life are plotted as a set of ascending and descending stairs (Cole, 1992). Shakespeare in *As You Like It,* provided a particularly grim image of man in the seventh age: "Last scene of all, / That ends this strange eventful history, / Is second childishness and mere oblivion; / Sans teeth, sans eyes, sans taste, sans everything" (act 2, scene 7).

Although today, this image would be attacked as hopelessly ageist, is it not possible that it rather reflected a general reality about old age in the early modern period, especially among the poor? And what would it be like today, if we could more bluntly accept change, but with less judgment?

In the ages and stages imagery, virtues and voices were commonly assigned to each stage and the expectation was that life functioned as a "career" (Cole, 1992). "From late antiquity throughout most of the [M]iddle [A]ges, aging and old age were conceptualized within a morally ordered view of the life course, with distinct expectations of how individuals were to conduct themselves and distinct ontological interpretations associated with each particular age grouping" (Gilleard, 2002, p. 25). The life course, ordained by God, was the natural order, a morality tale reflecting the moral order of the universe, "of which aging and old age form an integral part" (Gilleard, 2000, p. 29).

But there was also a saving grace that the alternative conception of life as a journey represented. Though from one point of view older people, bent and gray, stood at the lowest rung of the ladder, medievalists offered an alternative vision—life as a positive ascent, a sacred pilgrimage, a journey to God; hence it was simultaneously possible to physically decline and spiritually ascend (Cole, 1992), an image often lost today when the 80-year-old on skis is contrasted to the 80-year-old in a wheelchair (Rowe & Kahn, 1987). Lost is the possibility that the latter may possess spiritual wisdom and the former may suffer from spiritual emptiness (Holstein & Minkler, 2003). As religious and spiritual values infuse gerontological thinking, we may once again be able to reintegrate physical decline and spiritual growth.

Florida Scott Maxwell (1968–1979), the Jungian analyst writing in her 80s, suggested that the essence of old age was the chance to own one's whole self—to make whatever one has been and now is into an integrated whole; the journey toward old age ends in wholeness. Historically, these iconographic images of the journey—and the possibility of spiritual growth and an afterlife—helped people manage what was often a very difficult life, much as the Black churches did in the pre–civil rights era. When life and death seemed haphazard and few assumed that a bent back and changed appearance were anything other than unavoidable features of old age, when death could come randomly and at any age, it was wise counsel to be prepared at all times.

Religious thinking has been among the most important sources of continuity for the journey metaphor because it can embrace ambiguity and does not call upon individuals to do what they can no longer do. The Hebrew Scriptures may be the earliest known commentary on aging and old age. Though we are most likely familiar with the patriarchs and some matriarchs (e.g., Sarah) living to very ripe old ages, those ancient stories are not really commentaries on old age. Instead we look to the familiar biblical prescriptions: "Rise before the hoary head"; "Honor thy father and thy mother" (suggesting that dishonor might have been a problem); and hear the psalmist's plea that echoes through the centuries: "Do not cast me off in old age, when my strength fails and my hairs are gray, forsake me not, O God"{{AQ7}}

In the wisdom literature, "age-centered teachings are a tool to express the writers' search for theological answers and their personal quest for the good life" (Dulin, 2001; the following account relies on Dulin's thoughtful observations of Ecclesiastes). The original "fiddler," he clearly saw "on the one hand, on the other hand." Utilizing the stages metaphor, Ecclesiastes graphically spoke of an old man as "bent as an ape." Unable to take easy comfort in faith, Ecclesiastes challenged the possible meaningless of human life: What real value is there in anything under the sun? But recognizing the power of pleasure, he advised men to eat and drink and enjoy themselves. How modern he seems in all ways but one—how willing are moderns or postmoderns to accept the realities of the degradations that often accompany age? The essential tension that Ecclesiastes embraces is the tension that Barbara Myerhoff (1978) addressed in *Number Our Days*. This tension, however, is difficult to maintain in the age of the definitive diagnosis and the world of the body shops that tells us we can fix what ails us either physically or psychically. By denying the reality of senescence, it is unnecessary to live with the tension that Ecclesiastes so eloquently describes. In a lovely passage, he advises, "Go, eat your bread in gladness and drink your wine in joy" (9.7). To live fully, even if in the end all is futile, is the second half of the equation that existentialism did not embrace.

Capturing both the stages of life iconography and the journey metaphor, Pirkei Avot, (5:24—Ethics of the Fathers), the classical Hebrew text compiled in the second century, states: "At five years old, one begins the study of Torah; at 10 the study of Mishnah; and at 13 is ready to obey the commandments. At 15, he begins the study of Gemara; at 18 he married; at 20, he enters the chase; and at 30, he is at full strength. At 40, he gains the power of understanding and at 50 he can begin to give advice to others. At 60, he enters old age; at 70, he turns gray; at 80, he becomes full of vigor; and at 90, he is broken down. At 100, he is like a dead person who has passed away and faded from the world" (quoted by Goelman, 1997, p. 28).

These statements serve both normative and descriptive ends and like all Hebrew texts call for interpretation. In a tradition that makes obligation a central feature of both the religious and the moral life, one must assume normative intentions, but, as we noted above, the moral life must be possible for us; we cannot hold ourselves morally accountable for what we cannot do. The descriptive is not the normative but rather is the foundation for normative possibilities, a step that is often missing in contemporary discourses about aging. To take one example, the "successful aging" paradigm presumes that the possibilities to age in the lauded way (after all, the very word *successful* implies praise) are basically about choosing throughout one's life to engage in certain healthful practices. Although it is good to aspire to such practices, to actually engage in them is not equally available. Hence to "fail" to age successfully may have more to do with where you live—in a troubled neighborhood where walking is unsafe or where fresh vegetables are costly and hard to find—and the job that you have rather than the behavioral choices that you have made (Holstein & Minkler, 2003).

So we return to the Pirkei Avot and take a brief look at how the 16th-century scholar Ibn Machiri interpreted this passage. At age 40 begins the journey toward spiritual growth so familiar in the wisdom traditions; though physical powers are still present, we will be asked to account for our lives, "Not in terms of material growth and physical pleasure but rather in terms of spiritual knowledge and understanding" (Goelman, 1997, p. 32). Our spiritual growth continues as we examine our lives, repent for mistakes made, and use our understanding to guide others: "Recognizing the truth within us and offering truth to others as instruction are the challenges beginning at age 50" (p. 33). While preparing for death, as we enter our 60s, we deepen our wisdom and continue to examine, fix, and improve what is left of our lives. With escalating urgency, the path of reflection and repentance continues, ripening in our 80s, a gift of life that comes only as the result of overcoming adversity and living with fortitude and discipline. By 90, bent and broken down, we still are obliged to tell the story of our lives and how we reached this great age—we must teach so that others may learn. In this worldview there is loss and pain, but life is a gift that we must not squander by living it unreflectively. In closing his commentary, Ibn Machiri does what he has not done before and advises taking this journey with another, a "suitable" friend, in community. And so this is one version of the stages of life that gives a rich content of what is expected of us along the way.

Although the stages and journey tropes have many manifestations, the few that we have offered suggest how individuals might find them useful as they try to situate themselves in the cosmos and in their neighborhoods. Today, with the near certainty of formal retirement, the stages metaphor has become institutionalized as part of the life course. Only recently has the postmodern assault on the institutionalized life course and the practical concerns about supporting an expanding aging population come together to destabilize this institutionalized life course. This destabilization stemmed from two primary sources: a postmodern belief in life as a process of self-creation in which norms lost their familiar sanctions and what some considered a practical necessity—to postpone retirement to ever older ages because of the apocalyptic increase in the number of aged individuals. So far, this move toward "post-traditional" aging is either a hope for the future or a privilege of the affluent.

"QUASI"-NORMATIVE IDEAS ABOUT AGING: ANCIENT, MEDIEVAL, AND MODERN

Manheimer (1993) suggests that there are three paradigmatic viewpoints about old age: "the transformed/contributive, resigned/disengaged, and active/engaged" (p. 79). Less traditional but currently in vogue is the liberated/deconstructed view. We add, and as we shall discuss below, however, formulaic solutions are less apt to incorporate the vicissitudes of old age than a relational view of the virtues such as feminist philosopher Sara Ruddick (1999) proposes. Unlike traditional theories developed by well-born men for other well-born men, Ruddick and other contemporary philosophers are enmeshed in the possibilities that are available to each of us regardless of gender or status. This, we shall argue, is essential for any effort to address "enduring questions." But first, a brief sketch of time-honored philosophical thinking about aging.

Like Ecclesiastes, ancient Greek and Roman philosophers and other humanistic writers, especially playwrights, were conflicted about old age. Its physical manifestations challenged ideals of wisdom, and the aged were often depicted on stage, especially in the comedies, as weak and foolish. Yet, on occasion, a mysterious kind of beauty and wisdom was ascribed to at least some individuals of advanced age; witness Sophocles' depiction of Oedipus at Colonus. Plato seemed sensitive to such ambiguities, acknowledging the physical beauty, strength, and sexual appeal of youth and middle age, while at the same time trying to articulate an affinity for nonphysical beauty and truth that was perhaps accessible to the elderly in ways that it was inaccessible to the young. His student, Aristotle, was perhaps more ambivalent. On the one hand, advancing age did mean the possibility of advancing wisdom; but as a naturalist, Aristotle also seemed to regard many of the bodily and mental changes in older ages as declines, as movements away from the ideal of human flourishing.

Three centuries later, Cicero, particularly in *De senectute [On Old Age]*, a treatise that assumed an audience of upper-class men, advised stoicism in the face of loss, and recommended philosophical or spiritual activities and age-appropriate behavior (Troyansky, 2004). Anticipating philosophical naturalism, Cicero advised that no one be asked to do what he or she cannot do. Moral obligations exist in a realm of background conditions that are not easily, if at all, changeable. Hence, although Cicero acknowledged the physical degradations of age, to which he advised resistance through good self-care, he found many reasons to be optimistic, for he, like many moderns, was able to find the gift of wisdom a useful attribute and the chance to teach the young a worthy goal, even while physical strength declined. New learning was possible, "for in my old age I have learned Greek, which I seized upon as eagerly as if I had been desirous of satisfying a long-continued thirst . . . " (from *De senectute,* quoted in Cole & Winkler, 1994, p. 50). Thus Cicero advises, "Let every man make a proper use of his strength and strive to his utmost, then assuredly he will have no regret for his want of strength" (p. 50). Like Plato, Cicero delighted in the elimination of sensual pleasure, which leads us to many different unwise actions, including treason and the overthrow of states, and although he knows that few can forgo all pleasure, he advises temperance above all. Cicero is most definitely not in the camp of many who celebrate the sexuality of old age, but we might take counsel from him nonetheless because sexuality, though now so "in" as a desirable part of old age, can also be oppressive, an unintended consequence that enthusiasm tends to blur (Holstein, 2003; Katz, 2003). And, above all, Cicero exalts a leisured old age. Leisure frees us to study; without the obligations that constrain us in our earlier years, we can continue to contribute in whatever way we can. Old age also allows us to face a death that comes from ripeness, as the D. H. Lawrence poem with which we opened suggests.

Cicero did not alone speak for Roman views of aging. Seneca's less idealized vision recognized that how individuals experience old age had much to do with physical and mental health. For Seneca, then, suicide was a viable option if mind and body start to fail. For the satirists like Juvenal, images were far from the classic notion of the retired but still noble statesman. Not unlike today, these different social images contained idealizations of old age and implicit instructions about how to live. Yet ribald humor also freely mocked the depredations of age. We wonder how the saving grace of humor might liberate today's discussions about old age

With just these few examples we put to rest the belief that there was once a golden age in which elders were widely respected and honored; we fear instead that this wish represents a very human yearning that is nonetheless a myth. The "belief that the status of older people is always declining has a very long history. The longevity of this narrative trope in the discussion of old age suggests that it expresses persistent cultural fears of aging and neglect, and real divergences in most times and places, rather than representing transparent, dominant, reality" (Thane, 2003, p. 6). The Romans, for example, shared our fear of being put out to pasture at the same time that they advised staying physically and intellectually active in retirement. Also, not unlike modern discussions about aging being a roleless role, in ancient Rome the state's response to its oldest members was exemption from duties rather than the bestowal of privilege. Ancient representations of old age gave the proverbial mixed message to anyone paying attention.

With the advent of what we now call the "modern" age, aging increasingly became a technological problem. The "new science" conceived of the world as an orderly, scientifically understandable thing. As our scientific understanding of nature increased, so would our ability to manipulate nature to serve human ends. Thus the new science was not confined to something like astronomy or theoretical physics, but by the 18th century there was active and fruitful study of agriculture, economics, and medicine. The medieval fatalism about nature and health was supplanted by a science-facilitated project to improve our lot. Old age was reconceived not so much as a religious-moral problem (preparation for the life hereafter) but as a problem for the medical sciences. And antiaging medicine had its modern beginnings.

OLD AGE BECOMES A PROBLEM

This 18th-century beginning carried through into the 19th century as old age became less of a subject for philosophical analysis and more a problem demanding medical attention. The body became the focus of attention, and with that the unattractive features of old age—Juvenal's view rather than Cicero's—also became more dominant, a not surprising phenomenon, as the people writing about old age were primarily physicians who treated the sick and the poor. Narrowly attending to the physiology and pathology of a body that no longer worked very well did little to bring honor to the old. Simultaneously, the continued medicalization of old age, enmeshed in the emerging middle-class culture, to the relative exclusion of other interests was taking shape. Much as we now accuse biomedicine of focusing on the parts and not the whole, our 19th- and early-20th-century predecessors microscopically searched for the signs of aging. Severe osteoarthritis was located solely in the joints and not in the psyche of the 80-year-old woman who was so bent over that she was unable to walk the hills of her neighborhood to go to the grocery store. And like today, this bent over old woman failed to meet cultural ideals of activity and vitality (Cole, 1992). "In the bourgeois world of civilized morality, the old came to signify dependence, disease, failure and sin" (Cole, quoted in Haber & Gratton, 1994, p. 359). This is not a group about which one attends to philosophically.

Popular medical manuals reinforced the neediness of the aged and supported the ministrations of health and social service professionals. To forestall death, the old body needed all the help it could get (Haber, 1983). Thus began the modern preoccupation with health that today's norm of "successful aging" updates but leaves basically unchallenged. So the task of aging well became to stay as healthy as possible without any examination of the ends good health ought to serve. Though distinctly unhelpful in helping people decide how to live, it did contribute to the identification of the elderly as a class in need of social intervention, what Binstock (1977) labeled "compassionate ageism." Such defining of the old as needy and dependent gave implicit messages about how one ought to live; little was expected or offered that would encourage a socially reinforced self-worth. This negation was reinforced by the coming of formal retirement in the 1930s.

Only in the past 30 years have the humanities, which insist on the importance of thinking about ends and purposes, claimed space in the gerontological landscape. From the past, then, we have some ideas of what elite groups viewed as the meaning and purpose of old age (though how the poor, the uneducated, and the marginalized might have conceived old age is much less known to us). At times those views took seriously the key questions of how we ought to live and what a good life in old age is, but more often, particularly in the 20th century, the emphasis was on "problems" of old age and how society might respond to a group defined as dependent and in need. More recently, as a greater number of anthropologists and qualitative researchers have asked questions about aging cross-culturally, we have begun to gain some insight into the meanings of old age in different cultural traditions.

CONTEMPORARY GERONTOLOGICAL IDEALS:
IMPLICIT AND EXPLICIT

In the past 20 years or so, mainstream gerontology has altered much of its thinking about aging and old age, offering implicitly normative answers to archetypical philosophical questions. One difficulty with such implicit norms, however, is that unintended consequences are left unexamined. In particular, the transition from a decline and loss paradigm to an enthusiastic embrace of positive views of old age has dominated today's cultural ideals of aging. Joined with ideas that emerge from applied ethics and from other scholarship in the humanities, we can glimpse the contemporary situation as it relates to philosophical understandings of old age.

Age integration, ageism, and the concepts of "productive" and "successful" aging encouraged a different way to think about that period in life once known as old age. The late Bernice Neugarten (1982) segmented old age into three categories based on levels of functionality, suggesting that we were not really old until we reached the "old-old" category. Conceptually and perhaps unintentionally, age integration and the categorization of old age in chronologically identified groupings are suggestive of normative goals, namely, be in old age as you were in middle age, until you become so old that your health begins to fail. Hence a positive value ascribed to middle age and its typical lived experience is revered, in contrast to an implicit devaluing of old age and its typical lived experience.

Similarly, vanguard adjectives of *productive* and *successful* impose a more explicit but, we believe unintentional, normative ideal for what old age ought to be. These ideals carry forth the broader theme that aging is about liberty, freedom to construct whatever life one wants—the postmodern "turn." We think that as normative ideals these fail: They do not take seriously the fact of inevitable finitude; they do not situate the individual within a macro social-political-economic context that shapes the conditions of possibility for the micro-experiences of old age; and they impoverish rather than enrich the potentialities of old age. If continuity and change both operate in late life as in other stages, the pendulum has so strongly turned toward continuity and even old age valetudinarianism that it becomes easy to lose sight of the both/and that writers as diverse as Ecclesiastes and Cicero so eloquently described. Age is both a subjective and an objective experience; by focusing on the former, we cannot erase the latter (Andrews, 2000). Yet efforts at such erasure in the name of promoting agelessness denigrates the aging body, thereby compounding the effects of social devaluation that aging people experience in their day-to-day lives because their bodies are aesthetically displeasing to the youthful gaze. Moreover, we disregard the uncertainties that easily arise when the "personal identities and normative systems" that older people have developed exist in a "cultural sphere that no longer exists" (Rentsch, 1997, p. 8).

Like earlier middle-class ideals of activity, youthful vigor, and economic engagement, dominant gerontological views negate the many features of old age that are shaped by biology and psychology. The body, as in the 19th century, is a machine that we oil, exercise, tend to by eating properly and engage actively, but except in the work of feminist gerontologists (Calasanti & Slevin, 2001; Ray, 1996) and philosophers (Bordo, 1993; Furman, 1999; Harper, 1997) and some few others, the body is denied as our most immediate access to the world. When it works less efficiently no matter how well we have tended to it, our relationship to the world changes, and our self-understanding alters. To make meaning of this new body is a philosophical and not a biological question, yet biology dominates the gerontological discourse about the body. Even more importantly, perhaps, are the hidden class and race biases that these views contain. Not only do opportunities to engage in the practices that support "successful" aging differ by one's economic status and one's life chances, but it presumes, as did Cicero, that the audience is like the researchers—high-status individuals who evaluate their lives by measures contained in the now-popular adjectives.

To revisit briefly the older notion of "productive" aging, which reached its apogee in the early 1990s, we suggest that it too shared these class and race biases. Productive aging had two often contradictory goals; it was, in part, intended to show that older people, rather than being a drain on the economy, actually contributed a great deal through intergenerational exchanges and caregiving responsibilities that if monetized would amount to billions of dollars. Other messages, however, focused on the health of older people and their continued ability to work and engage in other productive activities. Although this view was meant to refute ageist claims that older people had little or nothing to contribute to the general good, it also unintentionally did two other things. It raised questions about people who no longer wished to work or actively engage in "productive" activities, while it undercut the previously prevailing reasons for Social Security and other forms of income support. The danger is that the more economically secure need not worry about this undercutting, whereas those who are barely able to make ends meet see continued work not as a choice but as a mandate. Ideology thus joins economic necessity. Poorer women are most likely to be in this group, the same women who might have scrubbed floors or worked in factories or low-wage service work and who, if given the chance, might enjoy being nonproductive, especially if their lifetime of work has had serious health repercussions (for an extended feminist critique of productive aging, see Holstein, 1993). One need only recall the challenge to old age legitimacy that came in the mid-1980s with the advent of Americans for Generational Equity (AGE). Instead of portraying older people as dependent and in need, this organization offered a vision of "greedy geezer," a phrase that has continued long beyond the life of AGE.

Taking these displeasing features of what often happens in old age in another direction, philosopher C. G. Prado (1990) advised preemptive suicide prior to the onset of disabilities. Perhaps like preemptive war, such suicide addresses what Prado views as an imminent harm—the degradations and deprivations of age. No Ciceronian stoicism if we can take control and choose the moment of our own death when we are still at the height of our powers. Though in a minority, Prado's postmodern view is on a continuum with those that reduce the goals for people with disabilities; these views seem to marginalize if not eliminate the ambiguities that the ancients wrestled with and that Ecclesiastes accepted as inevitable in old age. Rather than make meaning from disabilities, we are to hide them from view by segregation or suicide.

Another relatively recent trend—the attention to the ethics of aging— sheds further light, albeit indirectly, on philosophy and aging (Jecker, 1992; Moody, 1994). Applied ethics—the effort to work our way through real problems that we encounter in clinical and related settings—contributed a good deal to recognizing that older people are not simply passive recipients of ministrations by the medical profession or social workers but that they have the primary voice in deciding what treatments they would accept, where they would live, and how they wished to weigh matters such as safety and risk.

The immediate focus was on autonomy understood as self-determination. With autonomy as the trump, paternalism (or maternalism) was eclipsed. Not only did this discourse on ethics assume that ethics was about making choices—decisions—in a bracketed moment of time, but correlatively, it framed ethics in terms of dilemmas or conflicts between equally good (or equally bad) options and held that the best way to resolve such situations was procedural—weighing deductively derived, universally applicable principles against the specific facts of the case. This method seemed to provide secure action guides capable of directing thinking in conflictive situations. In particular, these action guides invited terms like *autonomy* and *best interests* into our everyday vocabulary. Autonomy—for better or worse—became the new version of the golden rule, and the most common value dilemma was framed as autonomy versus best interests. Simultaneously, procedures to ensure confidentiality, privacy, informed consent, treatment termination, or continuity were adopted. These procedural rules applied no differently to elderly patients than to anyone else unless they—again, like everyone else—were cognitively impaired or otherwise unable to make decisions. Then another person—their proxy—decided for them, but only as they would have decided if they still had the capacity to decide. Substituted judgment was a higher standard than best interests for such proxy decision making. The focus of applied ethics was on decision making, treatment, and place of residence, especially transfer issues, advance planning for disability, and end-of-life care. It did not address philosophical questions about aging or old age; such discussions were, in part, a casualty of the emphasis on making decisions. If decisions are the primary end of ethical reflection and autonomy the central value, the idea that these decisions ought to rest on some thoughtful appraisal of what old age ought to be about received little attention except from philosophers such as Daniel Callahan, to whom we will turn below.

The stress on autonomy also mapped comfortably onto social work norms that emphasized client self-determination and fit well within a society that stressed individualism and highlighted self-interested behavior (unless it directly harmed another). American society has tended to be most comfortable with liberty as nonintervention than a more activist notion of providing the conditions that would make freedom possible (see Berlin, 1969). It is for similar reasons that Americans find it easier to focus on rights rather than the good life, individual well-being over communal welfare.

The narrowness of this view has had interesting philosophical ramifications. Autonomy works, as philosopher George Agich (1993) pointed out, only when there are preconditions that allow people to make meaningful choices. It does little good to give someone a choice over options to which he or she cannot relate. A lifelong contract bridge player will find little meaningful in a choice between bingo and rummy in a nursing home activities program. Labeling this concept interstitial autonomy, Agich suggests that we rarely face large life-determining choices, but we do decide everyday when to get up or go to sleep, when to have breakfast or a cup of tea. What we owe people is ensuring that they have the chance to live meaningful lives in which their identities are preserved in forms they themselves recognize. Although this endorses an individualistic version of what it means to live well, it does call for more significant social obligations than the simple, albeit important, provision of choice. Choice itself does not mean that people can live their lives in ways that make sense to them, that supports continuity amidst change. As a surrogate for dignity and respect, choice or self-determination became the primary means to indicate respect for the individual. In contrast, a sturdy notion of dignity recognizes a dense moral universe, as our dignity rests on at least some important other who values us and what we do (Flanagan, 1991). This latter view of dignity is then quite particularistic; although we may all support the Kantian end—that each person is an end and not a means—we must go beyond that and learn what *this* older person, with whom we are in a relationship, means by dignity and how we might honor that.

This emphasis on autonomy raises other important questions about basic and enduring philosophical questions. It implies a voluntaristic model of human relationships, and a conception of the self as detached and self-interested. Yet caring for the dependent among us requires a response to the vulnerability of others, which may not be in our self-interest. This fact of life calls for an understanding of autonomy as relational, which views us all as "beings-in-relationship" (Mackenzie & Stoljar, 2000; Parks, 2003). Relational autonomy is important for understanding how older people, especially as age-related changes increase our needs for others, can flourish even in conditions of frailty, dementia, fear, poverty, and vulnerability. This view challenges the received view of autonomy as independent self-governance. It also takes nonvoluntary relationships of care as foundational to human relationships. Not only, as the saying goes, is one not able to choose one's family, but one is often unable to choose other relationships in which one becomes involved.

Entangled with public policy debates about care is the glaring cultural discomfort with dependency. Americans try not to notice dependency or the situations of exploitation that such dependency can create. Philosopher Eva Feder Kittay (1999) observed:

> The occlusion of dependency work combines with the inattention to dependency workers to make our obligations to those in need of care part of a system of exploitation, one which diminishes the moral worth of the caregiver as well as the person cared for. A society in which such a system of exploitation is the norm cannot be said to be a society in which equality, as both a moral and social value, thrives. (p. 28)

Yet how different the fact of dependency could be if it were endowed with its own accounts of practices and virtues—like gratitude—unique to the experience of dependency. Such an account would add to our knowledge of what it means to live a fully human life.

Autonomy as a central value does not easily inform public policy. Health care offers a prime example. Ought we receive whatever health care is available that may be beneficial no matter our age? If the answer is no, then we must consider rationing—the denial of potentially beneficial care. When philosopher Daniel Callahan (1987) posed this question in the late 1980s, he was greeted with a firestorm of opposition (e.g., Binstock & Post, 1991; Homer & Holstein, 1990). But, in Setting Limits, Callahan also raised questions about the meaning of old age. Without such a theory, there would be no grounding for his prescriptive public policy proposals. Introducing the concept of the natural life span, Callahan suggested that by age 80 or so we have done most of what we have wanted to do; hence we need to limit our wants, especially for medical care, and make room for the next generation. Yet Callahan's concept of the natural life span, an idea worth considering in its own right (Holstein, 1990), became totally enmeshed in his central concern, which was the seemingly unstoppable escalation in the costs of medical care.

Virtue ethics focuses on character and not decision-making, hence it does not fit easily with the contemporary focus on autonomy and choice as the most important ethical values decision making, open a useful approach to thinking about old age. More than 2 decades ago theologian William F. May (1984) wrote about the virtues and vices of aging, taking as his starting point that, as members of the moral community, elders have obligations as well as rights. More recently, however, in an explicitly normative argument, Sara Ruddick (1999) has begun to explore virtues that ought to be identified with aging and old age. The virtues, though not so identified, slip in through adjectives like *productive* or an emphasis on activity or sexuality. To be virtuous is to be all those things. In this way they hold out subtle and not so subtle demands but do not detract from where we opened—no matter how old we are, we want to "maintain conceptions of ourselves as good people" (Ruddick, 1999, p. 46). Ruddick seeks to identify virtues that do not impose intimidating ideals and take into account that decline is predictable, although its particular form is not. Taking as a given that most will experience multiple losses, Ruddick lists the following: "curiosity, a capacity for pleasure and delight, concern for near and distant others, capacities to forgive and let go, to accept, adjust, and appreciate; and 'wise independence,' which includes not only the ability to plan and control one's life but also the ability to acknowledge one's limitations and accept help in ways that are gratifying to the helper" (p. 50). Managing pain, mourning, and integrating the loss of those close to us must also be considered virtues. Instead of insisting that we are only as old as we feel, we need to learn to face disabilities without bitterness. But a cautionary note: Like successful aging, for each virtue there is a vice; so Ruddick wants to do more than identify what she describes as individualistic virtues and turn instead to virtues that are "an ongoing and relational process" (p. 51). "Being virtuous," says Ruddick, "is something one *sometimes* does, not something one is" (p. 53). Ultimately, however, Ruddick finds that virtue is created in relationships with others—those with whom we share a sunrise or confront our pain or dying—and it is not possible for us all the time, or it too would become a burden. Many years ago, philosopher William May (1984) called upon us to "live up to the occasion of our own death"; that is what Ruddick warns against—to be held so accountable even at the end. In contrast, Ruddick's suggestions encourage us try to overcome bitter regret over our own choices and perhaps those of the people we love. Finally, Ruddick turns to relationships of care where outlaw emotions—impatience, resentment, anger, and so on—are permitted while we adjust and adapt to changing circumstances. Above all, Ruddick grounds her thinking about the virtues of age in the "is"—in the inevitable vicissitudes of aging and the painful mood shifts and regrets and real hurts that are not eliminable. In this way, Ruddick, herself an aging person, tries to find a way to identify virtues of age that do not impose oppressive standards.

Rentsch (1997) has also sought to offer a philosophical ethics of old age. He asks: "What does it mean for a finite being to age but still lead a good life" (p. 263). Rentsch accepts the special conditions that old age presents, namely, finitude and vulnerability. Summoning Aristotle's idea of happiness, or *eudaimonia,* Rentsch argues that the "ethic of the good life cannot apply to man [sic] in general, but must instead refer to a concrete man in order to gain valuable insight into the possibility of happiness" (p. 263). From this starting point he focuses on the ethical meanings of finitude. Instead of seeking ways to tame finitude through advance planning, Rentsch emphasizes its radicalism and the lack of predictability that it represents. The consciousness of time becomes an ever-present reality in old age. We suggest that much in contemporary gerontology works against taking time as a critical variable in how we live. We are seemingly resistant to "numbering our days so we may have a heart of wisdom," the advice of the psalmists and the theme of an evocative work in cultural anthropology (Myerhoff, 1978).

CONCLUSION

We acknowledge that there are pressing and inescapable issues surrounding aging and social policy and medical ethics. We contend, however, that, although these questions will endure, their resolution will depend both on the specific circumstances of societies and the way societies make sense of aging as an existential and lived experience. Similarly, as we individually try to live our lives, including old age, with elements of conscious choice, we too must employ some notions of the nature and meaning of old age.

A postmodern view may argue that norms, which define what old age ought to be, are merely prejudices foisted upon us. But we remain convinced that, although there is some measure of plasticity in human nature, including old age, there are also common and natural realities. Any serious thought about old age must take these realities into account, for an awareness of what is possible influences the "ought". As Ruddick (1999) so clearly affirms, norms ought not be oppressive, but without a vision of what a good old age might be, we are left to improvise when we have little time to repair errors. The nature of old age is, then, an enduring philosophical question. It is enduring because of its importance, and enduring in the sense that any satisfactory answer will require a continuing dialogue.

If our lives in our advancing years, in our old age, are to have meaning, if they are to be regarded as worthy to ourselves and others, if they are to be thought of as well-lived or not, then we must not distance ourselves from old age itself. We must become intimately acquainted with it, in all its ambiguity and mystery, and rather than endlessly strive to defeat it, a struggle we shall lose, we must learn to redeem it so we can see and value its reality.

REFERENCES

Agich, G. (1993). *Autonomy and long-term care*. New York: Oxford University Press.

Andrews, M. (2000). Ageful and proud. *Aging and society, 20*, 791–795.

Atchley, R. (1987). *Aging: Continuity and change*. Belmont, CA: Wadsworth.

Berlin, I. (1969). *Four essays on liberty*. Oxford: Oxford University Press.

Binstock, R. (1977). The aged as scapegoat. *The Gerontologist, 23*, 136–143.

Binstock, R.H., & Post, S. G. (Eds.). (1991). *Too old for health care: Controversies in medicine, law, economics, and ethics*. Baltimore: Johns Hopkins University Press.

Binstock, R. H., Post, S. G., & Whitehouse, P. J. (Eds.). (1992). *Dementia and aging: Ethics, values, and policy choices*. Baltimore: Johns Hopkins University Press.

Bobbio, N. (2000). Old age. *Diogenes, 48*(190), 74–83.

Bordo, S. (1993). *Unbearable weight: Feminism, Western culture and the body*. Berkeley: University of California Press.

Bruner, J. (1990). *Acts of meaning*. Cambridge: Harvard University Press.

Calasanti, T., & Slevin, K. (2001). *Gender, social inequalities and aging*. Walnut Creek, CA: AltaMira Press.

Callahan. D. (1987). *Setting limits: Medical goals in an aging society*. New York: Simon & Schuster.

Callahan, D. (1996). Can the moral commons survive autonomy. *Hastings Center Report, 26*, 41–42.

Cicero. (trans. 1994). *De senectute* [On old age]. In T. R. Cole & M. G. Winkler (Eds.), *The Oxford book of aging* (pp. 48–53). New York: Oxford University Press.

Cole, T. R. (1985). Thoughts on old age and the welfare state. Political economy, history, and health policy. *Journal of the American Geriatrics Society. 33*(12), 869–873.

Cohen, E. (1988). The elderly mystique: Constraints on the autonomy on the elderly with disabilities. *The Gerontologist, 28*(Suppl.), 24–31.

Cole, T. R., & Gadow, S. (Eds.). (1986) *What does it mean to grow old? Views from the humanities*. Durham, NC: Duke University Press.

Cole, T. R. (1992). *The journey of life: A cultural history of aging in America*. New York: Cambridge University Press.

Cole, T. R., & Holstein, M. (1994). Interpreting the formative literature of gerontology and geriatrics: A view from American cultural history, 1890–1930. In C. Conrad & H. J. von Kondratowitz. (Eds.), *Before and after modernity: Toward a cultural history of aging*, Deutsches Zentium für Altersfragene. e.V., Berlin. iii, 177P.

Moody, H. R. (1989). Why dignity in old age matters. *Journals of Gerontological Social Work*; *29*(213): 13–38.

Moody, H. R. (1992). *Ethics in an aging society*. Baltimore: Johns Hopkins University Press.

Moody, H. R. (1994). The meaning of life and the meaning of old age. In T. R. Cole & S. A. Gadow (Eds.), *What does it mean to grow old?* (pp. 9–40). Durham, NC: Duke University Press.

Moreno, J. (1995). *Deciding together: Bioethics and moral consensus*. New York: Oxford University Press.

Myerhoff, B. (1978). *Number our days*. New York: E. P. Dutton.

Nelson, J. L., & Nelson H. L. (1996). *Alzheimer's: Hard questions for families*. New York: Doubleday.

Neugartern, B. (Ed.). (1982). *Age or need? Public policies for older people*. Belmont, CA: Sage.

Parks, J. (2003). *No place like home: Feminist ethics and home health care*. Bloomington: Indiana University Press.

Phillipson, C. (1998). *Reconstructing old age: New agendas in social theory and practice*. London: Sage.

Prado, C. G. (1990). *Last choice: Preemptive suicide in old age*. New York: Greenwood Press.

Rachels, J. (2003). The *elements of moral philosophy* (4th ed.). Boston: McGraw-Hill.

Ray, R. (1996). A postmodern perspective on feminist gerontology. *The Gerontologist, 36*(5), 674–681.

Rentsch, T. (1997). Aging as becoming oneself: A philosophical ethics of late life. *Journal of Aging Studies, 11*, 263–271.

Rowe, J. W., & Kahn, R. L. (1987). Human aging: Usual and successful. *Science, 237*, 263–271.

Ruddick, S. (1999). Virtues and age. In M.W. Walker (Ed.), *Mother time: Women, aging, and ethics* (pp. 45–60). Lanham, MD: Rowman & Littlefield.

Taylor, C. (1984). *Sources of the self*. Cambridge, MA: Harvard University Press

Thane, P. (2003). Social histories of old age and aging. *Journal of Social History, 37*(1), 93–111.

Troyansky, D. (2004). Growing older with Cicero (and others): A review of Tim Parkin, Growing older with Cicero (and others): Old age in the Roman world, a cultural and social history. *The Gerontologist, 44*(2), 279–282.

Walker, M. U. (1998). *Moral understandings: A feminist study in ethics*. New York: Routledge.

CHAPTER 8

Historical Gerontology

It Is a Matter of Time

W. Andrew Achenbaum

Since ancient times chroniclers have been preserving memories of the past by constructing narratives for their contemporaries. Their latter-day counterparts by and large share their assumption that "past is prologue." So historians still craft stories that highlight continuities and changes in the human condition that occur over time.

Life experiences no less than professional expertise make historians keenly aware of the various temporal forces that shape human nature and societal interactions. The best practitioners become attuned to the ironies that inhere in unfolding developments within individuals, institutions, and nations. With maturity, most historians accentuate those contingencies that by turns subtly and dramatically alter the course of history, whether it be written on a large canvas or with pointillist precision.

It should be noted at the outset that "theory building" is not generally a major disciplinary priority. (As we shall see, this affects historians' relationships with other academics.) Some historians borrow theories (or propositions) from other disciplines, notably the social sciences, adapting them for their conceptual framework. Most professionals, however, are inclined to deduce generalizations from the data they gather. This is why historians are as likely to share space on campus with artists and experts in the humanities as they are to associate with social and behavioral scientists.

Despite differences over the importance of theory, the fit between history and gerontology is potentially quite complementary: Both fields of inquiry are preoccupied with the passage and impact of time on human growth, development, and decline (Hendricks, 1987, 1995; Kubler, 1963;). Historians need gerontological insights into the promises and problems that encompass the latter half of the human life course. Gerontologists need historians to describe (and, ideally, to explain) what is novel and what is not in the present day.

Historians are trained through apprenticeships. Some mentors assign dissertation topics. For the most part, as is the case in other disciplines, historians tend to pick a "problem" (e.g., determining the causes of the American Civil War), or an "area" (e.g., 18th-century British history), or a "method" (e.g., historical demography) while in graduate school. They then spend the rest of their careers building their reputations by specializing in that domain. Lucky are the men and women who in their 20s choose a topic that still engages them several decades later; if really fortunate, their issue remains central to the concerns of the gatekeepers of the discipline.

Whereas mathematicians and "hard" scientists typically peak before they are 40, mastering the historical craft takes years of practice: Historians' most recent books are usually better than their previous publications. And it is books that count in this discipline; few achieve fame on the basis of essays or articles. This is because historians require many words to contrast adequately the past from the present. Remembering people and events that might otherwise be forgotten, as well as weaving facts and images into a meaningful context, requires historians to produce what Clifford Geertz (1973) characterized as "thick description."

Historians of aging, the subset of academics highlighted here, learn their trade and do history as do other members of their tribe. Historical gerontologists are taught to master a chronological segment of the past in terms of its own distinctive structures, patterns, and dynamics. (Insofar as some historical gerontologists seek to distinguish current circumstances from antecedents, they differ from "traditional" historians who rarely tackle topics in the recent past.) Like their peers, historians of aging delight in teasing out "critical moments," in illuminating the thoughts, feelings, and actions of men and women (long gone), famous and ordinary.

A striking paradox characterizes the contributions of the first wave of professionally trained historical gerontologists thus far. Since the 1970s most history graduate students in doctoral programs have chosen to explore the temporal dimensions of "race," "sex," "ethnicity," "region," or "sexual orientation" for their dissertation topic. Very few made "age" the focus of their doctoral studies. In large measure this explains why the number of professional historians who pursue careers in gerontology remains modest. That said, this small cadre of scholars has produced a dazzling variety of ways of writing history and of representing the past through art, medicine, or econometrics. Differences notwithstanding in period, analytic approach, or interpretive voice, historical gerontologists find common ground in a desire to be as "objective" as possible while stirring readers' imaginations, particularly scholars in other disciplines. To wit:

1. *Historians of aging write surveys of the subfield.* In the absence of much concrete data, historians have tried to fill gaps in our knowledge by carefully reconstructing the past. As they mine bits of data, most scholars interject a theme, a red thread, to link the pieces together. In creating the historical backdrop, historical gerontologists pay attention to the rhythm of "time." They look for turning points in the ways older people lived. They debate when—and to what extent— images of late life have differed by race, gender, class, or historical era. As we shall see, most of the historical surveys to date have been confined to studying continuities and changes in the United States and western Europe (Haber & Gratton, 1994; Stearns, 1977).

2. *Historians of aging write biographies.* Writing a definitive history of someone rich or famous once was the way to achieve status in historical circles. Biographies have gone out of fashion within professional circles, though they sell better than most monographs. That said, historical gerontologists have been more inclined than other professionals to write biographical sketches. This is because they recognize the paucity of individual case studies, especially those that probe the interiority of senescence. Historians of aging have limned portraits of pioneers in gerontology (Achenbaum & Albert, 1995). In addition, they have used diaries, letters, and official documents to trace the journeys of "anonymous" individuals into maturity and late life. For instance, scholars have studied groups of people, such as women in the early American Republic (Premo, 1990).

3. *Historians of aging engage in multidisciplinary studies.* Doing the spadework described in items 1 and 2 has paid off. Historical gerontologists have demonstrated that aging has many pasts, which differ dramatically from present conditions. Other scholars have come to see the value in such historical data for their own investigations. Thus historical gerontologists have joined social scientists, artists, and medical researchers in putting issues such as "wisdom," "retirement," "family," "life expectancy," and "Alzheimer's disease" into frameworks that are sensitive to temporal dynamics (Gubrium & Charmatz, 1992; Pifer & Bronte, 1986). Historians help other

experts to appreciate how key words, underlying assumptions, and serendipitous discoveries in past times often alter the ways people nowadays perceive age and the aged (Achenbaum, Weiland, & Haber, 1996).

4. *Historians of aging engage in policy studies.* U.S. officials and scholars have been publishing historically grounded "welfare" studies since New York's secretary of state J. V. N. Yates issued his critique of public relief in 1824. On both sides of the Atlantic, a present cohort of historians has been revisiting the raison d'être and pragmatics of poor laws, pension benefits, and of specific policies such as Social Security and the Beveridge Plan. Very often historians collaborate (and challenge) studies by political scientists and sociologists, who themselves seek to explicate the importance of understanding the origins and shifts in policies affecting the aged (Achenbaum, 1986; Thomson, 1996).

5. *Historians of aging do "public history."* In the 1980s, when the job market was tight, history departments launched graduate programs to train fledgling graduate students for careers in museums, archives, corporations, and government. Consistent with this tack, historical gerontologists wrote histories of nursing homes, often selecting ones that catered to minority groups. They studied the patients and programs of veterans' homes, especially after the Civil War (Cetina, 1983). They joined anthropologists in surveying modern-day retirement communities. They worked with medical care personnel in nursing home settings.

6. *Historians of aging engage in biomedical ethics.* In an area where philosophers, physicians, and lawyers might be expected to dominate, historians have been invited to participate in academic symposia and blue-ribbon commissions. They have argued fiercely over the relevance of "autonomy" in making end-of-life decisions. They have joined the debate over the relevance of "age" in allocating limited resources (Holstein & Cole, 1985).

7. *Historians of aging have joined artists and librarians in recapturing the faces and voices of older people in past times.* Historians once spent most of their time recounting the accomplishments and foibles of the rich and famous. In the late 1960s, with the rise of the new social history, itself a reflection of worldwide democratization, came a renewed interest in popular culture. Empowering older men and women to speak for themselves, to represent their lives generations

after they have died, has become a large priority (Achenbaum & Kusnerz, 1978; Spicker, Woodward, & Van Tassel, 1977).

8. *Historians of aging have engaged in applied as well as basic history.* Gerontologists who teach senior citizens how to do life reviews have much in common with historians (Butler, 1969). The shape of time is critical to both specialties. Life reviews help people to remember their pasts, to reflect on critical junctures in their lives. Older participants track ebbs and flows in relationships with family members, colleagues at work, neighbors, and others who have shaped their identities. Life review gives men and women the chance to evaluate what they have accomplished thus far. Equally important, the study of successive generations indicates, is the permission bestowed upon elders to prioritize how to live the years remaining to them (Chudacoff, 1989).

Some of the projects mentioned above emanate from a "traditional" style of doing history: Scholars primarily gauge the contrast between past and present. In an effort to recover the lessons of the past, such projects reflect a genuine appreciation that "it is a matter of time" that links history and gerontology. Some of the partnerships have been serendipitous, others pragmatic. Yet all underscore the power of historical perspectives and narratives to lay a solid contextual foundation for contemporary gerontology.

THE ORIGINS OF HISTORICAL GERONTOLOGY

The present cadre of professional historians now in their 40s and 50s did not invent historical gerontology. Their work builds on other people's scholarship—though there is a fundamental difference in the interpretive voice of the two sets of works. I have already intimated that those historians of aging with professional training tend to write books that are comprehensive (within the parameters of the enterprise) and thematic. They ask questions, they clarify misconceptions. The pioneers of historical gerontology, in contrast, tried to be encyclopedic in scope—without pretending to exhaust the historical landscape. More significantly, the trailblazers piled fact upon fact, rarely imposing a critical judgment on what they had discovered. The facts, they believed, could speak for themselves. Thus John Durand (1948), M. D. Grmek (1958), and F. D. Zeman (1944–1947) published longitudinal analyses of labor force participation and geriatrics, leaving it to readers to make explicit the historical inferences in their work.

An example of this mode of doing history is the work of Gerald Gruman, who painstakingly documented the views of philosophers, physicians, and other scientists from ancient times in *A History of Ideas about the Prolongation of Life* (1966). Gruman culled historical sources from Western and Eastern traditions that advanced (or challenged) prevailing notions about old age and aging. Gruman's research remains so meticulous that Springer Publishing recently reprinted the monograph. Yet one could not deduce from Gruman's scholarship his views on the benefits of extending the life span. Nor could one guess his heroes. Gruman wrote a compendium, as "objective" (i.e., opinion-free) as possible. Besides writing historical bio-sketches of pioneers in gerontology, Joseph Freeman (1979) compiled the first comprehensive bibliography of historical and literary works on aging. Like Gruman, Freeman had no desire to share his opinions or prejudices in his compilation. He wanted to gather in one place key citations that others could use in advancing the field of aging.

Because Gruman and Freeman were so self-effacing, their work more closely resembles other pioneering "amateurs" (in the best sense of the term) than the current wave of professional historians. In the early 20th century, well-known investigators and critics cited historical materials for their own sake as a way to embellish their scientific and literary assertions about aging at the time. Nobel laureate Elie Metchnikoff (1908) accentuated the novelty of his optimistic model of aging by contrasting it with 19th-century theories that equated old age with disease. I. L. Nascher (1914) established geriatrics as a medical specialty that dealt with age-specific etiologies requiring distinctive care by differentiating his clinical studies from classics that had focused on pathological aspects of aging. At 78, psychologist G. Stanley Hall completed his last major work, *Senescence* (1922). Eclectically devoting several chapters to the history of old age, Hall asserted that the 20th century, unlike previous eras, afforded unprecedented opportunities for capitalizing on the potentials of the second half of life. Simone de Beauvoir recounted a darker story in her bestseller, *The Coming of Age* (1972). Historical records, in her opinion, dwelt on perduring physical, mental, social, and economic vicissitudes of advancing years. Immensely influential upon publication, scholars have since demonstrated how selectively Beauvoir culled evidence to support her bias.

"Professional" historical gerontology took root as *The Coming of Age* made the bestseller lists. Philippe Aries's *Centuries of Childhood* (1962) set the stage for all that followed. First, he demonstrated that various stages of the human life course were "invented"—in this instance, parents in early-modern Europe began to dress their very young as children in clothes that distinguished them from boys and girls over the age of nine. This meant, second, that the chronological boundaries of the life course were malleable, subject to historically grounded values, interventions, and exigencies. Joseph Kett demonstrated in *Rites of Passage* (1977) that G. Stanley Hall (1904) was correct when he declared that a new stage of life, adolescence, came into being on both sides of the Atlantic in the latter third of the 19th century. Other academics bolstered Kett's scholarship by demonstrating that novel institutions, such as a juvenile court, arose in the same period. Historical circumstances, in short, made the life course malleable.

Some investigators have not been content to analyze just one stage of life. John Demos, for instance, studied generational dynamics family life in Plymouth colony. *A Little Commonwealth* (1970) rested on an analysis of primary documents (wills, estate inventories, legal documents) and a clever use of material artifacts. In keeping with the "new social history" then coming into vogue, Demos presented a theoretical model to grid his analysis. Demos borrowed insights from major historians, anthropologists, and psychologists. After discussing Pilgrim household structures, Demos turned to "themes of individual development." He wrote brilliant expositions of infancy, childhood, and youth, and a less compelling characterization of middle age. He devoted a mere seven pages to "later years." Plainly, insofar as *A Little Commonwealth* was cutting edge, "old age" was ready for the same sort of historical inquiry as earlier stages of life.

The academic birth of historical gerontology occurred at a colloquium at Case Western Reserve University organized by David D. Van Tassel, a master at moving the profession in new directions. (He was an early advocate of incorporating quantitative techniques into historical methods and of training historians for nonacademic jobs.) Van Tassel secured funding from the National Endowment for the Humanities to promote humanistic perspectives on aging. Keynote speakers included Erik Erikson and Joan Erikson (who discussed director Ingmar Bergman's *Wild Strawberries*), Leon Edel (who illuminated Henry James's later years), Juanita Kreps (who would serve as secretary of commerce in the administration of President Jimmy Carter), British historical demographer Peter Laslett, and pathologist Robert Kohn. All agreed that an infusion of humanistic perspectives would enrich gerontology. (Their essays appeared in Van Tassel's collection, *Aging, Death, and the Completion of Being,* 1979.) In their estimation, historians—with their long-standing ties to both the humanities and the social sciences—were likely to serve in the vanguard in broadening gerontology's purview.

The second phase of Van Tassel's project provided an opportunity for intellectual and institutional outreach to researchers on aging. Van Tassel had selected 18 assistant and associate professors of art, classics, communications, drama, English, history, and religious studies to write age-related essays that might inspire their disciplinary colleagues to follow their example and do research in gerontology. The authors were to present their papers at the 1976 meeting of the Gerontological Society of America (GSA). Van Tassel reckoned that his authors would be willing to move beyond their modus operandi, but not too far. He knew that his fellow historians would think about "age" in disciplinary ways; still, he hoped that their final product would pique the interest of physicians, social workers, psychologists, and others in GSA.

Results were mixed. As he anticipated, most authors did not venture far from their tribal boundaries (Spicker et al., 1977). Nonetheless, because they produced solid work, their scholarship advanced ideas and raised questions that would be useful for other researchers on aging to pursue. The project produced a laundry list, not an agenda. Disappointingly, although Van Tassel hoped that his rising stars would continue to do research on aging, few ever wrote on the subject again. Gerontology did not stir their imaginations.

Meanwhile, at the same meeting, GSA's governing board created a secondary committee on the "humanities and arts." Council's action fulfilled a goal long championed by Joseph Freeman, who owned one of the world's finest collections of historic gerontological texts. Gerald Gruman and Van Tassel, both good friends of Dr. Freeman's, worked behind the scenes to secure the council's approval for the committee. Thus 1976 marked the beginning of an academic affiliation among clinicians and nurses, biological and behavioral scientists, social welfare practitioners, artists, and experts in the humanities. This institutional alliance afforded historians and gerontologists common ground for possible multidisciplinary partnerships.

But the affiliation with GSA did not put historical gerontology on the map. Rather, it took an intradisciplinary fight to attract the notice of scholars across the academy. Intellectual fights (preferably with a few ad hominem barbs) advance a subfield, particularly if the debate is as substantial as it is volatile. In this case, historians heatedly debated whether there had been a dramatic shift in attitudes toward the elderly in the United States. There were three conflicting opinions.

David Hackett Fischer argued in *Growing Old in America* (1977) that a "revolution in age relations" occurred between 1780 and 1820. Whereas people had exalted gray heads from the colonial era until the revolution, an age bias against the elderly was palpable in the antebellum period; it became more pronounced over time, well into the 20th century. To document his argument, Fischer elaborated a series of temporal tests (e.g., changes in seating patterns in meetinghouses, alterations in word usage, and shifts in fashion) to measure the direction and rate of change in the status of being old—hardly scientific instruments, but more quantitative than found in most historical monographs.

Growing Old in America was an instant hit: It was written in a sprightly manner and had no competition. Better yet, Fischer relished in provoking polemical arguments. (He had ripped to shreds the major works of the nation's leading historians, including his own mentor, in *Historians' Fallacies*, 1970.) Those who were not trained as historians thought that Fischer had set forth fresh data in a field where so little was known. The evidence seemed overwhelmingly to corroborate his argument.

Not everybody was impressed: Princeton's Lawrence Stone trashed the thesis of *Growing Old in America* in the *New York Review of Books*. The dean of British historians took particular delight in demolishing Fischer's tests that purported to document a historical tidal wave coinciding with the American Revolution. I, too, thought that many of Fischer's "measures" proving that there was a "deep change" in attitudes toward old age between 1780 and 1820 were wrongheaded (Achenbaum, 1978a). Gerontophagia—the eating of the monographs of one's elders—is a way to get ahead professionally. To put it less cynically, history is only as good as the evidence that supports its argument. The verisimilitude of the historical data necessary to sustain a cogent temporal argument improves revision by revision, critique by critique.

I presented my temporal baseline in *Old Age in the New Land* (1978b). Surveying the decades between 1790 and 1970, my account differed from Fischer's in several ways. First, I detected a shift in perceptions (I was not sure how to measure historical "attitudes") between the Civil War and World War I. I avoided terms such as *deep* and *revolutionary* in describing change. Instead, changes in the occupational structure, medicine, manners, and religion converged to make older men and women seem "obsolescent." This shift in the realm of images, however, was not accompanied by an alteration in the actual experiences of being old. The most dramatic demographic, social, economic, and political changes in the status of older Americans, I contended, occurred in the 20th century.

Carole Haber found fault with both Fischer's thesis and mine in *Beyond Sixty-five* (1983). Haber was impressed by the negative evidence she uncovered concerning views of the elderly and their treatment from the earliest days of U.S. history. The aged's race, gender, class, and health, in her view, were more important than age in ascribing positive attributes to the old, especially in the colonial period. Thus Haber was skeptical that there was any noticeable age-related shift in the historical baseline in either the revolutionary period or in the latter decades of the 19th century. Accordingly, Haber concentrated on specific institutions, such as the development of the old age home, and the transformation of medical practice.

The debate among Fischer, Haber, and me, which persisted (at least among the protagonists) for several years, was not resolved. It fizzled out. Fischer moved on to other historical projects. Haber and I softened our positions with time (after each of us had been tenured). Another debate arose among historians and economists. This one dealt with the timing and extent of the exodus of older men from the labor force, notably in the period between 1880 and 1930. This second controversy was more technically interesting than the earlier debate, because it hinged on how census definitions were read and the confidence scholars placed on data collected in certain years. It also drew economists and economic historians into the fray. Alas, this second debate did not generate as much controversy as the first (Schaie & Achenbaum, 1993).

Historical gerontology thereafter rested primarily on the quality of the scholarship its practitioners produced. Its future hung on its perceived usefulness to the discipline and (independently) to other researchers on aging. Thus it was important for the fledgling field that Thomas Cole's first book, *The Journey of Life: A Cultural History of Aging* (1992) was nominated for a Pulitzer Prize. Cole, moreover, did much to maintain ties to the experts in the humanities and to make overtures to the biomedical community. He edited two editions of the *Handbook of the Humanities and Aging* (Cole et al., 1992, 2000), as a way to consolidate the work of artists, critics, theologians, historians, and philosophers (scholars inclined to work alone on individual projects). He integrated history and gerontology by offering courses on life review; he revealed his maturation in autobiographical sketches. For nearly 2 decades, Cole has used his position in various medical centers to grapple with medical ethics from a spiritually grounded historical and humanistic perspective. He also has gone into anatomy labs and collaborated with nurses to illustrate suffering and death in late life.

Not all of the seminal work in this area has been accomplished by historians of aging.

Other contemporary U.S. historians have made important contributions, although they are not primarily known (nor do they wish to be considered) as historical gerontologists. The late Tamara Hareven, who launched family history as a branch of social history and wrote many articles and several books that included materials about the aged's place in household structures in the U.S. and Japan. Her *Family Time and Industrial Time* (1983) became a classic. William Graebner's *A History of Retirement* (1980) remains oft cited 25 years after publication. Charles Rosenberg highlights geriatrics in his medical histories (1987). Social welfare historians such as Edward Berkowitz (1991) and Walter Trattner (1994) analyze the economic and political conditions that caused the enactment and expansion of old-age entitlements.

European historians of aging enjoy interplay with their American cousins. Peter Laslett's historical work and pleas for greater opportunities for men and women in the Third Age inspired a generation of British scholars, such as Andrew Blaikie (1994), Michael Featherstone (1985), Paul Johnson (2001) and Pat Thane (2000). Michel Philibert (1968), a grand philosopher of the old school, had the same effect on French scholarship. Georges Minois (1989) surveyed the history of old age from antiquity to the Renaissance. Works translated into English by German scholars such as Christoph Conrad influence U.S. gerontology.

These historians—and other scholars not cited—have generated a plethora of "facts" about old age in past times that would have remained inaccessible to other researchers on aging. Their scholarship has posed enduring questions and generated fresh perspectives in gerontology. Let me highlight a dozen contributions, eight conceptual and four methodological, by historical gerontologists.

Conceptual

1. *Old age has always been a stage of life.* Historians, as we have seen, have shown that people in various eras segment the human life course in different ways (Aries, 1962; Kett, 1977). Social scientists speculate that another stage—adult children who return home, postponing marriages and delaying their careers—is unfolding. But old age has been perceived as a stage of life since the beginning of recorded history. It has always encompassed the years between the prime of life and death.

2. *Chronology has always defined the lower boundaries of old age.* Not only has old age always been defined as a stage of life, but its lower boundaries have remained remarkably constant despite amazing gains in life expectancy at birth since the earliest periods of recorded history. Median longevity was far lower in the Classical era than nowadays, but the ancients did not lower the bar to, say, 30 in designating someone as elderly. In ancient Sparta, a soldier had to be 60 to join the *gerusia,* literally the "council of elders." The Roman term *senator* is derived from the Latin *senex,* or "old man." In the United States, children born in 1790 had as much chance of living to their first birthday as those born in 1970 have of reaching 65.

The age of 65 has taken on great significance in modern times, thanks to Bismarck (though he initially established 70 as a threshold for receiving a pension) and to the provisions in the 1935 Social Security Act that set that age as a criterion for old-age assistance and old-age insurance (Achenbaum, 1986). Under Social Security today, 66, 68, 70, 72, and 75 are also relevant benchmarks. Indeed, it is fair to say that "old age" throughout American history began somewhere between 50 (when the American Association of Retired Persons entitles you to membership) and 80 (which was the marker used by Benjamin Rush, physician to the U.S. founding fathers in late life). Or, one could agree with Bernard Baruch, who in his 90s said that old age was constantly 5 years beyond his reach. No other stage of life has such an elastic threshold, especially since the age of death at advanced years varies.

Old age's wide boundaries have prompted researchers to subdivide the stage. Bernice Neugarten's distinction (1974) between the healthy, wealthy "young-old" and the dependent "old-old" quickly became age graded: the former, 55 to 75, the latter 75 plus. Only her terms were new: Writers in the Classical era distinguished between a "green" old age, supple in its ripening, and "second childhood" or "decrepitude," wherein winter's chill became paramount.

3. *The most dramatic changes in the history of old age have occurred recently.* By any measure, the middle third of the 20th century marked a "deep change" in the meanings and experiences of old age, particularly in advanced industrial countries. Demographically, three quarters of all increases in life expectancy at birth and in adult longevity have occurred since 1900. Children are more likely to have at least three grandparents alive in their formative years than ever before. Economically, "retirement" became the norm for more and more workers, not just the rich. Socially, divorce, same-sex partnerships, and new living arrangements have altered the family structures and household residencies. Politically, older people and their advocates have mobilized to demand "entitlements" from a variety of public and private sources.

4. *Ageism is virulent and prevalent.* Robert Butler wrote in 1969 that "ageism" was analogous to "sexism" and "racism," but in fact an animus against old age can be traced back through history. Rich, well-positioned personages had enough prestige and control to inure themselves from abuse: They could solicit support or threaten to disinherit

their detractors. The majority of older people, alas, were not so fortunate. Late-life frailty handicapped them. Old-age poverty was treated out of a sense of obligation rarely leavened with compassion. Fears of abandonment and contempt were understandable.

5. *Sexism and ageism has always provoked double jeopardy.* Until recently, most societies were patriarchal: Older men wielded more power and controlled greater wealth than women. Scripture attests to the vulnerability of widows in biblical times. U.S. historians (Premo, 1990; Scandron, 1988) effectively described the plight of widows on the East Coast and in the Southwest.

6. *Ethnicity/race typically result in triple jeopardy—with a spin.* Especially in the United States, immigrants arrived young and either returned to their homeland or died on average at a younger age than native Americans. They faced social, economic, and political prejudice. Slave owners often freed African American elders when they no longer were economically productive. Blacks on average still have higher morbidity rates and lower life expectancies than Whites. Yet within their respective communities, the old were accorded respect. They determined marriage patterns and resolved kinship disputes. Younger people in their network, not society at large, heeded their sage experience.

7. *Class counts.* European and Asian historians take this as axiomatic, but Americans, proud of their middle-class traditions, must be shown that the rich truly are different than the poor, especially at advanced ages. That roughly 40% of all men died intestate before the Civil War gives a sense of economic marginality. Disability and premature deaths (often from accidents) always limited working-class careers, though farmers usually could keep the books when they no longer could toil the earth. Age discrimination became manifest after the Civil War. Only executives before 1929 could anticipate pensions, and even these were viewed as gratuities. Unions, eager to gain members, demanded bread and butter issues for younger, not older, workers until after World War II. Lack of resources makes a good old age harder to attain.

8. *Older Americans are a key constituency of the welfare state.* Families and local communities since the colonial era have been primarily concerned with the welfare of children, youth, and their mothers. Relief was provided on an ad hoc basis to older people, along with the sick, insane, and criminals. In the 19th century states dealt with old age through public health measures and then (in the early 20th century) through old-age assistance expanded coverage, but few judged

old-age dependency a serious problem before 1929. Since the Great Depression, the federal government has been a major provider of income security, health care, and social services—often through state agencies. Roughly 100 organizations have emerged in the private sector to advocate as a "gray lobby" for elders in need.

Methodological

9. *The limits of scientism.* To be viewed as credible by "hard" scientists, gerontologists and geriatricians have hewed to prevailing standards of theory building, of collecting and measuring data, and of testing the validity of assumptions. Historians initially found scientism off-putting; gerontologists dismissed history as soft. Disciplinary transformations over the past 3 decades, however, have resulted in more tolerance for methodological variety. Historians and other experts in the humanities have demonstrated some value in alterative approaches to doing research on aging. Life review is a prime example. So is the theoretical respect accorded "critical gerontology," which relies in part on qualitative analyses and interpretive "turns."

10. *The importance of studying values, especially in medical ethics.* Once researchers in gerontology acknowledge that "scientism" is not invariably objective, then it becomes possible to tease out the contingent, ambiguous, countervailing values that inhere in society as well as research paradigms. Historians have joined philosophers in documenting that such normative analysis is a practical undertaking. They have joined the debate over the future of the antiaging movement and questions of resource allocation in geriatrics (Holstein & Cole, 1995).

11. *Individual and population aging necessitate institutional adaptation.* Institutions are situated in the middle ground between micro- and macro-analyses. Too often we ignore the fact that institutions change, as the times change, albeit not in the same ways. Yet retirement pensions have taken on profoundly different shapes in the transatlantic community (Hannah, 1986; Sass, 1997). So have hospitals and other health facilities (Rosenberg, 1987).

12. *Images as windows on the mind.* The "aging body" since ancient times has inspired painters, photographers, sculptors, athletes, and dancers. Usually words are employed to describe the ravages and ravishing qualities of advancing years. But "the mind's eye" apprehends what words cannot convey. Hence historians, particularly those

interested in popular culture, have paid critical attention to image making as a methodological tool to complement quantitative analyses and narrative discourses (Blaikie, 1999).

ENDURING ISSUES AND BROADER PERSPECTIVES IN HISTORICAL GERONTOLOGY: AN AGENDA

Although historians and researchers in aging have accomplished much to create a time line with which to situate current gerontological trends into perspective, much remains to be done. What follows is one scholar's five-item agenda for filling gaps in our knowledge base. It will take the imagination and perseverance of another generation of scholars to accomplish what I propose. In the process, new issues and questions will arise, as practitioners would hope and expect in a vibrant field of inquiry.

First, the best historical work on aging to date analyzes developments in western Europe and the United States. To comprehend the diverse dynamics of human senescence, historical gerontologists must join their disciplinary colleagues in doing "world history." Over the past decade historians have been crafting new techniques and models for executing comparative, cross-national studies of demographic, economic, social, and political trends associated with empire building. Others examine the cross-fertilization that results from changing migration patterns of peoples and jobs in a global economy. Similarly, U.S. gerontologists, who have been leaders in organizations such as the International Association of Gerontology, are producing case studies of health care patterns in the East and developing nations. U.S. gerontology has been insular in focus; historians, collaborating with social and behavioral scientists, can blaze new frontiers.

Emphasis, in my opinion, should be placed on older people who have spent most of their lives south of the equator. Although issues surrounding children and youth, poverty, genocide, and disease preoccupy most academics, it is important to remember that there are already more older people in developing countries than in advanced-industrial nations. We are remarkably ignorant about the history of age and aging in Latin and Central America, India and the subcontinent, Africa, and China. Basic information is critical if we are to grasp the variations and scope of population aging.

Second, within the Western world, there are huge lacunae in the history of aging. Good work has been done on growing older in the Classical era, but far less is known about the status and duties of elders in biblical times or in religious communities associated with Judaism and the Jesus movement to Constantine. There is, to my knowledge, no monograph or exhaustive article that reports basic demographic, cultural, socioeconomic, or political realities affecting the aged from the 4th century CE to the Middle Ages. Our knowledge of developments between 1500 and 1800 is sketchy. No one has studied the history of age and aging in the Balkans, Baltic countries, the Iberian peninsula, Greece, or Russia. Rounding out the early-modern periods will not improve demographic projections of the 21st century. Yet mapping this terrain will enable us to make more nuanced observations about what are novel today in the realm of human emotions and late-late relations.

Third, historical gerontologists might join forces with social scientists in exploring specific classes of institutions and individuals. The to-do list seems daunting because so little has yet been done. With political scientists historians of aging should consider case studies and comparative analyses of veterans' programs, especially in Europe, Asia, and south of the equator. Our knowledge of private and public pension plans remains largely limited to North America, western Europe, and Oceania, with an occasional nod to Chile and Cuba. Given the interdependencies of the global economy, it is hazardous to speculate about trends in the absence of basic data. We know even less about similarities and differences in origins and development of medical care (institutional and home-based) for the elderly in all but a few countries. Historian gerontologists should recruit medical historians, anthropologists, and sociologists to reconstruct changing notions of the whole range of chronic impairments and acute diseases that afflict the elderly.

Even in U.S. surveys the stories of diverse demographic groups from the first settlements to present times have yet to be incorporated into the historical narrative of old age. White old men still dominate the literature of historical gerontology. The best information on African Americans in late life is to be culled from books on slavery and Reconstruction. Unfortunately, women's historians have paid less attention thus far to older women than to young activists. This is surprising because historical gerontology offers so many possibilities for testing feminist theories. We know virtually nothing about tribal differences among Native Americans. There is much to be investigated about the convoys of aging immigrants who arrived from different countries to these shores in the 1830s and 1840s, between 1880 and 1920, and since 1965. Asian Americans are particularly underrepresented. In an era of multiculturalism, we need to recapture our pluralist heritage, especially the legacies of those who lived to a ripe old age.

Fourth, gerontologists need access to life reviews of men and especially women in past times to complement their field studies. Prosopographies should reconstruct the lives of ordinary citizens in past times to learn more about the trials and tribulations, as well as the joys and contributions, of farmers, clerks, laundresses, and miners. Welfare scholars and political analysts depend on historians to write biographies of social advocates and activists who established the ways that we have come to assist and empower the elderly.

Ultimately, this exercise should help historians and gerontologists alike probe the inner voices of aging, a task that particularly intrigues sociologists, psychologists, and artists. What did it mean to grow older at given points in time? How did people feel about long-standing ties with kin and friends? Did new forms of intimacy emerge? Did religious beliefs and spiritual yearnings sustain elders as they faced death? How much variation exists by age, ethnicity, gender, race, region, and religion?

Finally, historians interested in the media should collaborate with artists in showing us the faces of age, especially since World War II. The images of middle-class aged men have been better documented than older women, but the aged remain largely invisible. Few depict portraits of age that take account of race and ethnicity. Far more attention should be paid to (the paucity of) images of age on television, radio, films, and recent technological innovations.

Other scholars doubtless would amend and expand this agenda. Suffice it to say, however, this list attests to the vast amount of work in historical gerontology that remains to be done. Some will be disciplinary in nature, executed by scholars with no formal training in gerontology. Much of this agenda lends itself to multidisciplinary endeavors if the conditions are suitable. Frankly, I find the challenge exciting, but I realize that completing any agenda acceptable to both historians and gerontologist is complicated by conceptual and methodological differences between the two tribes.

THE CHALLENGE

"Time" has always been the link between history and gerontology in academic circles. In his introduction to the 1939 edition of Edmund Cowdry's *Problems of Ageing,* John Dewey stressed that "the underlying problem, both scientifically and philosophically, it seems to me, is the relation of ageing and maturing." Dewey wanted scholars to attend to temporal differences in the dynamics of nature, society, and culture on the biological, physical, and mental aspects of aging. T. Wingate Todd's essay on the "Skeleton, Locomotive System, and Teeth" alluded to the importance of biological time (Cowdry, 1939, p. 278). In his essay on the psychological aspects of aging, Walter Miles stressed the subjectivity of time and mental longevity (Cowdry, 1939, p. 564).

James Birren, one of the major architects of contemporary gerontology, has long been interested in how experts in the humanities insinuate "time" into gerontology. In his *Handbook of Aging and the Individual* (1959), Birren included a lengthy piece on "the place of time and aging in the natural sciences and scientific philosophy" (pp.43–81). The piece distinguished between the subjective experience and objective properties of time: its metric, directional, and metaphysical properties, but also its applications to age and aging. Later in his career, Birren became a chief proponent of autobiographies and life review. More recently, gerontologists have explicated the meanings of time to research on aging. Jon Hendricks (1987, 1995), for instance, offered valuable insights in the first two editions of the *Encyclopedia of Aging*. Hendricks emphasized different types of constancies and change, and explicated various rhythms of time.

Because they understand the complexities of time, historians have potentially much to offer researchers on aging in synthesizing and analyzing multifaceted gerontological data. Scholars in both tribes are interested in interpreting continuities and changes over the time course in particular milieu. Both have been receptive, and successful, in engaging in multidisciplinary projects that unify gerontological knowledge. "Interpretation," observed Edward O. Wilson (1998, p. 320), "is the logical channel of consilient explanation between science and the arts."

The handbooks of aging produced by gerontologists and historians have been similar in format. Editors increasingly include representative works by scholars from far-flung fields of endeavor; the gesture attests to a genuine effort to broaden theoretical, methodological, and canonical traditions within a field that has been more multidisciplinary in rhetoric than practice. Points of convergence work both ways. Social scientists and medical researchers rely more than before on narrative discourse in presenting their work. Historians who delve into medical ethics and ethnographic studies are competent to critique the literature written in other fields. But openness to divergent ways of thinking is not enough to advance research on aging.

Fundamental differences nevertheless impede progress. Science orients gerontology; historians rarely incorporate multivariate analyses in their monographs. The reward structures differ. Historians, unlike biochemists, do not expect to circulate their articles over the Internet before they are actually published. No one denies that R01's major proposals form the National Gerontological Health are difficult to obtain, but competition is even fiercer among historians fighting to get modest stipends so that they can partially pay for a leave of absence to do research. Yet the National Institute of Aging has approved scientific grant support to a few historians. Pulitzer Prize winner Robert Fogel was successful because his proposal promised epidemiological applications of interest to basic scientists. Therein lies a strategy for increasing the visibility of historians in the field.

History has long been nurtured by the humanities and social sciences. Thus far historical gerontologists have largely banded with other experts in the humanities in trying to gain a place at the gerontological table. Perhaps they should concentrate more effort building alliances with medical researchers, biological scientists, behaviorists, and social scientists who know how to get support from Big Science. *The Forgetting* (2001) by David Shenk attests to the value of having anthropologists, biologists, and physicians study Alzheimer's disease together. The cost of adding historians to such a research team would be nominal: They do not require labs; the books and data that they need are in libraries or online; they generally have lower salaries.

Even if historians were to forge different sorts of partnerships, a major obstacle remains: Doing research on aging has not appealed much to young historians. In 30 years, I have directed many dissertations, but only one that was truly gerontological (Bradley, 1994). Historical gerontology lacks a critical mass of scholars. There are probably no more than six men and women in the United States who (1) identify themselves primarily as historical gerontologists and (2) have written two books on the subject. There are more scholars in Europe, but their numbers are miniscule compared to the ranks of social scientists who have created subfields in their disciplines as well as participate in multidisciplinary projects. The failure to produce a rising cohort of researchers is a great disappointment. It will impede advances in a discipline in which debate requires a large number of diverse opinions.

Part of the problem lies in the halls of graduate schools. Writing a history dissertation on Blacks, women, or gays is far more appealing than studying older people. Ageism is rampant among students and faculty. Graduate students find the topic depressing and alien.

Ironically, the penchant of historians like Tom Cole, and other experts in the humanities, to engage in multidisciplinary studies may have hurt them when their disciplinary peers evaluate their work. Even if "gerontology" were more respected among historians, it simply does not fit the grid used in making appointments. Also, GSA gatekeepers are wary to allow newcomers from the humanities too much space, lest they disrupt the status quo. Untenured historians can try to satisfy two different audiences—historians with some publications, gerontologists with others—but that gets fatiguing.

In the future, historians interested in gerontology will remain contrarians, pursuing careers as they see fit. They will take advantage of multidisciplinary opportunities that present themselves. Foundations and government agencies might stir interest by providing funds for travel and sustained scholarship. Ultimately, the degree to which they become bona fide members of the gerontological community will depend on the degree to which they recognize that historians can show them when, if, and why time matters. And historians, long taught to treat the past on its own terms, must be willing to tease out the varieties of time to imagine how they might contextualize present circumstances in fresh ways.

REFERENCES

Achenbaum, W. A. (1978a). From womb through bloom to tomb. *Reviews in American History, 6,* 178–184.

Achenbaum, W. A. (1978b). *Old age in the new land: The American experience since 1790.* Baltimore: Johns Hopkins University Press.

Achenbaum, W. A. (1983). *Shades of gray: Old age, American values, and federal policies since 1920.* Boston: Little, Brown.

Achenbaum, W. A. (1986). *Social security: Visions and reviews.* New York: Cambridge University Press.

Achenbaum, W. A. (1995). *Crossing frontiers: Gerontology emerges as a science.* New York: Cambridge University Press.

Achenbaum, W. A., & Albert, D. M. (1995). *Profiles in gerontology: A biographical dictionary.* Westport, CT: Greenwood Press.

Achenbaum, W. A., & Kusnerz, P. A. (1978). *Images of old age in America, 1790 to the present.* Ann Arbor: Institute of Gerontology.

Achenbaum, W. A., Weiland, S., & Haber, C. (1996). *Keywords in sociocultural gerontology.* New York: Springer.

Aries, P. (1962). *Centuries of childhood.* New York: Knopf.

Beauvoir, S. de (1972). *The coming of age.* New York: G. P. Putnam's Sons.

Berkowitz, E. D. (1991). *America's welfare state from Roosevelt to Reagan.* Baltimore: Johns Hopkins University Press.

Birren, J. E. (Ed.). (1959). *Handbook of aging and the individual.* Chicago: The University of Chicago Press.

Blaikie, A. (1999). *Ageing and popular culture.* Cambridge: Cambridge University Press.

Bradley, D. B. (1994). *Constructing state old-age policy: A Pennsylvania perspective.* PhD dissertation, Carnegie Mellon University.

Butler, R. N. (1969). Ageism—another form of bigotry. *The Gerontologist, 9,* 243–246

Celina, J. (1977). A history of veterans names in the U. S., 1811–1930. Case Western University.

Chudacoff, H. (1989). *How old are you?* Princeton, NJ: Princeton University Press.

Cole, T. R. (1992). *The journey of life: A cultural history of aging.* New York: Cambridge University Press.

Cole, T. R., Kastenbaum, R., & Ray R. E. (Eds.). (2000). *Handbook of the humanities and aging* (2nd ed.). New York: Springer.

Cole, T. R., Van Tassel, D. D., & Kastenbaum, R. (Eds.). (1992). *Handbook of the humanities and aging*. New York: Springer.

Conrad C. & Kessel, M. Kultur & Geschechte. Stuttgart: Redam, 1988.

Cowdry, E. V. (Ed.). (1939). *Problems of ageing*. Baltimore: Williams & Wilkins.

Bismarck, O., In Achenbaum, W. A. (1986). Social security: *Visions and Revisions*. New York: Cambridge University Press. 212.

Demos, J. (1970). *A little commonwealth*. New York: Oxford University Press.

Disney, R. and Johnson, P. A. (eds.) (2001). Pension Systems and Retirement Incomes across OECD Countries. Cheltenham, U. K.: Edward Elgar.

Durand, John D. (1948). *The labor force in the United States*. New York: John Wiley.

Featherstone, M. & Wernick, A. (eds.) (1995). Images of Aging. New York: Routledge.

Fischer, D. H. (1970). *Historians' fallacies*. San Francisco: Harper & Row.

Fischer, D. H. (1977). *Growing old in America*. New York: Oxford University Press.

Fogel, R. (2004). *Escape from Hunger and Premature Death*. New York: Cambridge University Press.

Freeman, J. T. (1979). *Aging: Its history and literature*. New York: Human Sciences Press.

Graebner, W. (1980). *A history of retirement*. New Haven, CT: Yale University Press.

Geertz, C. (1973). *Interpretations of Cultures*. New York: Harper Torchbooks.

Grmek, M. D. (1958). *On ageing and old age: Basic problems and historical aspects of gerontology and geriatrics*. The Hague: Uitgeverij Dr. W. Junk.

Gruman, G. J. (1966). *A history of ideas about the prolongation of life*. Philadelphia: American Philosophical Society.

Gubrium, J. F., & Charmatz, K. (Eds.). (1992). *Aging, self, and community*. Greenwich, CT: JAI Press.

Haber, C. (1983). *Beyond sixty-five*. New York: Cambridge University Press.

Haber, C., & Gratton, B. (1994). *Old age and the search for security*. Bloomington: Indiana University Press.

Hall, G. S. (1904). *Adolescence* (2 vols.). New York: D. Appelton.

Hall, G. S. (1922). *Senescence*. New York: D. Appelton.

Hannah, L. (1986). *Inventing retirement*. Cambridge: Cambridge University Press.

Hareven, T. K. (1983). *Family time and industrial time*. New York: Cambridge University Press.

Hendricks, J. (1987, 1995). Time. In G. L. Maddox (Ed.), *Encyclopedia of aging*. New York: Springer, 669–670.

Holstein, M., & Cole T. R. (1985). Long-term care. In L. McCullough & N. Wilson (Eds.), *Long-term care decisions* (pp. 15–34), Baltimore: Johns Hopkins University Press.

Kett, J. (1977). *Rites of passage*. New York: Basic Books.

Kubler, G. (1963). *The shape of time*. New Haven, CT: Yale University Press.

Laslett, P. (1991). *Fresh Map of Life*. Cambridge, MA: Harvard University Press.

Metchnikoff, E. (1908). *The nature of man: Studies in optimistic philosophy*. New York: G. P. Putnam's Sons.

Minois, G. (1989). *History of old age: From antiquity to the renaissance.* Chicago: The University of Chicago Press.

Nascher, I. L. (1914). *Geriatrics.* Philadelphia: P. Blakiston & Sons.

Neugarten, B. L. (1974, September). Age groups in American society and the rise of the young-old. *Annals of the American Political and Social Sciences, 320,* 187–198.

Pifer, A., & Bronte, L. (Eds.). (1986). *Our aging society.* New York: W. W. Norton.

Premo, T. (1990). *Winter friends.* Urbana: University of Illinois Press.

Rosenberg, C. E. (1987). *The care of strangers.* New York: Basic Books.

Sass, S. A. (1997). *The promise of private pensions.* Cambridge, MA: Harvard University Press.

Scandron, A. (1988). *On their own.* Urbana: University of Illinois Press.

Schaie, K. W., & Achenbaum, W. A. (Eds.). (1993). *Societal impact on aging: Historical perspectives.* New York: Springer.

Shenk, D. (2001). *The forgetting.* New York: Doubleday.

Spicker, S. F., Woodward, K. M., & Van Tassel, D. D. (Eds.). (1977). *Aging and the elderly: Humanistics perspectives on aging.* Atlantic Highlands, NJ: Humanities Press.

Stearns, P. N. (1977). *Old age in European society.* New York: Holmes & Meier.

Stone, L. (May 12, 1977). Walking over Grandma. *New York Review of Books, 24,* 26–29.

Thane, P. (2000). L'echelle des ages. Paris: Le Senil.

Thomson, D. (1996). *Selfish generations?* Cambridge: White Horse Press.

Trattner, W. I. (1994). *From poor law to welfare state* (6th ed.). New York: Free Press.

Van Tassel, D. D. (Ed.). (1979). *Aging, death and the completion of being.* Philadelphia: University of Pennsylvania Press.

Wilson, E. O. (1988). *Consilience.* New York: Vintage.

Zeman, F. D. (1944–1947). "Life's later years, ser." *Journal of Mount Sinai Hospital.*

CHAPTER 9

The Purview and Sweep
of Aging Policy

Phoebe S. Liebig

The field of aging is less than 100 years old. Its major impetus began in the mid 1940s and 1950s, shaped by gradual recognition of the increased numbers and proportions of older people. While research on aging was spearheaded by the core disciplines of biology, psychology, sociology, and medicine, the policy sciences—political science, public administration, and economics— explored the dimensions and implications of the demographic transition somewhat later, largely during the mid 1960s and 1970s. Of particular interest was an examination of the political activity and economic status of older adults and, as more public policies and programs were enacted, on the administrative and regulatory aspects affecting the elderly, as well as the impact of those policies on the larger society.

The purpose of this chapter is to examine the extent to which gerontology has utilized the theories, concepts, and approaches of the policy sciences to pose questions about the nature of aging; what contributions gerontology has made, in turn, to those disciplines; and what untapped "growth" areas in the policy sciences might foster new perspectives in gerontology. Like other social science disciplines, research orientations of the policy sciences in aging are problem-driven rather than theory-driven (Myers, 1996). However, unlike the core disciplines, the intellectual "meat" of the policy sciences is, per force, highly sensitive to and often shaped by decisions being made in Washington, DC, state capitals, and the boardrooms of corporate America. Still, new questions have arisen as perspectives have changed. In the past decade or so, the policy sciences, especially economics, have focused on international aspects of policy as multinational corporations locate their operations around the globe and the World Bank issues policy recommendations and makes loans contingent on compliance. The macrolevel challenges posed by population aging have gained the attention of policy makers worldwide, with increased attention to the economic, health, and social welfare challenges of providing for the needs of current and future older adults (Schulz, 1996).

THE POLICY SCIENCES: THEORY AND PRACTICE

The goal of the policy sciences is to describe, explain/predict, and assess the actions of government by analyzing why and how policies are made and succeed/fail. The focus includes examining the policy process: public sector decision making, the policy tools used to implement those decisions (e.g., taxes), and actions to redress policy problems due to changes in the national mood and other factors (Kingdon, 1995). In essence, the policy sciences strive to answer the political question posed by Lasswell (1936): Who gets what, when, how?

Political science is the study of political conditions as they are, with critical examination of the gap between the formal provisions of government and its actual practices and a focus on public opinion and public policy (Lowi, 1992). One major area of inquiry has been political attitudes and behavior of individuals, especially their participation (e.g., voting, contacting public officials) (Verba & Nie, 1974). Included are studies of declines in participation (except for the elderly) and voting and citizen preferences of various groups (e.g., the elderly, baby boomers, Hispanics). The other major area of inquiry in the United States and elsewhere has centered on the roles of social movements and interest groups working on behalf of specific agendas (Berry, 1984; Binstock & Day, 1996; Nayar, 2003; Pinner, Jacob, & Selznick, 1959; Pratt, 1993).

Three primary concepts have undergirded this inquiry: pluralism, constitutionalism, and federalism. Pluralism embraces the notion that the public interest or social justice is served via conflicts and compromises among organized groups rather than individuals (Binstock, 1972; Lowi, 1992). Interests competing for power and influence proliferate, in part due to government largesse, leading to an "interest group society" (Berry, 1984; Salisbury, 1990; Walker, 1983). However, those with clout in one policy domain (e.g., the American Association of Retired Persons [AARP] in aging) do not necessarily exercise power and influence in other areas (Peters, 2004). Some have greater power and influence as members of dominant coalitions (Hula, 1999) or of policy subsystems (e.g., "iron triangles") that include select legislative committees and bureaucrats (Gais, Peterson, & Walker, 1984; Pratt, 1976). Their resources (e.g., access to policy makers, size) help determine their levels of influence (Day, 1990; Kingdon, 1995). Additionally, some groups move beyond legislative policy making to use of the courts (Caldeira & Wright, 1998), or ballot initiatives (Cronin, 1989), providing fertile ground for other studies. Other investigations have focused on the dimensions and effectiveness of state-level interest groups (Thomas & Hrebnar, 2004).

An alternative to pluralism and interest group theory is political economy. This macrolevel framework (Binstock & Quadagno, 2001) or interpretative theory (Marshall, 1996) challenges democratic nostrums. It posits that social policy is the result of economic, political, and sociocultural forces and processes (Estes, Linkins, & Binney, 1996). These include the national and international context of the economy, labor market conditions, the role of the state, and the web of social and cultural factors that emphasize class, gender, race, and age divisions within society (Marshall, 1996). They mold outcomes for the sake or detriment of subsections of the population. The goal of social control and the mechanisms for addressing social problems reflect the system of social and power relationships in society (Piven & Cloward, 1971), leading to examinations of how policy elites shape policies for elders and others (Anderson, 1979; Kingdon, 1995; Minkler & Estes, 1984); for example, see Pynoos (1984) on elderly housing and Vladeck (1999) on Medicare. A primary contention of advocates of the political economy perspective is that policies and practices seldom aim at redistributive justice; instead they help to maintain existing arrangements.

Constitutionalism, a system of fundamental principles of government, emphasizes the institutional roles of the three branches of government and how they affect the policy process. It forms the basis for the institutional theory of policy making (Anderson, 1979). Constitutionalism, with its separation of power doctrine, is designed to keep government power in check. The "actors" inside government (executive, legislative, judicial, and bureaucracy) have legitimacy and power. They play different roles in various stages of the policy process—formulation, adoption, implementation, and evaluation—based on constitutional and traditional powers and informal arrangements developed over time (Anderson, 1979; Kingdon,1995). "Outsiders," such as interest groups, think tanks, and the mass media, try to influence the insiders (Kingdon, 1995).

Whereas policy formation studies have continued to emphasize legislative actions, research on the roles of other actors has increased. The power of the president to place issues on the public policy agenda has become a major area, reflecting the increased power of the presidency vis-à-vis Congress (Kernell, 1993; Light, 1991). Trial balloons by the White House often precede attempts to change existing policies, for example, labeling Social Security as in a "crisis." Similarly, how unelected officials shape policy at different stages of the policy process has expanded research on bureaucracy, as it has grown in size and professionalism (Meier, 1993; Wilson, 1989). The policy-making stature and powers of the courts, particularly the U.S. Supreme Court, in reviewing actions of administrative agencies, protecting individual rights, and preserving the federal relationship (e.g., Glick, 1994; Humphries & Songer, 1999; Wise, 1998) have become yet another fertile research area. Similar analyses have been conducted of the roles of governors, legislatures, courts, and bureaucrats at the state level (Gray & Hanson, 2004).

Lastly, federalism is the theory and practice of governing in which a national government and one or more subnational levels of government, each with substantial policy-making powers, enter into arrangements for jointly and separately working out solutions and adopting policies; the resultant sharing of authority and policy making is neither simple nor static (Nathan, 1990). Designed to decentralize power in the United States and other nations (e.g., Canada and India), it provides opportunities for "venue shopping"; that is, policy proposals that are not successful at the national level may achieve success at the state level (e.g., physician-assisted suicide) and vice versa (e.g., civil rights).

Responsibilities and powers of the two levels of government often are spelled out in national constitutions, for example, Article X of the U.S. Constitution and the State List in the Indian Constitution (Gokhale, 2003). Shifts occur in national-state government power relationships, alternating between devolution of responsibilities (with or without additional funding) and refederalization and/or preemption of powers once exercised by the states (Nathan, 1990; Zimmerman, 1991). Under the rubric of federalism, individual states are sources of innovation later adopted by other states (diffusion) or bubble up to the national level (Gray & Hanson, 2004; Lammers, 1989; Walker, 1969). The states' ability to fill the gaps in national policies—"compensatory federalism"—has been examined in several areas, for example, health care financing and delivery in Medicaid and the Children's Health Insurance Program (Holahan, Weil, & Wiener, 2004; Thompson & DiIulio, 1998). A heavier reliance on subnational governments, however, can lead to geographic disparities and inequities in policies and programs benefiting the elderly.

PUBLIC ADMINISTRATION AND LAW

Legislatures at the national and state levels pass broadly written laws, with details about implementation and enforcement delegated to bureaucracies: administrative and regulatory agencies. Those agencies generate rules and regulations specifying how a law will be carried out, through the administrative law-making process that includes public hearings. A similar process occurs at the local level, after ordinances have been enacted. Government agencies are not passive actors in the policy process; they often act as policy entrepreneurs in initiating/strengthening programs (Doig & Hargrove, 1987). Bureaucratic policy making is dominated by the ideas, norms, routines, and choices of nonelected public officials; resources include expertise, legislative authority, and leadership. Public administrators are subject to oversight by their respective legislatures and the courts (Humphries & Songer, 1999; O'Leary & Wise, 1991). Still, because Americans are suspicious about public authority, U.S. civil servants are generally viewed with disdain and sometimes outright enmity. This contrasts with the respect accorded their counterparts in other countries, such as Britain, France, and Japan (Doig & Hargove, 1987).

The growth of governmental activity since the 1930s has led to more public employees at all levels of government. Despite various attempts since the 1980s to shrink government, especially at the national level (Osborne & Plastrik, 1997), intergovernmental programs and grants have boosted the numbers of state and local administrators. Intergovernmental management of policies and programs, such as Medicaid (Holahan et al., 2003), nursing home regulation (Kelly, 2004), the Older Americans Act (Holt, 1994), and services in general (Thompson & Elling, 1999), has become a major research focus to identify the differing patterns of federal and state responsibilities and actions and to determine where accountability lies.

Still another area of inquiry has been the nonprofit sector, a substantial source of service delivery to the aged. U.S. nonprofits increased from 309,000 in 1967 to 1 million 30 years later (Weisbrod, 1997). Known as nongovernmental organizations (NGOs) in nations like India (Gokhale, 2003), nonprofits perform the kinds of functions often identified with government, for example, providing social services, hospital care, and housing to the aged and other groups. They have impacts on private firms, government, consumers, and other nonprofits. They encounter charges of being unfairly competitive with the for-profit sector (e.g. nonprofit museums run gift shops), but they also enter into joint ventures with private firms. Nearly every major university has joined forces with large multinational firms, such as the pharmaceutical industry (Weisbrod, 1997). Nonprofits have negative effects on government revenues because they are tax-exempt, but they also substitute for government service provision, reducing the need for a larger public work force. Consumers, especially in countries with diverse populations, can benefit from nonprofits providing culturally sensitive services to elders and other groups. Finally, nonprofits also create for-profit subsidiaries. Though not illegal, these ventures blur the lines between nonprofits and private firms. The upshot is that the nonprofit sector is entwined with the rest of the economy and is likely to become even more so in the future (Weisbrod, 1997).

Economics, sometimes known as "the dismal science," deals with the production, distribution, and consumption of wealth. Mainstream economics in the United States has its roots in utilitarian philosophy and laissez-faire capitalism, based on the principles of self-interested, rational decision making ("economic man"), that the greatest good of the greatest number provides the greatest net benefit to society in satisfying its material needs, and that the free market operates best with minimal government interference. Broadly speaking, topics of interest include economic cycles and market fluctuations, economic growth and productivity, savings and investment, inflation and interest rates, structural changes in national economies and rates of employment, supply and demand, economic choices, opportunity costs and trade-offs (e.g., work vs. leisure), income distribution and poverty rates, and international markets. The concepts of market failure, public goods (e.g., national defense), and externalities (e.g., spillover costs of pollution) are tied to delineating appropriate roles for government(s). Defining public sector limits vis-à-vis the market parallels political concerns about limited government, emphasizing individual rather than collective responsibilities.

Economic policies of governments also receive scrutiny, the results of which are often tied to conflicting ideologies about the roles government should play. Keynesian economics came into prominence during the Great Depression, as a means of priming the pump of private enterprise via public spending. Because economic problems were viewed as springing from inadequate demand, public budgets were designed to regulate effective demand via deficits to stimulate economic growth and reduce unemployment; to counter inflation, governments would run a budget surplus. A challenge to the Keynesian approach has been "supply-side" economics, in which a lack of supply, especially investment in labor and capital, is defined as the major problem. A U.S. dearth of savings and investment compared to other industrialized nations has been a major issue and increasingly has framed the Social Security debate (Arnold, Graetz, & Munnell, 1998; Feldstein, 1975). Echoing 19th-century economics, government and high taxes are seen as a major barrier to economic growth, especially if the public sector competes with the private sector for savings and in delivering services. Calls for privatization, whether of garbage collection or Social Security, reflect a growing dominance by "classic" and supply-side economics.

Instruments of economic policy, all affecting elders directly or indirectly, are multidimensional (Peters, 2004). Fiscal policy uses the budgetary process to allocate resources between the private and public sectors; however, even the best budget planning cannot adjust deficits or surpluses precisely (Peters, 2004). Monetary policy centers on the Federal Reserve Board monitoring the amount of money in circulation to control economic fluctuations, by expanding the supply to lower interest rates and tightening it to slow inflationary pressures. Regulations are designed to foster competition, both internally and globally, or to protect consumers. Public support for business consists of grants for modernization and expansion of industry, trade policy (e.g., tariffs and free-trade agreements), deregulation, and regional policy to counteract the effects of declining industry in different geographic areas. Public ownership, especially by state and local governments, of economic functions (e.g., electricity, gas, transportation, and insurance) is yet another economic management approach. Incentives, usually through the tax system, are used by all levels of government to make it easier and profitable for industry to invest or relocate and for consumers to save/create assets. Finally, moral suasion or "jawboning" is used by presidents (Kernell, 1993) and other elected officials to persuade businesses and industries to change their behavior. All in all, management of the economy has continued to be a governmental concern; historically, the U.S. government has supported private business and industry (Beard & Beard, 1960; Peters, 2004).

ENDURING QUESTIONS IN AGING POLICY

The key theories, concepts, and concerns of the policy sciences described above have helped shape ongoing questions about the nature of aging and aging policy. As discussed below, not all policy sciences have been accorded equal status in gerontological inquiry. In addition, the contributions of gerontology to the policy science disciplines have been somewhat limited. Finally, even within the areas investigated by those disciplines, several important topics have not been addressed in depth on the gerontological side of the fence.

The Politics of Aging and Aging Policy

The political science and public administration approaches to aging have yielded several enduring questions:

- What is meant by aging policy? Why do we get the aging policies we have?
- What are the roles played by the elderly in the policy process? What effects do they have as individuals and as group members?
- What is the reality of "senior power" now and in the future?

Although these questions have formed the basis for U.S. gerontological research, with population aging occurring worldwide and more rapidly in several countries, they have become more salient in industrialized nations, such as Canada and Britain (Pratt, 1993), and increasingly, in developing nations, such as India (Nayar, 2003). The development of Golden Age clubs for recreation in America in the 1940s and 1950s are similar to those found in Japan and India today. They provide nonpolitical forums for airing grievances and opportunities to link age status with political variables (Wallace & Williamson, 1992). The United Nations' focus on world population aging and its promotion of national policies for older persons (Gokhale, 2003), as well as the World Bank's proposals for "multipillared" pension systems (Schulz, 1996), are further evidence that these questions are increasingly global.

What Is Aging Policy?

In its aging policy, the United States has taken a different tack from the social policy of western Europe of class-based politics and social citizenship (Hudson, 1997). Provisions benefiting older Americans have been part of the policy landscape since state old-age assistance laws were enacted in the 19th and early 20th centuries, followed by Social Security in 1935, all based on age as a proxy indicator of need. However, when the U.S. Social Security Act was passed, it was not labeled "aging policy"; the aged were not its only beneficiaries. Perhaps successive White House Conferences on Aging in 1961 and 1971 can be viewed as placing age center stage as a policy variable and defining "aging policy." The Older Americans Act (OAA) of 1965 expanded the dimensions of a national aging policy to encompass wide-ranging goals (e.g., income, health, employment, housing, and social services). Certainly, the passage of Medicare in that same year, primarily for elders, made "aging policy" a greater reality, as did Medicaid, although the elderly were only one eligible group. The folding in of the national old-age assistance program and other programs into the Supplemental Security Income (SSI) program further extended the reach of aging policy. Similarly, the 1981 White House Conference on Aging expanded aging policy several-fold, with a focus on private-sector roles. In many respects, the period of 1935–1985 can be regarded as the golden age of U.S. aging policy, or more appropriately, of U.S. policy for the aged (Marshall, 1996). However, aging policy has primarily been defined as national policy, with far less scrutiny of state policies (except Medicaid), until fairly recently.

Gerontologists using the policy sciences as an analytic template are indebted to Robert Hudson, who laid out a framework for aging policy: age-based and age-related (Hudson, 1995, 1997). Age-based policies use chronological age as the primary eligibility criterion, that is, the universal policies of Social Security, Medicare, and the OAA. Social Security and Medicare are highly visible to the American public as "aging policy" due to their widespread impact and because the media have heightened awareness of their costs to society (Samuelson, 1978, 1990). Age-related policies, by contrast, may use age as one criterion, but low-income and asset levels are primary determinants in income-tested/means-tested programs, such as SSI, Medicaid, housing and veterans' health benefits. Beneficiaries are the poor or near poor of all ages, usually viewed as "undeserving." Elders and veterans generally have been exempted from that label.

Tax incentives by all levels of government to benefit current and future elders (e.g., individual retirement accounts, sales tax exemptions, and property tax assistance) do not fit easily into Hudson's framework. Some are targeted specifically for retirees, sometimes regardless of income (e.g., non-taxation of pension benefits). Some inadvertently benefit elders more than other age groups (e.g., sales tax exemptions for prescription drugs), and others are income-tested and age-related (certain property tax policies). In general, these policies get passing mention in the gerontological literature (Campbell, 2003; Crown, 2001; Hudson, 1995). In one sense, many tax expenditures are truly "aging" policies, as opposed to policies for the aged, in that they help younger persons prepare for their retirement years. Either way, these off-budget items obscure the true public costs of social welfare and of an aging society (Howard, 1997; Liebig, in press).

Hudson's prescience (1978) about how a growing percentage of the federal budget for aging programs might affect aging policy was picked up by other gerontologists in the 1990s who wrote about a "new" aging policy (Steckenrider & Parrott, 1996; Torres-Gil, 1992). They described a far harsher landscape for aging policy compared to 1935–1985 (Binstock & Quadagno, 2001, however, suggest that earlier period may have been an anomaly in U.S. social policy.). An era of "compassionate ageism" for the elderly as "the deserving poor" (Binstock, 1983) turned into one of "greedy geezers," "doing too much for the elderly" and "entitlement politics" (Moon & Mulvey, 1996; Smith, 2002), with the aged blamed for economic upheavals in the larger society (Minkler & Estes, 1991). This reconsideration of aging policy was part of a much larger debate over the legitimate role of government in society (Hudson, 1997; Smith, 2002). Aging policy became the focus of something more fundamental in American political values: the size and scope of government and individual versus collective responsibility for personal welfare (Achenbaum, 1983; Burke, Kingson, & Reinhardt, 2000; Cutler, 1977).

Why Do We Get the Aging Policies We Have?

The answers to this question have centered on pluralism, alternative explanations are less prominent. However, a model of policy making for the elderly proposed by William Lammers (1983) helps explain the shift in the political climate for aging policy since the 1980s. His emphasis on systemic factors included the role of societal attitudes: views of the aging and views of the public sector (similar to Kingdon's "national mood," 1995), as well as their impact on what the elderly get. In addition, Lammers pinpointed the importance of policy characteristics: cost, impact, and visibility, as crucial aspects of policy formation in determining policy outcomes. Written before the 1983 Social Security reforms were enacted, his insights continue to be valuable in answering Why do we get the aging policies we have?

Institutional policy making has received little attention in gerontology, compared to mainstream political science, despite the greater importance of presidential agenda setting and the role of the courts. A few authors have examined the interactions between Congress and the White House on aging issues (Lammers, 1983; Wisensale, 1996) and the role of the courts in areas such as right to die and guardianship (Glick, 1994; Kapp, 1996; Smith, 1996). However, analysis of court rulings on various aging issues (e.g., age discrimination, retiree health benefits, aging in prisons, and grandparents' rights) is largely the province of law review articles.

Furthermore, few gerontologists (Vinyard, 1972, 1983) have examined institutional models of policy making by studying the special institutions that provide a forum for aging policy formation, such as the Federal Council of Aging, the White House Conferences on Aging, and the Special Committees on Aging at the federal level. The impact and effectiveness of the White House conferences have been debated since the 1970s (Pratt, 1978; Vinyard, 1979); the 1995 conference in particular was regarded as little more than a holding action (Scharlach & Kaye, 1997). The "silver-haired legislatures," which exist in about half the states, deliberate on state policy affecting the elderly and make recommendations to their official state legislatures that may represent what their fellow elders want. They have virtually been ignored, perhaps because they are perceived as an example of symbolic politics, designed to avoid offending seniors but without giving them any real power.

By contrast, the concept and practice of federalism have received greater attention by gerontologists, especially after devolution became more pronounced (Estes & Gerard, 1983, and, more recently, Caro & Morris, 2002). Lammers and his colleagues were among those examining state-level policies in depth. In the 1980s, they addressed interstate differences in innovation, policy effort on behalf of the elderly, pension regulation, and state health and long-term care policies, as well as the factors influencing those differences (Lammers, 1989; Lammers & Klingman, 1984; Lammers & Liebig, 1990; Liebig, 1983). Other examples of comparative state policies for the elderly have included supportive housing (Pynoos, 1999; Pynoos, Liebig, Alley, & Nishita, 2004), long-term-care (Benjamin, 1986; Kane, 1998; Miller, 2002; Pandey, 2002; Wiener & Stevenson,1998), technology (Sheets, Liebig, & Campbell, 2002; Shrewsbury, 2002), Alzheimer's disease (Kaskie, Knight, & Liebig, 2001), and nursing home regulation (Harrington, Mullan, & Carrillo, 2004; Kelly, 2004; Walshe & Harrington, 2002). However, relatively little has been written about state tax policy. Interstate tax comparisons have been addressed by the National Conference on State Legislatures (Mackey & Carter, 1994) and in single states, such as Massachusetts, by Reschovsky (1989) and Kiesel (2002).

Despite the importance of implementation in determining the shape and impact of aging policies, research on intergovernmental management has been sparse because too little attention has been paid to the numerous national programs requiring subnational administration (Liebig, 1994a). Additionally, policy formation, rather than implementation, has been emphasized in aging policy. Capacity building in the aging network in carrying out the OAA received some attention, with contributions made by Brown (1983), Cutler (1984), and Hudson (1986), but little has been done since then. Although fragmentation of services, partly due to a lack of interagency cooperation, is acknowledged widely, fewer studies than are warranted have examined this vital concern (Myrtle & Wilber, 1994; Sheets et al., 2002). The same is true for in-depth examinations of private-public partnerships and nonprofits and their capacities (however, see Bradley, Patch & Gwyther, 2006, Meiners, McKay, & Mahoney, 2002). Instead, gerontologists have explored the roles of the older voter and age-based interest groups as the major reasons for the aging policies we have, but this viewpoint has not been without controversy.

What Are the Roles and Effects of the Elderly on the Policy Process?
This overarching query sprang from the dominant political science focus from the1940s to the 1970s on attitudes, voting behavior, and interest group roles. The older voter and senior interest groups provided examples to test dominant theories and concepts. In general, research in this area has exemplified the application of existing theories in political sciences to aging rather than contributing new theories. The main contribution has been the concept of life-cycle political engagement and participation.

Voting behavior and political participation of the aged have attracted attention among gerontologists and others, especially the media, since the 1960s. Although elders voted at lower rates from the 1950s through the 1970s than the middle-aged, they have always voted more than the young (Campbell, 2003), even with education and income controlled for (Verba & Nie, 1974). In the 1980s, they surpassed the middle-aged as well, just when aging policy was being examined more critically than it had been in the past. Cross-sectional studies of presidential elections show a consistently higher voting rate for elders than other age groups (Binstock, 2000; Binstock & Day, 1996; Campbell, 2003; Strate, Parrish, Elder, & Ford, 1989). Seniors' voting rates are now at a historical high, even in midterm elections; other age groups are at a historical low (Campbell, 2003). The proportion of seniors contacting elected officials has grown to 13%, but it rose to 20% in 1983 when Social Security and Medicare were both threatened. Although their engagement levels in campaign work are roughly equal to other age groups, 14% now contribute to political campaigns, surpassing both young and middle-aged voters (Campbell, 2003); however, this does not tell us the dollar amount given nor what happens beyond the national level.

State-level voting behavior and political participation of seniors have received minimal attention, but some studies have focused on the local level. Rosenbaum and Button (1989) examined the level and outcomes of senior political activism (i.e., school bond voting) in several Florida counties and municipalities, summarizing their findings in three hypotheses about the likelihood of increasing political power among the aged. Andel and Liebig (2002), based on a case study of a city dominated by seniors, found that when a crisis arises, higher income and better educated elders (Hudson's, 1988, "able elders") may be very influential. On the other hand, Boswell (2000) has suggested that elders may be less influential in municipal planning processes because they are often ignored by planners. A parallel view is expressed by Jirovec and Erich (1992) about political participation among the urban elderly. The issue of senior power and advocacy in state and local politics requires more attention.

Reasons for high levels of senior activism and the possibility of their decline or increase have also been explored. Age consciousness/age solidarity surrounding political interests has been one explanation. Pinner et al. (1959) and Piven and Cloward (1971) identified the Townsend movement as the beginnings of age solidarity, and Rose (1965) insisted that the elderly would become a subculture and a voting bloc. Cutler (1977) and Hudson (1988) suggested that growing participation and the possibility of bloc voting might increase elders' ability to influence politics. But since then, age consciousness as a driving force in senior activism has been downplayed. Elders coalesce around the issues of personal financial interest, but otherwise their opinions on any given issue are highly diverse; their focus is on objective economic and health issues that are not necessarily age-related (Binstock & Day, 1996; Wallace & Williamson, 1992). Social and economic class or political party affiliation (Binstock & Day, 1996; Campbell & Strate, 1981; Wallace, Williamson, Lung, & Powell, 1991) may be better predictors of how seniors vote; older people do not become politically homogenized when they turn 65 (Binstock, 2004). However, in the future, government efforts to cut entitlements may generate heightened age-consciousness and greater political cohesion, but Campbell (2003) points out this could be destroyed if Social Security is reformed in a way that pits better-off elders against the poor aged, as occurred with the Medicare Catastrophic Care Act (MCCA).

Other scholars have sought to address other reasons why elders are so highly engaged politically. Earlier scholars noted a heightened interest in politics among the aged (Glenn & Grimes, 1968) and their being better informed (Dobson, 1983; McManus, 1996), because they have more leisure time (Binstock & Day, 1996). Furthermore, this interest is sustained over time. Strate et al. (1989) concluded that interest and political knowledge increase with age and decline only slightly in advanced age; the young-old/able elderly are particularly active (Campbell, 2003; Hudson & Strate, 1985). Due to larger numbers of better educated, healthier baby boomers, it is anticipated these patterns will be more pronounced in the future (Williamson, 1998).

In a related fashion, life span civic development and political socialization of today's elders during their formative years have been identified as a major factor in elders' participation (Cutler, 1977; Putnam, 1995), leading to higher levels of civic education and politically relevant skills (e.g., letter writing) than younger cohorts (Campbell, 2003; Nie & Verba, 1974). And although formal education and adult household incomes are lowest among today's seniors, they have a huge stake in government programs that increase their interest and activity (Day, 1990). Despite the conventional wisdom that the poor are less politically active, this is belied by the participation rates of poorer elders (Campbell, 2003). Still, Binstock (2000) concludes that the aged have benefited from "electoral bluff" because of their relatively high voting turnout. Given this equivocation concerning the impact of older voters, gerontologists have focused on organized groups of seniors as major participants in shaping aging policy.

Although organized political action in the United States began in the 1930s with the Townsend movement, it died out after Social Security was enacted. Aging interest groups as stable structures emerged in the 1940s, first with the American Geriatrics Society and the Gerontological Society of America (GSA), followed by the National Retired Teachers Association and, later, the American Association of Retired Persons (now called AARP). Old-age groups in the United States and in industrialized nations around the world have proliferated since the mid-20th century (Binstock & Quadagno, 2001), with U.S. groups numbering over 100 with thousands of local chapters and state affiliates (Day, 1990; Van Tassel & Meyer, 1992). They include mass membership groups (e.g., AARP, National Council for Senior Citizens [NCSC]), organizations representing special older constituencies (e.g., Older Women's League, National Hispanic Council), and others representing professional and trade organizations (GSA, American Association of Homes and Services for the Aging) (Binstock & Day, 1996; Torres-Gil, 1992). Taken as a whole, advocacy groups for elders constitute an "aging enterprise" (Estes, 1979) and a "gray lobby" (Pratt, 1976).

These organizations have proliferated for several reasons: Expansion of government aging programs have led politicians and bureaucrats to mobilize political support for legislation and programs; similarly, threats to existing programs have produced new groups (e.g., Save Our Security). Grants from government and foundations also have played a role, as have the incentives offered to members (Binstock & Day, 1996; Binstock & Quadagno, 2001; Day 1990). These include material (e.g., travel benefits), solidarity (e.g., social events), and purposive incentives (e.g., improving the status of minorities) (Day, 1990). Individuals can and do belong to multiple organizations, however, many are not age 65 plus and/or do not engage in political activism.

Aging interest groups have several important resources to enhance their political influence. These include expertise in particular areas (e.g., long-term care and pensions), legitimacy with policy makers and, therefore, access and national media attention, large memberships (e.g., AARP) and geographic diversity, and the ability to mobilize campaigns to contact elected officials. Perhaps more importantly, they are perceived as powerful, especially by the media and social commentators, because they are numerous and well organized (Morris, 1996; Peirce & Chohari, 1982; Price, 1997). Although gerontologists first identified the potential for intergenerational conflict (Cain, 1975; Foner, 1974), this idea of young versus old has been co-opted by the media. With the ranks of the elderly being swelled by 76 million better educated baby boomers, these writers assume even higher levels of participation, so that the size and political vigor of greater numbers of elders may thwart efforts to implement policies that disadvantage the elderly. Among political economists in aging, this is seen as a social construction of an intergenerational problem, rather than a reality (Walker, 1993).

Additionally, proliferation of aging groups is not an isolated phenomenon; it has occurred with all other interest groups. This "crowding" has its downside, often resulting in less clout for all groups (Salisbury, 1990). In addition, no one organization can represent the diverse elderly; the concerns of low-income elders often get lost, raising questions about how representative aging interest groups are (Binstock, 2004; Wallace et al., 1991). Furthermore, aging constituencies often are divided on specific policies. Two coalitions have been created to enable these groups to "speak with one voice": the Leadership Council of Aging Organizations and Generations United; the latter was created to meet the challenges of generational equity. However, coalition effectiveness is often limited due to internal divisions, as occurred with the MCCA and President Bill Clinton's health plan (Liebig, 1994b). Similarly, coalitions with nonaging groups but with similar interests (e.g., disability advocates) can break down as well (Torres-Gil & Pynoos, 1986). Because most attention has been focused on the national level, we know little about the activities and impacts of senior interest groups at the state level which are of growing importance due to decentralization and devolution of aging policy (Liebig, 1992, 1994b).

What Is the Reality of Senior Power?

In general, most gerontologists believe that aging interest groups have been limited in their impact on aging policies, senior power best summed up as ambiguous (Campbell, 2003). Aging interest groups had little to do with passing Social Security and Medicare and subsequent amendments; those major programs were largely the work of insiders: the president, Congress, and bureaucrats with their own social policy agendas (Binstock & Day, 1996; Binstock & Quadagno, 2001). Although aging interest groups have grown more prominent since then, they are rarely "agenda setters" (Kingdon, 1995) and seldom able to dictate policy outcomes. For example, in the recent enactment of the Medicare Modernization Act, AARP (not all aging groups) served as a tipping point but not an initiator, and despite Social Security being dubbed "the third rail of politics," major reforms were enacted in 1983, with negative effects on the elderly. Similarly, since the 1990 debates over the role of government, aging advocates have largely defended existing policy, as exemplified by the top resolutions emanating from the 1995 White House Conference on Aging. In short, the expansion and contraction of the welfare state have not been under the control of the elderly as group members or voters.

Additionally, it is hard to discern who can "deliver" the "senior" vote; approximately half of AARP members are under age 65, and many join for nonpolitical reasons (Day, 1990). Indeed, Binstock (2000) opines that the aged have largely benefited from an "electoral bluff." Given their voting rates, seniors can influence electoral outcomes, but there is no guarantee that those will have an important bearing upon solving the group's problems. It is hard to trace the impacts of seniors' political activism on specific policy outcomes that would validate the "senior power" model (Binstock, 2000, 2004).

The political economists in aging in particular look askance at the concept of "senior power," suggesting they are really lambs in wolves' clothing (Wallace et al., 1991). They would subscribe to Heclo's view that "the elderly is really a category created by policy analysts, pension officials, and mechanical models of interest group politics" (1988, p. 393). The very presence and absence of issues on the policy agenda are shaped by strategically located interests and classes to define the problem of aging, with an emphasis on "crisis" leading to action (Estes et al., 1996). Crisis is a recurring theme with regard to the aging and the economy, and is tied to threats to Social Security and Medicare and the generational equity debate over whether the elderly are getting more than their fair share of national resources and children are getting too little. This "kids versus canes" debate has been shown to be a uniquely U.S. phenomenon (Cook, Marshall, Marshall, & Kauffman, 1994), and is linked to the elderly as the "800-pound gorilla" of American politics, with negative effects on government budgets and the American dream (Howe, 1997; Samuelson, 1978).

The concept of intergenerational interdependence has been put forth to counter the ideas of intergenerational conflict and generational equity (Kingson, Hirshorn, & Cornman, 1986), but it did little to defuse the arguments that the costs of the aged to society were hard to justify.

The Economics of Aging and Aging Policy

As population aging became more apparent in the 1960s and 1970s, its implications for all societies began to receive greater attention. Although some of the ensuing focus in the United States accompanies the rapid expansion of Society Security benefits in those decades, attention was enhanced by the creation of the National Institute on Aging, the White House conferences of 1971 and 1981, and the work of bureaucrats, such as Dr. Paul Haber of the Veterans Administration (VA), who drew attention to the impact of a growing number of aging veterans on the VA health system.

On a global level, the United Nations, through the World Assembly on Aging in 1982, promoted discussions about the needs of growing numbers of older persons, especially in developing nations such as China and India. Projections of the numbers and proportions of the elderly worldwide in the twentieth first century led to heightened concerns about the costs of supporting ever larger numbers of longer-lived, physically frail, and often impoverished elders through the efforts of smaller numbers of younger workers. The impact of population aging on national economies in the first stages of development has also been addressed by the World Bank. The United States, in common with most industrialized nations, particularly those with higher proportions of the aged (e.g., Italy) or faced with very rapid aging (e.g., Sweden and Japan), has had to examine what the costs of an aging society are now and in the future. Many of these concerns are tied to key topics in economics: economic growth and productivity, savings and investment, inflation, employment, and income distribution and poverty rates. A major contribution has been the life-cycle hypothesis: Consumption needs and income are unequal at various points over the life span (Ando & Modigliani, 1963).

The major questions in the economics of aging have been

- What is the economic status of the elderly? How well-off are they?
- What are the sources and shares of income for elders?
- How much aging can we afford? Are we doing too much for the aged?
- Are the boomers saving enough?

What Is the Economic Status of the Elderly? How Well-off Are They?
The contributions of gerontologists to economics initially centered on the economic status of older adults, with a focus on poverty. When Social Security was passed, approximately 50% of the elderly were below the poverty line. Juanita Kreps and James Schulz in the 1960s and 1970s, subsequently followed by others, also examined the major sources of income available to the elderly, the changes over time as both public and private retirement income programs took effect, and the income of elders compared with other adults,

as well as among subgroups of the aged. More recently, these investigations have become more global, with cross-national comparisons of income and wealth (Crown, 2001; Pampel, 1998; Schultz, 1996).

Well-being of the aged, however, is dependent on more than just income. Mental and physical health, social relationships and living arrangements, attitudes, assets, and needs are also important variables. Economic (or financial) well-being can be measured in several ways; annual money income and differences by income class; poverty rates; and adequacy relative to some standard of living, that is, the ability to make necessary purchases (e.g., housing, food, and medical care). In-kind benefits (e.g., housing subsidies and Medicare) and tax subsidies also contribute to economic well-being of the elderly. Although annual income has continued to be an important indicator, measures of wealth or net worth have been used more recently to define the financial well-being of those age 65 and over.

Annual Income Incomes of the elderly have increased since the 1960s and 1970s. In 1974, median (pretax) household income (stated in 2002 dollars) was $16,882; it grew to $23,152 in 2002 (Federal Interagency Forum on Aging-Related Statistics [FIFARS], 2004). But without some comparison to income levels of different age households, this information is not very meaningful. Median income for the elderly ages 65 to 74 is about the same as for ages 15 to 24, while the median income of elders age 75 plus is less than all other households of any age (Clark et al., 2004).

A different story, however, is told by tracking trends in median incomes of older and younger households from 1967 to 1999. During this period, U.S. median incomes adjusted for inflation rose by 24%, for all ages. Whereas median income gains for younger households (ages 25–44) were less than that figure, increases for those ages 55 to 64 were 40% and 80% for persons age 65 plus (Clark et al., 2004). Although most of these gains for elders occurred by the late 1980s, their incomes increased significantly in the last third of the 20th century, in absolute terms, when adjusted for inflation, and in comparison with the rest of the population, a testament to the effectiveness of Social Security. However, some of these gains have been reduced by federal tax treatment of the elderly becoming less favorable since the 1980s, resulting in a slight shift in the tax burden from younger households to the elderly (Crown, 2001).

In addition to differential tax treatment of the elderly, in-kind benefits affect their economic well-being. The treatment of Medicare benefits as an income equivalent has been controversial, because it makes elders appear better off. Counting Medicare reimbursements as income has the perverse effect of making older persons with costly illnesses seem wealthy (Crystal, 1996). However, these imputations do not take into account the greater health care needs of elders and the growing out-of-pocket costs for health care and long-term care nor, in comparison with younger households, the value of work-related health insurance (Crystal, 1996).

A further note of caution is sounded by Crown (2001, p. 360), who suggests it is not totally valid to compare family incomes across different age groups, due to differences in life-cycle consumption needs and household size. It is more appropriate to describe the economic status of the elderly as being similar to younger persons. Some are poor, some are wealthy, with the majority in between. In 2002, people in the middle-income group (measured as 200% to 399% of poverty) were the largest income category of the aged (35%), a slight increase over 32.6% in 1974; during the same period, the proportion of low-income elders shrank from 34.6% to 28% (FIFARS, 2004). The proportion of elders with high income (> 400% of poverty) has risen, from 18% in 1974 to 26% in 2002 (FIFARS, 2004). This rise in income inequality parallels that in the general population, but it is higher among aged households. Still, Social Security plays an important role in reducing this inequality (Crown, 2001); without it, the income gap between high- and low-income elders would be even more pronounced.

These increases in income, however, need to be examined in the light of purchasing power and expenditure patterns. Although senior consumers' expenditures are 70% of expenditures made by all consumers, they spend relatively more of their income on property taxes (109%) and a whopping 155% more on medical care, despite Medicare coverage (Campbell, 2003, p. 43). Seniors also spend somewhat more of their incomes on food and utilities than all other consumers. Housing expenditures are more equivocal. Although seniors expend less on mortgage payments (25% of what other consumers pay), examining overall housing expenditures (i.e., mortgage payments, rent, utilities, property taxes, and insurance) by seniors provides a different perspective. Between 1987 and 2002, the proportion of expenditures for housing rose among all older American households in each of five income groups, with the lowest quintile paying 40% of their income for shelter-related expenses (FIFARS, 2004). These intragenerational differences in housing reflect the wide range of economic well-being among the elderly (Liebig, 1996).

Disaggregation of data on the economic status of the elderly provides additional insights. Due to age, incomes vary considerably within the age 65+ group, with those age 75 plus generally less well-off. In 1999, the young-old had median incomes of $27,000; those age 75 plus had median incomes of

$19,000. However, 13% of young-old households and nearly 19% of those age 75 plus had incomes of less than $10,000. At the other end of the spectrum, 24% of those age 65–74 and 12% of age 75 plus had incomes over $50,000 (Clark et al., 2004). Still, the latter group is more likely to be in the lower end of income distribution among the elderly; this is especially true for the oldest old.

Median incomes of the elderly also vary by marital status and race. From the mid 1960s through the mid 1990s, the median income of older married couples grew from $15,845 to $27,944, although gains in 1990 (to $28,033) were followed by reductions in 1992 and 1994. Nonmarried persons' median income rose from $6,125 to $11,302; the losses in the early 1990s were less severe than for married couples (FIFARS, 2004). Different patterns also exist for race. From the mid 1960s to the mid 1990s, median income for Whites grew from $8,935 to $16,954, compared with Blacks, from $6,314 to $9,649. Average incomes for Black and Hispanics ages 65 to 74 are about two thirds of Whites; in the 75 plus age group, the proportions are somewhat higher (70%, FIFARS, 2004).

Wealth A final measure of the economic well-being of the elderly is household wealth: the total market value of such items as home equity and other real estate, stocks and bonds, and savings accounts. A related measure, net worth, subtracts outstanding debts (e.g., mortgage balances). Wealth and net worth are important indicators of economic security. In keeping with the life-cycle hypothesis, they represent a household's ability to maintain a standard of living when income falls due to health problems, as well as the capacity to finance future consumption (e.g., long-term care) by drawing on those resources. For most older households, the major source of net worth is the equity in homes. Since the 1980s, public policies (e.g., reverse annuity mortgages) have allowed elders to convert that equity into income for various purposes.

The median net worth of older households in 2001 (excluding pension wealth) grew since the mid 1980s, from $98,900 to $179,800, an 82% increase (FIFARS, 2004). However, differences exist among subgroups of the elderly. The median net worth of older married couples was nearly triple that of unmarried persons age 65 plus ($291,000 vs. $100,800), with older White households having a net worth 5 times larger than elderly Black households ($205,000 compared with $41,000). Older White households experienced an 81% gain in net worth from 1984 to 2001, compared with a 60% increase for Black households. Furthermore, more educated households (with at lest some college education) had a higher net worth, more than 6 times larger than those headed by elders without a high school diploma ($360,500 vs. $57,300).

Over the past several decades, gerontologists and other researchers have established that the financial status of today's elderly in terms of income and wealth is much improved, compared with earlier cohorts of retirees. For example, the total household income per adult equivalent (IAE), which reflects impacts of earnings on living levels and changes in the number and age composition of dependents in the household, shows that the economic status of retirees born before World War II is the highest of any cohort that has retired (Easterlin, 1996). These documented gains have generated a new stereotype of all elders doing well, replacing the earlier stereotype of all aged being poor. In turn, this good news about elders' financial well-being has led to new policies based on differences in the economic status of older Americans (e.g., taxation of Social Security benefits for those above certain income levels and targeting of OAA programs). These statistics also have been amplified by the media and have helped fuel the "kids versus canes" debate, despite a lack of "citizenship-based" policies for children and their welfare (e.g., publicly subsidized child care) of the sort found in Europe. However, improved economic well-being does not hold true for all persons age 65 and over. Pockets of economic distress among older Americans remain.

Poverty rates among the elderly are one way to measure economic well-being, a major emphasis in the economics of aging for several decades. The U.S. Census Bureau compares annual money income with a set of poverty thresholds that vary by family size and composition, adjusted yearly by the Consumer Price Index (CPI). In 1959, 35% of the elderly lived below the poverty threshold (FIFARS, 2004). In that year, the aged had the highest poverty rate, compared with children (27%) and with those of working ages (17%). This trend continued through much of the 1960s and the early 1970s, laying the foundation for concerted advocacy on behalf of the elderly and a rationale for "compassionate ageism" (Binstock, 1983). Since 1982, the poverty rate for elders has been lower compared with the population as a whole, following major Social Security benefit boosts in the 1960s and 1970s. In the year 2002, 10% of the aged were poor, equal to the working-age poor, but less than children (17%; FIFARS, 2004). If in-kind benefits and taxes are factored in, the aged poverty rate is cut by half (Clark et al., 2004).

However, aggregate data tell only part of the story. Poverty rates among the elderly differ by age, gender, race, and other factors. Those age 75 and over (12%) have higher rates than people ages 65 to 74 (9%), with older women (12%) more likely to live in poverty than older men (8%, FIFARS, 2004). Aged women also are poorer than their male counterparts at all ages: 10% for those age 65 to 84 compared with 8% for men in the same age group and 15% for those age 85 (Clark et al., 2004). Furthermore, race and ethnicity are related to poverty among the aged: 8% of non-Hispanic Whites compared with 24% of older Blacks and 21% of older Hispanics. Higher rates of poverty in old age are associated with discontinuous labor force attachment because receipt of Social Security and pensions in the United States is determined by work history; this is not the case in Europe (Pampel, 1998). All these factors lend credence to the concept of "cumulative disadvantage" (Calasanti & Slevin, 2001; Crown, 2001). Living arrangements also are a crucial factor. Elders who live alone are far more likely to be poor, 21% of older women and 16% of older men, compared with the poverty rate (5%) for older married couples (FIFARS, 2004). In particular, much older women who are Black and live alone are the poorest of the poor, the victims of "triple jeopardy."

However, when examining these poverty statistics, two issues deserve consideration. One is how poverty is measured, the other is the disproportionately higher numbers of elders among the near poor. The U.S. poverty index is based on increases in the cost of living over a baseline established in the 1960s for a minimum food budget; poverty thresholds for the aged and other types of households are increased annually by the CPI to maintain a 1963 level of purchasing power. The current index does not include clothing, shelter, or other common, everyday needs. A revised index encompassing these items was recommended by the National Academy of Sciences in 1995, but it was not adopted.

Proposals have been made to tie the U.S. poverty line to increased prices and rising median incomes, due to greater inflation and real national productivity. If adjustments were made to reflect price changes and the increased standard of living since the 1960s, the measured poverty rates of young and old Americans would be much higher (Clark et al., 2004). This would bring U.S. measures more in line with European poverty indices. The decision not to do so is politically motivated, as was the creation of the original index during President Lyndon Johnson's "War on Poverty" and more recent explorations of income definitions that include in-kind benefits, capital gains, and an imputed return on home equity. These adjustments would disproportionately favor the elderly who receive Medicare, are home owners (80% own their own residences), and are more likely to have nontaxable income (e.g., municipal bonds; Clark et al., 2004). Furthermore, proposals to recalibrate the CPI also have encountered difficulties. The results of an elder-specific CPI in the 1980s were problematic, and had the recommendations of a 1990s commission that found the CPI overstated inflation by 1.1% annually been embraced by policy makers, future cost of living adjustments for Social Security, SSI, veterans' benefits, and government pensions would have been reduced.

The second issue is that poverty among the elderly is a subsistence adequacy measure (Crown, 2001). A substantial proportion of elders are not "officially" poor but are so economically vulnerable that one illness or reduction in interest income payments (as has happened for the past several years) can have severe repercussions. These persons, known as the "tweeners" (Smeeding, 1986), are not poor enough to be eligible for means-tested programs, but they do not have adequate resources to live above a subsistence level. Tweeners' incomes fall between 100% and 150% of the poverty level; 16% of elders' incomes are at 125% of poverty, the same figure as the general population. However, 23% of the aged have incomes of 150% of poverty, compared with 21% of the general population. If the upper limit is raised to 199% of poverty, 28% of the elderly fall into this low-income group. Although the proportion of this group has declined since 1974 (FIFARS, 2004), 38% of today's near-poor elders still live precariously, in part because their sources of income differ greatly from those of their higher income counterparts.

What Are the Sources and Shares of Income for Elders?

Most older Americans are retired from full-time work, necessitating other sources of income. Income of the elderly is derived from five sources: Social Security, created as a "floor" of protection, supplemented by private and public employer pensions, asset income, earnings, and other sources (e.g., public assistance). As of 2000, over 90% of elderly households received some income from Social Security, with nearly three fifths getting some asset income. Employer pension benefits go to about 40% of retired households, and 22% have earnings income, followed by public assistance (5%) and veterans' benefits (4%; Clark et al., 2004). However, sources differ according to age cohort: Of households headed up by someone age 62 to 64, 62% have earnings income. Forty-four percent of those age 65 to 69 have earnings income, compared with 4% of those age 85 plus. The drop in earnings among those in their 60s reflect the effects of Social Security availability on labor force decisions of older workers (Crown, 2001). Pension receipt also declines with age, dropping from 44% at age 70 to 74 to 33% at age 85 plus, probably a cohort effect, that also is reflected in smaller amounts of asset income for the oldest old (Clark et al., 2004). Thus Social Security is particularly important for the oldest-old.

A focus on the relative importance of those different income sources, or shares, provides important information; however, identifying shares does not tell the complete story because the among of income is not considered (Clark et al., 2004). Since the early 1960s, Social Security has provided the largest share of aggregate retirement income, now at 39%. The automatic indexing of benefits in 1972 to the CPI during retirement and the tying of benefit levels to increases in earnings over time underscore how vital Social Security is for older households. Earnings continue to be important, accounting for 25% of income compared with 30% in the 1960s (Crown, 2001). Employer pensions and income from assets account for 19% and 14%, respectively. Pension coverage expanded dramatically in the 2 decades after World War II, primarily due to substitution of fringe benefits when wartime policies forbade wage increases. Since then, coverage of workers has been stable at about 50%, although there has been a shift to defined contribution plans that entail higher risk for employees. The proportion of workers in defined benefit plans has declined steeply, from 80% in 1985 to 33% in 2003 (FIFARS, 2004). In general, women and minorities are less likely to enjoy pension coverage because they work for employers who do not provide such benefits (Calasanti & Slevin, 2001). Asset income peaked in the mid 1980s and has declined since, whereas earnings have shown the opposite trend, having declined until the mid 1980s and subsequently increased since then, reflecting somewhat higher labor force participation among older women (FIFARS, 2004).

Again, it is useful to disaggregate the data to examine the differences in shares of income among subgroups of the aged. First, there are differences by age: Those ages 65 to 69 rely most heavily on earnings and Social Security, whereas the rest of the young-old get most of their income from Social Security, followed by earnings. Among the old-old, the primary income sources of those ages 75 to 79 are Social Security, earnings, and pensions, contrasted with 80- to 84-year-olds, who rely most on Social Security, pension, and asset income. The oldest-old derive their largest shares of income from Social Security and asset income (Clark et al., 2004). The biggest contrast among age groups 65 plus is the relative importance of earnings for the young-old, compared with the bigger role played by Social Security among the old-old and the oldest-old.

Differences also are revealed by examining income quintiles. The lowest 20% of older households subsist almost entirely on government sources, Social Security, and SSI, with only 7% from all other sources. Among the next quintile, asset income and earnings provide about 12% of their income, with heavy reliance on Social Security. For these two lowest income groups, two legs of the "three-legged stool" (Social Security, pensions, and savings) are missing. Among persons in the third quintile, Social Security provides two thirds of their income (Clark et al., 2004). Even in the fourth quintile, nearly half of those households receive more than half of their I ncome from Social

Security. Among the top 20%, earnings are most important, providing one third of all money income, followed by asset income (25%), and Social Security and employer benefits at 20% each (Clark et al., 2004). For this income group, privatization of retirement income is already a fact.

Clearly, Social Security is the bedrock for all older Americans, except the mostaffluent. This is a key consideration when evaluating whether American society can afford its aging population. Similar questions are being raised by other industrialized nations around the world; the answers, however, are not the same as those provided in the United States, the nation with the most restrictive social welfare policies among industrialized nations in the world.

How Much Aging Can We Afford? Are We Doing Too Much for the Aged?
These questions were first raised by nongerontologists, but they were soon taken up by researchers in aging (Aaron, Bosworth, & Burtless, 1989). Somewhat perversely, the work of gerontologists and others documenting the improved economic status of today's aged over earlier cohorts of retirees led to questions as to whether we are doing too much for the elderly, "who don't really need help." These debates have raged since the 1980s, fueled by visions of apocalyptic demography (Howe, 1997) and a federal budget devoted increasingly to supporting ever growing numbers of retirees and far too little to building capacity in the American economy (Auerbach & Kotlikoff, 1993; Hudson, 1978; Samuelson, 1978). Similar arguments have been made about the impacat of aging on corporate America's bottom line (Walker Wyatt Worldwide, 2004; hereafter Walker, 2004).

This graying of federal and corporate budgets was blamed for the poor performance of the U.S. economy (Binstock, 1983; Minkler & Estes, 1991) and raised questions about the low rates of savings available for investment. Feldstein (1975), Auerbach and Kotlikoff (1993), and others identified Social Security as a drain on savings that otherwise would be allocated for private investment, a position challenged by Aaron et al. (1989) and Schulz (1996), among others. There is no guarantee that a rising savings rate will necessarily increase productive investment and economic growth (Schultz, 1996). This macrolevel analysis about the role of social insurance and savings has more recently been changed into discussions about the "rate of return" on individuals' Social Security "investment." This viewpoint, promoted by the Heritage Foundation and other conservative think tanks, has become the primary argument for private accounts in Social Security.

The dependency ratio, or the proportion of workers to nonworkers (children and all persons age 65 and over), has been cited as major burden, in part because Social Security taxes paid by today's workers support today's retirees. Counterarguments have been presented: A higher dependency burden occurred from 1870 to 1913, a time when the U.S. economy was far less robust (Walker, 2004). No change in the overall dependency ratio has occurred because, although there are more elders, fewer children are being born (Aaron et al., 1989), and measuring labor force participation solely by gross age parameters provides an imcomplete picture. Political economists (Minkler & Estes, 1991) stressed the contrived dependency of the elderly, and advocates emphasized the role of age discrimination and mandatory retirement. In turn, this led to "productive aging" as a way to combat the stereotype of "useless" or unproductive elders by focusing on both market and nonmarket contributions to society (Butler & Schechter, 2001; Hendricks, 2001).

In the meantime, labor force participation has changed since the end of the 20th century. Many more younger persons stay in school, in part due to child labor laws and age minimums (usually age 16) before they can quit. Many also pursue postsecondary education to meet demands of the job market, thereby delaying their entry into the work force. Similarly, the labor force participation of persons age 60 and over has changed since the 1970s, due to economic circumstances (Clark et al., 204), as the cost of living, especially health care, has gone up. The desire for a more financially stable retirement has led to worker concerns about achieving higher earnings replacement targets compared with their preretirement income (replacement ratios). In addition, the abolition of mandatory retirement for most workers has made it possible for older workers to work longer, should they so choose.

Those who retire often return to work, taking part-time jobs or becoming self-employed (Clark et al., 2004), and more older women are now working, reflecting an upsurge of women of all ages in the American work force. Nearly 40% of women ages 60 to 64 are working, compared with 33% in 1975; 18.4% of women ages 65 to 69 are working, compared with 14.5% in 1975 (FIFARS, 2004). In contrast, work patterns of men ages 60 to 64 have declined slightly (from 55.6% to 54.8%), but labor force participation of men 65 to 69 has grown since 1986, from 24.5% to 28.5% today (FIFARS, 2004). Although Social Security, early retirement, and employer pensions and "bridge" health benefits before Medicare eligibility occurs induce workers to leave the work force (Clark et al., 2004), the figures cited above indicate a shift in the dependency ratio. This may continue, as boomers indicate they expect/want to work longer.

Changes in Social Security will likely impact future labor force participation; many were designed to influence workers to continue working beyond age 62 or age 65. The penalties for taking early retirement were raised in

1983, and bonuses for delayed retirement were enacted, as were gradual changes in the normal retirement age; boomers will need to work longer to get full Social Security benefits. As as 2000, the "earnings test" was eliminated for persons age 65 and over and liberalized for those ages 62 to 64, so individuals can work and receive benefits with little or no penalty. Because current earnings of these "working retirees" are subject to the Social Security tax, they continue to pay into the system, and benefits are recalculated.

The dependency ratio issue morphed into the intergenerational equity debate, in which it was said that one group of dependents, the elderly, were getting more than their fair share of public resources, whereas children—our future—were being neglected. This, in turn, set off a flurry of "generational accounting" (Auerbach, Gokhale, & Kotilikoff, 1992), comparing the public costs of raising and educating children who would be productive in the future with the public costs of supporting "greedy geezers." Proposals were made to means-test Social Security—actually, an income test, as no assets calculations were involved. Taxation of Social Security benefits for higher income individuals and couples, first in 1984 and then again in 1994, helped accomplish this objective, with the revenues deposited I nto the Social Security trust fund. Gerontologists and advocates for the aged were quick to point out that supporting elders at the expense of children was not a deliberate policy trade-off; indeed, children of deceased or disabled workers were also beneficiaries of Social Security. If poor children were not getting sufficient support, income and health programs for poor families, funded by general revenues, were at fault.

Employers also began to reduce the costs of their voluntary retirement income and health benefits programs, recognizing that due to greater longevity, they would be paying out those benefits over longer time periods. Through these changes, employees became more responsible for their retirement years, a foreshadowing of the "ownership society" praised by President George W. Bush. Traditional defined benefits programs were first supplemented and then gradually replaced by defined contribution plans that only guarantee the amounts invested, not the amount of the retirement income benefit (Walker, 2004). Similarly, health benefits were reduced, by making them less open-ended, using health maintenance organizations (HMOs), eliminating retiree benefits for new hires, or discontinuing them entirely. Employers have used retiree health benefits as part of early retirement incentive packages for workers under the age of 65; often this "bridge" benefit is withdrawn after the retiree becomes eligible for Medicare. This differential treatment of newer worker cohorts could have been part of the generational equity debate, but it has been fairly low profile.

Older persons' access to Medicare, however, did become part of the debate. Under the fair share argument, advocates noted that children were a substantial proportion of the growing numbers of the uninsured, whereas the elderly enjoyed public support for their medical care (Auerbach et al., 1992; Lamm, 1999). The concept of limiting health care for the elderly based on the idea of a natural life span and medical goals of cure was accompanied by a proposal for age-based rationing (Callahan, 1987). With reports that Medicare costs of the last year of life were exorbitant, health care rationing advocates stated that medical resources should not be "wasted" on those, such as the aged, who would not benefit sufficiently from them. Again, the extent to which the "savings" achieved by not treating the elderly would be allocated to children without insurance was never articulated (Cook et al., 1994).

This debate raised on ethical and political firestorm (Binstock & Day, 1996; Binstock & Quadagno, 2001) extending to related issues of physician-assisted suicide (Clark & Liebig, 1996) and the right to die (Glick, 1994). Furthermore, the burgeoning costs of Medicare and employer-sponsored health benefits generated major concerns about the costs of health care for elderly boomers and the increasing share of the gross domestic product devoted to health care, now 15% and projected to be 19% in 2014. This realization also led to major changes in health care delivery (e.g., outpatient surgery and shorter hospital stays) and changes in public and private reimbursement systems. As out-of-pocket costs for today's elderly continue to rise—95% paid something for their health care from their own resources in 2001 (FIFARS, 2004)&mdaash;questions have been raised about the ability of boomers to save enough for their retirement years.

Are the Boomers Saving Enough?

Closely tied to the issues of generational equity and our ability to afford an aging society is whether the baby boomers are saving enough for retirement, with important repercussions for Social Security and Medicare as well as public and private employer pensions and retiree health benefit plans. Put another way, what will boomers' economic status be in old age, compared with their financial status as workers and to today's elderly? Much of this discussion stems from differences in the boomers' and their parents' work-life experiences. The flood of boomers into the labor market and consequent job competition, accompanied by a slowing economy in the 1970s, contrasted with the experience of their parents, the original "baby bust" generation who benefited from a rapidly expanded post–World War II economy and scarce labor supply (Easterlin, 1996).

This scenario has led to the view that the boomers will be the first U.S. cohort to be less well-off than their parents when they reach retirement age. However, it ignores the improved educational status of the boomer cohort and more favorable labor market situation for women, as well as certain demographic decisions, such as postponing or deferring marriage or having fewer children (Easterlin, 1996). All these factors have an impact on saving for retirement. In addition, the strength of the economy and assets markets, increased incentives for savings (e.g., IRAs and added incentives for those age 50 and over), timing of retirement, and the structure of employer and government programs (e.g., pensions and retiree health benefits, Social Security, and Medicare) will all affect the financial status of the boomers in retirement (Clark et al., 2004).

Despite the media doom and gloom, many economists and others share the view that many boomers are doing as well as or better than their parents were at the same age, relative to their current income and accumulated wealth (Clark et al., 2004). The life-cycle income profiles for earlier cohorts suggest that income differences earlier in life are linked to income differences in retirement. Comparisons of boomers with their parents at ages 25 to 44 show that, on average, they are currently about two-thirds better off (Easterlin, 1996, p. 86). Tax rate reductions of the early 21st century are likely to increase this advantage.

Another study (cited by Clark et al., 2004) showed that, depending on adjustments for household size, the boomers had 40% to 80% more annual income than their parents did at the same age. The gains over time were lowest in the bottom income quintile (despite higher incomes and higher income/wealth ratios than their parents) and highest at the top, indicating widening income disparities. In addition, the life-cycle hypothesis of savings and dissavings over the life course (Ando & Modigliani, 1963) would inciate that boomers, like their parents, would save in earnest once expenditures associated with family formation (e.g., home ownership and college education for children) are completed. Comparisons of the boomers' savings rates with their parents' indeed confirm the same patterns at the same life stage (Easterlin, 1996; Easterlin, MacDonald, & Macunovich, 1990). This appears to be true of the middle-aged worldwide (Cutler & Cregg, 1990). The current net worth of the boomers and the likelihood they will inherit substantial wealth from their parents are further indications that their economic status in retirement will be better than their parents' (Easterlin, 1996).

Still, because the earlier group of boomers has "done better" economically than the later group, some will have comfortable retirements; many others, however, will not (Clark et al., 2004). Several factors are operative.

Traditionally vulnerable groups, such as Blacks and those living alone (due to growing numbers of never-marrieds and childless individuals), are projected to grow among the boomers. This cohort also is less likely to enjoy in their retirement years the dramatic increases in real estate wealth of the 1990s and major increases in Social Security benefits in the 1960s and 1970s experienced by their parents or grandparents. Additionally, they are facing the prospect of benefit cuts/eligibility delays (e.g., a higher normal retirement age) in Social Security and Medicare, significant fluctuations in financial markets, and rapidly rising health care costs. Although their standard of living will be higher than their parents', their retirement resources may fall short of their own preretirement standards or expectations.

It is worth noting that the majority of the boomers (i.e., those born between 1946 and 1956) would not be affected by Social Security privatization proposals that specify workers age 50 and over would be exempt from establishing private accounts. The "tail end" boomers born between 1957 and 1964, already less well-off compared with their older brothers and sisters, would be eligible; however, it is not clear how many would select private accounts or the extent to which they would benefit from that action. The costs of the boomers' retirement that have driven intergenerational equity discussions and ideas about our inability to afford an aging society are not going to be solved by the Bush proposal. It also is clear that whether or not we can afford an aging society is not solely an economic issue, but one freighted with political and value issues about the appropriate role of government (Achenbaum, 1983; Arnold et al., 1998).

THE NEXT GENERATION OF ENDURING QUESTIONS

Some questions in the policy sciences in aging that have persisted in the past and exist today—How much aging can we afford as a society? How powerful are the elderly politically?—are likely to command attention over the next several decades. Many of the answers will be shaped not only by changes in policies that affect the elderly, but also by policies that "compete" for public and private resources, such as homeland security, energy prices, and war in the Middle East or other parts of the globe. How those questions are answered may also be affected by Americans adopting/attempting to adopt or rejecting solutions employed by other nations (e.g., Chilean retirement income policy).

The next generation of enduring questions can be roughly divided into two groups. One might be termed "new wrinkles" on old questions, that is, newer ways to reexamine questions that have dominated the policy sciences and aging in the past. The other can be defined as an intellectual "face lift," issues that have emerged in the policy sciences over the past several decades that deserve examination by gerontologists.

"New Wrinkles" in the Policy Sciences and Aging

Elder participation, whether as voters or members of interest groups, will continue to command attention. However, with significantly large numbers of older voters in the future, research should be conducted on teasing out variations by age, rather than aggregating all older adults into one group (age 65 and older) as we do now. Similar disaggregation in the realm of health has given us a far better picture of the physical and mental profiles of the elderly. Are there differences among older voters, for example, always-single older women or older widows, similar to different groups of younger voters, for example, "soccer moms"? Are there differences (e.g., party affiliation) among different cohorts of older voters who, with greater longevity, range from persons in their 60s to those in their 90s and beyond? To what extent do baby boomers continue the same patterns of political activism experienced by their parents or in which they were engaged when they themselves were younger? Are there different patterns among older voters based on the growing numbers of racial/ethnic minorities? Do older persons vote more conservatively than younger voters on ballot initiatives that increasingly encompass "hot button" social issues (e.g., physical-assisted suicide and gay marriage)? This inquiry would enable us to answer more fully the questions about the roles played by older voters.

Additionally, what the impacts of new ballot mechanisms (e.g., "permanent" absentee ballots and electronic voting) on voting by elders? (The case of "butterfly ballots" in the 2000 presidential election shows how unfamiliar methods can effectively disenfranchise older voters.) To what extent do older persons use new I nformation sources (e.g., bloggers and talk radio) to define their voting stance or make online contributions? How might this impact baby boomers' participation relative to that of their parents? These technological issues deserve attention.

Similarly, looking at presidential elections as the major measure of voting by elders provides only a limited picture, particularly when trying to characterize the impact of the "elderly vote." Some questions that might be addressed include To what extent do elders vote as a bloc in congressional elections at the district level? What is the voting behavior of the elderly on a variety of state and local issues affecting their well-being (e.g., zoning for granny flats, not just school bonds)? What is the impact of the "snowbird vote" in Sunbelt states or the impact of "silver-haired" legislatures on policies and programs affecting the elderly? Other state-related questions need to address the specific impact of aging interest groups in state politics, beyond a perception of their being rated as influential (Thomas & Hrebnar, 2004). State- and local-level case studies to flesh out the contentions made by political economists about policy elites also could provide fresh insights about this framework/interpretive theory.

Research on aging interest groups also requires more attention. Similar to case studies of policy entrepreneurs (Kingdon, 1995), we need more examples of successful and less successful actions that would enhance knowledge about the reality of "senior power." One example might be how aging interest groups use the courts, either as initiators of lawsuits or as supporters through filing amicus curiae briefs. Much has been written about the need to build coalitions (Day, 1990; Torres-Gil, 1992), but gerontological inquiry has not examined the kinds of coalitions entered into by advocates for the aged or ways to measure their success (Hula, 1999). For example, what are the long-range implications of events such as the repeal of the Medicare Catastrophic Care Act or the enactment of the Medicare Modernization Act on the solidarity among the aging advocacy groups?

Additionally, cross-national comparisons of aging interest groups need to be examined in several ways: the extent to which the American model of interest group theory fits other countries, especially in non-Western democracies. Because population aging is a global phenomenon, this research also should address the extent to which aging interest groups in other countries, especially in developing nations such as India, follow the same developmental paths experienced by their American counterparts (for an appraisal, see Nayar, 2003). Studies of this kind would help us better understand the roles played by and the impact of the elderly on the policy process in America and elsewhere.

Institutional policy making deserves far greater emphasis, whether documenting the impact over time of different White House Conferences or the roles played by special committees in state legislatures (e.g., aging and long-term care), similar to their congressional counterparts. More case studies should be undertaken of the presidential-congressional interactions on various policies affecting the elderly (e.g., privatization of Social Security, Medicare Part D) to validate theories/models of such interactions (Kingdon, 1995). Additionally, the roles of administrative and regulatory agencies in policy making, implementation, and evaluation, especially at the state level, require greater attention. Of particular interest is the ability and capacity of state and local agencies on aging to absorb new programs (e.g., the National

Family Caregiver Support Program) mandated under each new reauthorization of the Older Americans Act. Who wins and who loses with each new iteration? Also warranting research are "best practice" models and concepts of bureaucratic policy making, specifically intergovernmental management (e.g., enforcing age discrimination laws and nursing home regulation) and the ability of public and private agencies to overcome fragmentation of aging services in keeping with interorganizational models of behavior. Gerontologists need to be more "self-conscious" about adding to theory in this area, not just describing what happens.

The roles of nonprofits and nongovernmental organizations in the developed and developing nations are yet another area warranting inquiry. Different value systems (e.g., laissez-faire economics) often propel these organizations to the forefront in delivering services to the elderly and aiding their families. Although most gerontologists tend to assume that nonprofits are better/safer service deliverers compared to for-profits because they are not motivated by making money, little is known about their differential impact on elders, even among nursing homes or hospitals. The role of nonprofits as innovators and diffusers of innovation is another area requiring more attention. The roles played by corporate America in meeting the challenges of an aging society also deserve inquiry, especially as suppliers to older consumers of basic needs such as housing and pharmaceuticals. And though much has been said about the value of faith-based organizations in solving or ameliorating problems posed by society, little research has been conducted on their relevance to the aged.

Similarly, gerontologists have focused on the practice of federalism but have rarely sought to enhance theory in this area. The reasons is that few geronologists conduct research in this area, despite the fact that states and their localities are increasingly called upon to meet the challenges of population aging in the United States. Studies on the aging policies of individual states have been undertaken; cross-state comparisons organized around the federal principle have been more rare in this country then others (e.g., Canada, Germany, and Australia). Additionally, more needs to be written about intergovernmental relations, especially in finance, service delivery, and reglation, and about "horizontal" federalism, the diffusion of innovative ideas and solutions to the needs of older persons from one state to others. Replication studies in aging have generally been conducted at the agency rather than the state level. Multistate demonstration programs of the type funded by the Robert Wood Johnson Foundation (e.g., supportive housing and long-term care insurance) needs to be evaluated for their long-term impact. Research on cross-national comparisons of the practice and theory of federalism in aging policy domains

(Pynoos & Liebig, 1995) also is needed to help us better understand our own system and to identify promising areas that might be adopted or adapted by the United States.

"Affordable aging" is not only an American conundrum. Other societies that are aging far more rapidly than the United States are also faced with the challenges of population aging. One dominant American response to this question, however, seems to be that demography is destiny and that we cannot easily afford the "burden" of today's elderly and certainly not tomorrow's. It is difficult to understand how the richest nation in the world that prides itself on its "can do" attitude cannot somehow meet the challenges posed by an aging society that involves not just "taking care" of elders, but also ensuring the productivity of future workers of all ages. Research and analysis need to focus on what mix of educational, immigration, and technological policies are required to improve productivity. Additionally, what public and private investments need to be made in infrastructure to strengthen economic development and productivity? Other nations, such as India in its National Policy on Older Persons, have focused on elders as productive members of society, rather than as dependents. What policies, beyond the few employment programs primarily for low-income elders, can be put in place to ensure/enhance that productivity? What types of economic policy instruments (Peters, 2004) can be used?

Additionally, the "affordability" of an aging society in America seems to be posed and answered as a public-sector budget issue, largely at the federal level. Yet many proposals to relieve the national budget look to the states, the private sector, and individuals. Reducing federal public outlays does not truly answer the question of how much aging we can afford or what the "true" costs of our aging society might be. For example, similar to "corporate welfare" policies, the roles played by federal, state, and local tax policies are not well understood among most professionals in the field nor by the general public. Better analysis and dissemination of those practices might reveal how much the costs, as well as the benefits, are spread across society and provide a basis for making difficult political decisions on how to distribute those costs and benefits.

A "Face Lift" for the Policy Sciences and Aging

Several emerging areas where aging and the policy sciences intersect merit examination; however, this chapter can only suggest a few that seem particularly important. It should be noted that these areas are not new in the policy sciences, but they are novel to those of us in the policy sciences and aging. Increasingly, the courts are engaged in interpreting/evaluating policies that affect the elderly, whether age-based policies such as age discrimination or age-related policies such as the right to die. Courts also oversee the activities of administrative agencies that affect older persons. Some areas, such as guardianship, have received attention, but in an ever-litigious society, gerontologists cannot afford to neglect this vital area of research, education, and advocacy. Those of us in academia perform an enormous disservice to the next generations of gerontologists by ignoring how court decisions affect the well-being and quality of life for many older adults.

Another area ripe for exploration is the domain of presidential power that has grown over the past decades. Presidents are major players in the policy process, as witness the *Presidential Studies Quarterly*. Although presidents are not always successful in achieving their policy goals, they often set the parameters of public debate. They have been major agenda setters (Kingdon, 1995) in primary policy areas (Social Security, Medicare, and Medicaid) and in less prominent policy domains, such as housing and SSI, that have lasting effects on elders' income and health care. In addition, presidents can be a major player in whether or not White House Conferences on Aging recommendations are implemented or ignored. Research is needed on presidents and their shaping of aging policy that adds to theories of presidential power and helps us to understand better how we get the aging policies we have.

In addition, the behavior and actions of agencies that provide programs and services to older persons, both nonprofits and governmental entities, are deserving of greater inquiry. How programs are implemented have implications for consumer satisfaction and policy makers' willingness to expand those programs. The links between resources and performance need greater scrutiny—another type of evidence-based outcomes. The roles of area agencies on aging and state units on aging, especially in their ability to broker and pool resources and to collaborate beyond informal mechanisms, merit attention, as does intergovernmental regulation in such areas as nursing home quality and age discrimination.

Similarly, because long-term care policy continues to be a central activity of the 50 states, studies should be undertaken on the why and how of policy formation, as well as the outcomes of policies after they are implemented. The roles of governors and state legislatures in creating aging policy deserve study, using the models of state policy making in the political science literature, several of which include economic factors (Gray & Hanson, 2004). Those models differ from the models that help explain how national laws are formulated (Kingdon, 1995). In particular, the diffusion of policy innovation across states warrants examination, because activity at the substantial level often gains prominence at the national level (Lammers, 1989). The role of dominance of different interest groups in state capitals in influencing policy outcomes also deserves attention as aging interest groups, particularly AARP, seek to have a greater impact.

A CAVEAT

These areas of research and similar inquiries, if undertaken, would help expand our understanding of aging policies substantially. However, they require a critical mass of researchers in aging who have been trained in these disciplines. Although the numbers of economists so trained have expanded over the last 10 to 15 years under National Institute on Aging training grants, few political scientists and a bare handful of public administration students have received fellowships. Similarly, elder law programs in the nation's law schools are limited, and multidisciplinary training programs characteristically lack a policy science emphasis. The small cadre of the earliest researchers in aging from the policy science disciplines are now in their late 50s, early 60s, and beyond, and the new PhD programs in aging, as well as long-established policy-oriented programs, such as those at Brandeis and Syracuse universities, are not providing an adequate supply of new manpower to undertake these crucial studies. Unless support can be found from other sources, such as foundations or other federal programs, the training of new investigators in the policy sciences and aging will fall even further behind. This is an issue worthy of being addressed by the major professional organizations in aging that have a major stake in research training.

A related issue is the relative lack of publication outlets for new and established policy scientists in aging. Only one journal in aging—the *Journal of Aging and Social Policy*—has a policy focus. Few of the other gerontological journals feature more than an occasional article dealing with the theory and practice of the policy sciences. Similarly, only a handful of other publications, such as newletters and special reports (e.g., GSA's *Public Policy and Aging Report,* analyses from the Center on Aging, and AAHSA's Institute for the Future of Aging Services) focus our attention on the policy sciences and their importance in the field of aging. Because policy issues and policies shape the possibilities for aging well, this situation needs to be rectified, if gerontologists are to exert sufficient influence on how America can meet the challenges of its aging society well into the rest of the 21st century.

REFERENCES

Aaron, H., Bosworth, B. P., & Burtless, G. (1989). *Can America afford to grow old?* Washington, DC: Brookings Institution.

Achenbaum, W. A. (1983). *Shades of gray: Old age, American values, and federal policies since the 1920s.* Boston: Little, Brown.

Andel, R., & Liebig, P. S. (2002). The city of Laguna Woods: A case of senior power in local politics. *Research on Aging, 24(1),* 87–105.

Anderson, J. E. (1979). *The study of public policy making.* New York: Holt, Rinehart and Winston.

Arnold, R. D., Graetz, M., & Munnell, A. (Eds.). (1998). *Framing the social security debate: Values, politics, and economics.* Washington, DC: Brookings Institution.

Auerbach, A. J., Gokhale, J., & Kotlikoff, L. J. (1992). Social security and Medicare from the perspective of generational accounting (Working paper 9206). Cleveland: Federal Reserve Bank of Cleveland.

Auerbach, A. J., & Kotlikoff, L. J. (1993). The impact of the demographic transition on capital formation. In A. M. Rappaport & S. J. Schieber (Eds.), *Demography and retirement: The twenty-first century.* Westport, CT: Praeger, 163–181.

Beard, C. A., & Beard, M. R. (1960). *The Beards' new basic history of the United States.* Garden City, NY: Doubleday.

Benjamin, A. E. (1986). State variations in home health expenditures and utilization under Medicare and Medicaid. *Home Health Care Services Quarterly, 7,* 5–28.

Berry, J. (1984). *The interest group society.* Boston: Little, Brown.

Binstock, R. H. (1972). Interest-group liberalism and the politics of aging. *The Gerontologist, 12,* 265–280.

Binstock, R. H. (1983). The aged as scapegoat. *The Gerontologist, 23,* 136–143.

Binstock, R. H. (2000). Older people and voting participation: Past and future. *The Gerontologist, 40,* 18–31.

Binstock, R. H. (2004). The prolonged old, the long-lived society, and the politics of age. *Public Policy and Aging Report, 14(2),* 1, 28–31.

Binstock, R. H., & Day, C. L. (1996). Aging and politics. In R. H. Binstock & L. K. George (Eds.), *Handbook of aging and the social sciences* (4th ed.). San Diego, CA: Academic Press, 362–387.

Binstock, R. H., & Quadagno, J. (2001). Aging and politics. In R. H. Binstock & L. K. George (Eds.), *Handbook of aging and the social sciences* (5th ed). San Diego, CA: Academic Press, 333–351.

Boswell, D. (2000, November). *Older citizens and the plan-making process.* Presentation at the Annual Conference of the Association of Collegiate Schools of Planning Atlanta, GA.

Bradley, D. B., Patch, M., & Gwyther, C. R. (2006). Factors that may limit the role of community philanthropy in developing nonprofit capacity. *Policy and Management Review.*

Brown, D. K. (1983). Administering aging programs in a federal system. In W. P. Browne & L. K. Olson (Eds.), *Aging and public policy*. Westport, CT: Greenwood Press, 201–229.

Burke, S., Kingson, E., & Reinhardt, U. (2000). *Social security and Medicare: Individual versus collective risk and responsibility*. Washington, DC: Brookings Institution.

Cain, L. (1975). The young and the old: Coalition or conflict ahead? *American Behavioral Scientist, 19*, 166–175.

Calasanti, T. M., & Slevin, K. R. (2001). *Gender, social inequalities, and aging*. Walnut Creek, CA: Altamira Press.

Caldeira, G. A., & Wright, J. R. (1988). Interest groups and agenda setting in the Supreme Court. *American Political Science Review, 82*, 1109–1127.

Callahan, D. (1987). *Setting limits: Medical goals in an aging society*. New York: Simon & Schuster.

Campbell, A. (1971). Politics through the lifecycle. *The Gerontologist, 11*, 112–117.

Campbell, A. L. (2003). *How policies make citizens: Senior political activism and the American welfare state*. Princeton, NJ: Princeton University Press.

Campbell, J. C., & Strate, J. M. (1981). Are old people conservative? *The Gerontologist, 21*, 580–591.

Caro, F. G., & Morris, R. (2002). Devolution and aging policy. *Journal of Aging & Social Policy, 14*(3/4), 1–14.

Clark, R. L., Burkhauser, R. V., Moon, M., Quinn, J. F., & Smeeding, T. (2004). *The economics of an aging society*. Malden, MA: Blackwell Publishing.

Cook, F. L., Marshall, D., Marshall, J., & Kauffman, J. (1994). The salience of intergenerational equity in Canada and the United States. In T. R. Marmor, T. M. Smeeding, & V. L. Greene (Eds.), *Economic security and intergenerational justice: A look at North America*. Washington, DC: Urban Institute Press.

Cronin, T. (1989). *Direct democracy*. Cambridge, MA: Harvard University Press.

Crown, W. H. (1989). Trends in the economic status of the aged and implications for state policy. *Journal of Aging & Social Policy, 1*(3/4), 89–128.

Crown, W. H. (2001). Economic status of the elderly. In R. H. Binstock & L. K. George (Eds.), *Handbook of aging and the social sciences*. San Diego, CA: Academic Press.

Cutler, N. E. (1977). Demographic, social-psychological, and political factors in the politics of aging: A foundation for research in "political gerontology." *American Political Science Review, 71*, 1011–1025.

Cutler, N. E. (1984). Federal and state responsibilities and the targeting of resources under the Older Americans Act. *Policy Studies Journal, 13*(1), 185–196.

Cutler, N. E., & Gregg, D. W. (1990). Financial gerontology and the middle-aging of populations around the world. Presentation at the annual meeting of the Gerontological Society of America, Boston.

Day, C. L. (1990). *What older Americans think: Interest groups and aging policy*. Princeton, NJ: Princeton University Press.

Dobson, D. (1983). The elderly as a political force. In W. P. Browne & L. K. Olson (Eds.), *Aging and public policy: The politics of growing old in America.* Westport, CT: Greenwood, 123–144.

Doig, J. W., & Hargrove, E. C. (Eds.). (1987). *Leadership and innovation: A biographical perspective on entrepreneurs in government.* Baltimore: Johns Hopkins University Press.

Easterlin, R. A. (1996). Economic and social implications of demographic patterns. In R. H. Binstock & L. K. George (Eds.), *Handbook of aging and the social sciences* (4th ed.). San Diego, CA: Academic Press, 73–93.

Easterlin, R. A., MacDonald, C., & Macunovich, D. (1990). Retirement prospects of the baby boom generation: A different perspective. *The Gerontologist, 30,* 776–783.

Estes, C. L. (1979). *The aging enterprise.* San Francisco: Jossey-Bass.

Estes, C. L., & Gerard, L. (1983). Government responsibility: Issue of reform and federalism. In C. L. Estes & R. J. Newcomer (Eds.), *Fiscal austerity and aging.* Beverly Hills, CA: Sage, 41–58.

Estes, C. L., Linkins, K. W., & Binney, E. A. (1996). The political economy of aging. In R. H. Binstock & L. K. George (Eds.), *Handbook of aging and the social sciences* (4th ed.). San Diego, CA: Academic Press, 346–361.

Feldstein, M. (1975). Toward a reform of social security. *Public Interest, 40,* 75–95.

Foner, A. (1974). Age stratification and age conflict in political life. *American Sociological Review, 39,* 187–196.

Gais, T., Peterson, M., & Walker, J. L. (1984). Interest groups, iron triangles, and representative institutions in American national government. *British Journal of Political Science, 14,* 161–185.

Gist, J. (1992). Did tax reform hurt the elderly? *The Gerontologist, 32,* 472–477.

Glenn, N. D., & Grimes, M. (1968). Aging, voting, and political interest. *American Sociological Review, 33,* 563–575.

Glick, H. G. (1994). The U.S. Supreme Court and the right to die. *Political Research Quarterly 47*(2), 207–222.

Gokhale, S. D. (2003). Towards a policy for aging in India. In P. S. Liebig & S. I. Rajan (Eds.), *An aging India: Perspectives, prospects, and policies.* New York: Haworth Press.

Gray, V., & Hanson, R. L. (Eds.). (2004). *Politics in the American states* (8th ed.). Washington, DC: CQ Press.

Harrington, C., Mullan, J., & Carrillo, H. State nursing enforcement systems. *Journal of Health, Politics, Policy and Law, 29,* 43–74.

Heclo, H. (1988). Generational politics. In J. Palmer, T. M. Smeeding, & B. Torrey (Eds.), *The vulnerable.* Washington, DC: Urban Institute Press, 381–411.

Holahan, J., Weil, A., & Wiener, J. M. (Eds.). (2003). *Federalism and health policy.* Washington, DC: Urban Institute Press.

Holt, B. J. (1994). Targeting in federal grant programs: The case of the Older Americans Act. *Public Administration Review, 54*(5), 444–449.

Howard, C. (1997). *The hidden welfare state: Tax expenditures and social policy in the United States*. Princeton, NJ: Princeton University Press.

Howe, N. (1997). Why the graying of the welfare state threatens to flatten the American dream–or worse. In R. B. Hudson (Ed.), *The future of age-based public policy*. Baltimore: Johns Hopkins University Press.

Hudson, R. B. (1978). The "graying" of the federal budget and its consequences for old age policy. *The Gerontologist, 18,* 428–440.

Hudson, R. B. (1986). Capacity building in an intergovernmental context: The case of the aging network. In B. W. Honadle & A. M. Howitt (Eds.), *Perspectives on management capacity building*. Albany, NY: SUNY Press, 312–333.

Hudson, R. B. (1988). Politics and the new old. In R. Morris & S. A. Bass (Eds.), *Retirement reconsidered: Economic and social roles for older persons*. New York: Springer, 59–70.

Hudson, R. B. (1995). The history and place of age-based public policy. *Generations, 19*(3), 5–10.

Hudson, R. B. (1997). The history and place of age-based policy. In R. H. Hudson (Ed.), *The future of age-based policy*. Baltimore: Johns Hopkins University Press, 1–22.

Hudson, R. B., & Strate, J. M. (1985). Aging and political systems. In R .H. Binstock & E. Shanas (Eds.), *Handbook of aging and the social sciences* (2nd ed.). New York: Van Nostrand Reinhold, 554–585.

Hula, K. V. (1999). *Lobbying together: Interest group coalitions*. Washington, DC: Georgetown University Press.

Humphries, M., & Songer, D. (1999). Law and politics in judicial oversight of federal administrative agencies. *Journal of Politics, 61,* 202–220.

Kane, R. L. (1998). Variation in state spending for long-term care: Factors associated with more balanced systems. *Journal of Health Politics, Policy and Law, 23*(2), 363–390.

Kapp, M. B. (1996). Aging and the law. In R. H. Binstock & L. K. George (Eds.), *Handbook of aging and the social sciences* (4th ed). San Diego, CA: Academic Press, 467–480.

Kelly, C. (2004). *The extent and effectiveness of nursing home regulation in the 50 states.* Unpublished dissertation, University of Southern California, Los Angeles.

Kernell. S. (1993). *Going public* (2nd ed.). Washington, DC: CQ Press.

Kiesel, K. (2002). Strengthening state tax credit programs in Massachusetts. *Journal of Aging & Social Policy, 14*(3/4), 141–160.

Kingdon, J. W. (1995). *Agendas, alternatives, and public policies* (2nd ed.). New York: HarperCollins.

Kingson, E. R., Hirshorn, B. A., & Cornman, J. M. (1986). *The ties that bind: The interdependence of generations*. Washington, DC: Seven Locks Press.

Lamm, R. (1999). Care for the elderly: What about our children? In J. B. Williamson, D. M. Watts-Roy, & E. R. Kingson (Eds.), *The generational equity debate*. New York: Columbia University Press, 87–100.

Lammers, W. W. (1983). *Public policy and aging.* Washington, DC: CQ Press.

Lammers, W. W. (1989). Prospects for innovation in state policies for the elderly. *Journal of Aging & Social Policy, 1*(3/4), 37–66.

Lammers, W. W., & Klingman, D. (1984). *State policies and the aging: Sources, trends, and options.* Lexington, MA: DC Heath.

Lammers, W. W., & Liebig, P. S. (1990). State health policies, federalism, and the elderly. *Publius: The Journal of Federalism, 20*(3), 131–148.

Lasswell, H. D. (1936). *Politics: Who gets what, when, how.* New York: McGraw-Hill.

Liebig, P. S. (1983). *Extent of disclosure by the public employee retirement systems (PERS) of the states.* Unpublished dissertation, University of Southern California, Los Angeles.

Liebig, P. S. (1992). Federalism and aging policy in the 1980s: Implications for changing interest group roles in the 1990s. *Journal of Aging and Social Policy, 4*(1/2), 17–33.

Liebig, P. S. (1994a). Decentralization, aging policy, and the age of Clinton. *Journal of Aging & Social Policy 6*(1/2), 9–26.

Liebig, P. S. (1994b). The aging coalition, advocacy, and health care reform. Presentation at the annual meeting of the Gerontological Society of America, Atlanta, GA.

Liebig, P. S. (1996). Housing for the elderly: Intragenerational issues and perspectives. In J. Steckenrider & T. M. Parrott (Eds.), *The new aging policy.* Albany, NY: SUNY Press.

Liebig, P. S. (in press). Tax policy. In R. Schultz (Ed.), *The encyclopedia of aging* (4th ed.). New York: Springer, 51–71.

Light, P. C. (1991). *The president's agenda.* Baltimore: Johns Hopkins University Press.

Lowi, T. (1992). Lowi and Simon on political science, public administration, rationality, and public choice. *Journal of Public Administration Research and Theory, 2*(2), 105–112.

Mackey, S., & Carter, K. (1994). *State tax policy and senior citizens* (2nd ed.). Denver: National Conference of State Legislatures.

Marshall, V. W. (1996). The state of theory on aging and the social sciences. In R. H. Binstock & L. K. George (Eds.), *Handbook of aging and the social sciences* (4th ed.). San Diego, CA: Academic Press.

McManus, S. A. (1996). *Young vs. old: Generational combat in the 21st century.* Boulder, CO: Westview.

Meier, K. (1993). *Politics and the bureaucracy* (3rd ed). New York: Harcourt Brace.

Meiners, M. R., McKay, H. L., & Mahoney, K. J. (2002). Partnership insurance: An innovation to meet long-term care financing needs in an era of federal minimalism. *Journal of Aging & Social Policy, 14*(3/4), 75–94.

Miller, E. A. (2002). State discretion and Medicaid program variation. *Journal of Aging & Social Policy, 14*(3/4), 15–36.

Minkler, M., & Estes, C. L. (Eds.). (1984). *Readings in the political economy of aging.* Amityville, NY: Baywood.

Minkler, M., & Estes, C. L. (Eds.). (1991). *Critical perspectives on aging: The political and moral economy of growing old.* Amityville, NY: Baywood.

Moon, M., & Mulvey, J. (1996). *Entitlements and the elderly.* Washington, DC: The Urban Institute Press.

Morris, C. R. (1996). *The AARP: America's most powerful lobby and the clash of generations.* New York: Times Books.

Myers, G. C. (1996). Aging and the social sciences: Research directions and unresolved issues. In R. H. Binstock & L. K. George (Eds.), *Handbook of aging and the social sciences* (4th ed.). San Diego, CA: Academic Press, 1–11.

Myrtle, R., & Wilber, K. (1994). Designing service delivery systems: Lessons from the development of community-based systems of care for the elderly. *Public Administration Review 54*(3), 245–252.

Nathan, R. P. (1990). Federalism: The great "composition." In A. King (Ed.), *The new American political system* (2nd ed.). Washington, DC: AEI Press, 231–261.

Nayar, P. K. B. (2003). Senior grassroots organizations in India. In P. S. Liebig & S. I. Rajan (Eds.), *An aging India: Perspectives, prospects, and policies.* New York: Haworth Press, 193–212.

Nie, N. H., & Verba, S. (1974). Political participation and the life cycle. *Comparative Politics, 6,* 319–341.

O'Leary, R., & Wise, C. (1991). Public managers, judges and legislators: Redefining the "new partnership." *Public Administration Review, 51,* 316–327.

Osborne, D., & Plastrik, P. (1997). *Banishing bureaucracy: The five strategies for reinventing government.* Reading, MA: Addison-Wesley Press.

Pampel, F. C. (1998). *Aging, social inequality, and public policy.* Thousand Oaks, CA: Pine Forge.

Pandey, S. K. (2002). Assessing state efforts to meet baby boomers' long-term care needs: A case study of compensatory federalism. *Journal of Aging & Social Policy, 14*(3/4), 161–180.

Peirce, N. R., & Chohari, P. C. (1982). The old as a political force—26 million and well-organized. *National Journal, 14,* 1559–1562.

Peters, B. G. (2004). *American public policy: Promise and performance* (6th ed.). Washington, DC: CQ Press.

Pinner, F. A., Jacob, P., & Selznick, P. (1959). *Old age and political behavior.* Berkeley, CA: University of California Press.

Piven, F. F., & Cloward, R. A. (1971). *Regulating the poor: The functions of public welfare.* New York: Vintage Books.

Pratt, H. J. (1976). *The gray lobby: Politics of old age.* Chicago: The University of Chicago Press.

Pratt, H. J. (1978, July–August). Symbolic politics and White House conferences on the elderly. *Society,* 67–72.

Pratt, H. J. (1993). *Gray agendas: Interest groups and public pensions in Canada, Britain, and the United States.* Ann Arbor: University of Michigan Press.

Pratt, H. J. (1997). Do the elderly really have political clout? In A. Scharlach & L. Kaye (Eds.), *Controversial issues in aging.* Boston: Allyn & Bacon, 81–91.

Price, M. C. (1997). *Justice between generations: The growing power of the elderly in America*. Westport, CT: Praeger.

Putnam, R. (1995). Tuning in, tuning out: The strange disappearance of social capital in America. *PS: Political Science and Politics, 28*(4), 664–683.

Pynoos, J. (1984). Setting the elderly housing agenda. *Policy Studies Journal, 13*(1), 173–184.

Pynoos, J. (1999). *Increasing housing options for frail older people: State roles and strategies*. San Francisco: American Society on Aging.

Pynoos, J., Liebig, P. S., Alley, D., & Nishita, C. (2004). Homes of choice: Towards more effective linkages between housing and services. *Journal of Housing for the Elderly, 18*(3/4), 5–49.

Reschovsky, A. (1989). State and local taxation of the elderly. *Journal of Aging & Social Policy, 1*(3/4), 143–170.

Rose, A. M. (1965). Group consciousness among the aging. In A. M. Rose & W. Peterson (Eds.), *Older people and their social world*. Philadelphia: Davis, 19–36.

Rosenbaum, W. A., & Button, J. W. (1989). Is there a gray peril? Retirement politics in Florida. *The Gerontologist, 29*, 300–306.

Rosenbaum, W. A., & Button, J. W. (1992). Perceptions of intergenerational conflict: The politics of young vs. old. *Journal of Aging Studies, 6*, 385–396.

Salisbury, R. H. (1990). The paradox of interest groups in Washington—more groups, less clout. In A. King (Ed.), *The new American political system*. Washington, DC: AEI Press, 203–229.

Samuelson, R. J. (1978, February 18). Busting the U.S. budget: The costs of an aging society. *National Journal*, pp. 256–260.

Samuelson, R. J. (1990, November 21). Pampering the elderly. *Washington Post*, p. A19.

Scharlach, A., & Kaye, L. (Eds.). (1997). *Controversial issues in aging*. Boston: Allyn & Bacon.

Schulz, J. H. (1996). Economic security policies. In R. H. Binstock & L. K. George (Eds.), *Handbook of aging and the social sciences* (4th ed). San Diego, CA: Academic Press, 410–426.

Sheets, D. J., Liebig, P. S., & Campbell, M. (2002). State rehabilitation agencies, aging with disability, and technology: Policy issues and implications. *Journal of Disability Policy Studies 12*(4), 243–252.

Silverstein, M., Parrott, T. M., Angelelli, J. J., & Cook, F. L. (2000). Solidarity and tension between age-groups in the United States: Challenge for an aging America in the 21st century. *International Journal of Social Welfare, 9*, 270–284

Shrewsbury, C. M. (2002). Information technology issues in an era of greater state responsibilities: Policy concerns for seniors. *Journal of Aging & Social Policy 14*(3/4), 195–210.

Smeeding, T. M. (1990). The economic status of the elderly. In R. H. Binstock & L. K. George (Eds.), *Handbook of aging and the social sciences* (3rd ed.) San Diego, CA: Academic Press, 362–381.

Smith, D. G. (2002). *Entitlement politics: Medicare and Medicaid, 1995–2001.* New York: Aldine de Gruyter.

Smith, G. P., III. (1996). *Legal and health care ethics for the elderly.* Washington, DC: Taylor & Francis.

Songer, D. R., & Sheehan. R. G. (1993). Interest group success in the courts. *Political Research Quarterly, 46*(2), 339–354.

Steckenrider, J., & Parrott, T. M. (Eds.) (1996). *The new aging policy.* Albany, NY: SUNY Press.

Thomas, D. S., & Hrebnar, R. J. (2004). Interest groups in the states. In V. Gray & R L. Hanson (Eds.), *Politics in the American states* (8th ed.). Washington, DC: CQ Press, 120–128.

Thompson, F. J., & DiIulio, J. J. (Eds.). (1998). *Medicaid and devolution: A view from the states.* Washington, DC: Brookings Institution.

Thompson, L., & Elling, R. (1999). Let them eat marblecake: Devolution and intergovernmental service provision. *Publius: The Journal of Federalism, 29*(1), 139–154.

Torres-Gil, F. M. (1992). *The new aging: Politics and change in America.* New York: Auburn House.

Torres-Gil, F. M., & Pynoos, J. (1986). Long-term care policy and interest group struggles. *The Gerontologist, 26*(5), 488–495.

Unah, I. (1996). The Supreme Court's institutional stature and role in public policy making. *Policy Studies Journal, 24*(4), 679–685.

Van Tassel, D. D., & Meyer, J. E. W. (Eds.). (1992). *U.S. aging policy interest groups.* New York: Greenwood.

Verba, S., & Nie, N. H. (1974). *Participation in America.* New York: Harper & Row.

Vinyard, D. (1972). The Senate Special Committee on Aging. *The Gerontologist, 12*(1), 298–303.

Vinyard, D. (1979). White House conferences and the aged. *Social Service Review, 53,* 655–671.

Vinyard, D. (1982). Public policy and institutional politics. In Browne, W. P., & Olson, L. K. (Eds.), *Aging and public policy.* Westport, CT: Greenwood Press, 181–199.

Vladeck, B. (1999). The political economy of medicare. *Health Affairs, 18*(1), 22–36.

Walker, A. (1993). Intergenerational relations and welfare restructuring: The social construction of an intergenerational problem. In V. L. Bengtson & A. Achenbaum (Eds.), *The changing contract across generations, 141–165.*

Walker, J. L. (1969). The diffusion of innovation among the American states. *American Political Science Review, 63,* 880–899.

Walker, J. L. (1983). The origins and maintenance of interest groups in America. *American Political Science Review, 77,* 390–406.

Wallace, S. P., Williamson, J. B., Lung, R. G., & Powell, L. A. (1991). A lamb in wolf's clothing? The reality of senior power and social policy. In M. Minkler &

C. L. Estes (Eds.), *Critical perspectives on aging: The political and moral economy of growing old.* Amityville, NY: Baywood, 95–114.

Wallace, S. P., & Williamson, J. B. (1992). *The senior movement: Reference and resources.* New York: G. K. Hall.

Weisbrod, B. (1997). The future of the nonprofit sector. *Journal of Policy and Management, 16*(4), 541–555.

Wiener, J. M., & Stevenson, D. G. (1998). State policy on long-term care for the elderly. *Health Affairs, 17*(3), 81–100.

Williamson, J. B. (1998). Political activism and aging of the baby boom. *Generations, 22*(1), 5–59.

Wilson, J. Q. (1989). *Bureaucracy.* New York: Basic Books.

Wise, C. (1998). Judicial federalism: The resurgence of the Supreme Court's role in the protection of state sovereignty. *Public Administration Review, 58*(2), 95–98.

Wisensale, S. (1988). Generational equity and intergenerational politics. *The Gerontologist, 28*(6), 773–778.

Wisensale, S. (1996). The White House and Congress on family leave policy: From Carter to Clinton. *Policy Studies Journal, 25*(1), 75–86.

Zimmerman, J. (1991). *Federal preemption.* Ames: University of Iowa Press.

EPILOGUE

Gerontology—Past, Present, and Future

James E. Birren

The study of aging is one of the most complex and important subjects facing science in the 21st century. It has implications for individuals, societies, and the professions that serve them. Despite its broad significance, gerontology as field of study did not exist 100 years ago. Although mankind has always speculated about longevity and death, the term *gerontology* was first proposed in 1903 by a biologist, Eli Metchnikoff, who was a professor at the Pasteur Institute in Paris. Gerontology evolved into an area of academic focus after 1950. Gruman (2003) reviews the history of prescientific concepts and beliefs about aging in detail. See also Achenbaum (1979, 1989) for more recent historical commentary.

During the second half of the 20th century, much has changed in the way we think about how we mature and become old. For example, the term "agequake" has been used more frequently to refer to the implications of the relatively recent changes in the demography of countries and the lengthening of life expectancy. It is quite possible that the anticipated agequake has encouraged the study of aging and it implications. Since the first meeting of the Gerontological Society of America was held in New York in February 1948, many changes have occurred in how we define and investigate questions related to aging. What follows is my view about the past, present, and future of gerontology from the vantage point of a researcher who presented research at the first meeting of the Gerontological Society of America and participated in the evolution of the field in the 20th century,

THE PAST

What follows is a brief description of the societal context in which the subject of gerontology emerged. In 1900 the United States was an agricultural country. Forty-seven percent of the labor force was employed in agriculture. Life expectancy at birth was about 46 years. Families on farms were large because children and older adults were useful for doing the many tasks in farm life. A man could cut a half acre of grain with a sickle or a full acre with a scythe. Then the steam engine came into use, and horses and human labor were replaced in plowing, reaping, and threshing. A steam engine reaper could cut 100 acres of grain in a day. Manpower on the farm was replaced, until today barely 2% to 3% of the labor force works in agriculture. Today the largest portion of the labor force is in the services industry.

What happened to the vast farm labor? It moved to cities to make steam engines and soon after, gasoline-powered cars. In the city, housing was more crowded and more expensive. Children and older adults were less useful for doing chores in city households than they had been on farms. Families became much smaller. More recently, society has moved from the industrial age into the information age, in which computers and robotics are reducing the need for manpower.

Gerontology in the First Half of the 20th Century

At the beginning of the 20th century, society was focused more on children, medicine on infectious diseases. In 1947 I was told by a professor of pediatrics at Johns Hopkins University that pediatrics emerged as a specialty in the early part of the 20th century when physicians in general practice realized that they were having common problems in advising parents about child feeding. Pediatric medicine has evolved into a contemporary profession with an impressive research base. The point is that the origins of professions and science can arise from the social pressures of very practical circumstances. This includes the emergence of gerontology, *geriatrics,* and the care and study of aging persons, in response to demographic change in the age structure of society.

A shift occurred in the study of aging in the late 1930s, when the population was beginning to have longer life expectancy. Chronic diseases associated with mid- and late life were beginning to receive attention in treatment and research, such as heart disease, cancers, and arthritis. During the earlier 20th century, when infectious diseases dominated public health efforts, the human organism was regarded as invaded by foreign agents, bacteria, and viruses. The invading agent had to be identified, and medical war had to be focused on the invader. In chronic diseases, however, the vulnerability of the host organisms contributed significantly to the onset and course of the diseases. The shift from the dominant focus on the infectious diseases to chronic diseases required a large reorientation of both medicine and basic research by requiring the development of a focus on the vulnerability of the host of the chronic disease and the contribution of social and behavior influences (Schroots, Birren, & Svanborg, 1988).

The first major step in reorienting scientists' views on aging was stimulated by a 1933 review of arteriosclerosis published by the Josiah Macy Jr. Foundation (Cowdry, 1933). That report summarized the findings of a small group of investigators who maintained that the processes related to aging were influencing the development of arterial disease. Today it is commonly accepted that an individual's diet, exercise, and behavior, along with stress, can contribute to the onset and course of the disease. That was a major shift in the paradigm of aging.

The emerging view of multiple causes of chronic diseases prompted the Josiah Macy Jr. Foundation to sponsor a conference on aging in 1937 at Woods Hole, Massachusetts. The findings of this multidisciplinary conference on aging were published as the groundbreaking book *Problems of Ageing* (1939), edited by E. V. Cowdry. The conference and the resulting publication had a strong effect in defining the problems of aging and encouraging research. Perhaps more importantly, the result was a multidisciplinary perspective on the processes of aging that has, fortunately, carried forward to this day. The behavioral and social sciences were included, along with biology and medicine, as relevant to the study of factors contributing to chronic diseases and to the processes of aging. This perspective has not been easy to adopt, and there was slow acceptance to the idea that environmental conditions influenced the course of aging.

Encouraging to a multifactorial, or ecological, view of aging was the National Health Survey of 1935–1936. During the Great Depression years, the Works Progress Administration provided funds to the U.S. Public Health Service to make a house-to-house canvas of health issues in 500,000 families, some 2.8 million persons in 84 cities and 223 rural areas in 19 states. Many reports were generated from the survey data. One important finding was the relationship between illness and unemployment. Unemployed workers were twice as likely to be disabled by illness on the day of the survey. It is interesting to read the conclusion of one of the reports these many years later that hint at the complex nature of disease, social and economic relationships, and aging:

It is impossible to escape the conclusion that because of the serious nature of the conditions from which they are suffering, many of those persons who reported they were seeking work will actually never be able to work again. It is also true that whether these diseases are cause or effect of being without a job, they tend to be concentrated among the unemployed and among those in the laboring classes, who are largely unable to obtain the adequate care necessary to promote recovery or to arrest the inroads of disease. (U. S. Public Health Service, 1938a, p. 11)

Another report indicated that pneumonia was twice as high in the lower economic group, those "on relief," as in the high-income group (U.S. Public Health Service, 1938b). Here was the emergence of evidence that health was, to a large degree, related to socioeconomic status. Apparently it takes a long time to assimilate evidence that runs contrary to the accepted paradigms of explanation of the time period. The growth of gerontology as a field of study was encouraged by a spreading recognition that health and illness are influenced by environmental and individual factors. In this regards, the researchers and scholars assembled by the Josiah Macy Jr. Foundation in the late 1930s stimulated the emergence of gerontology.

A further step in encouraging gerontology was taken in 1940 by Thomas Perron, Jr., Surgeon General of the U.S. Public Health Service. He appointed a National Advisory Committee to assist the newly formed Unit on Gerontology of the National Institute of Health (U.S. Public Health Service, 1943). Presumably, this was the first research unit of gerontology created in America and reflects the influence of the Josiah Macy Jr. Foundation. It is of interest that gerontology was encouraged by a group of researchers with a multidisciplinary view of health and aging. Behind this development appears to be the motivation that was created by the rising practical implications of chronic diseases and aging.

Another step to explore the issues of aging was taken in 1941. A conference on "Mental Health in Later Maturity" was held in Washington, DC, sponsored by the U.S. Public Health Service. The Surgeon General of the Public Health Service, Thomas Parran, in his address noted:

Because the effective control of the communicable and infective diseases of infancy and youth has permitted the survival of a greater proportion of the population than formerly, the disorders of later maturity take on greatly increased significance. . . . However, in order to solve the urgent clinical and sociologic problems introduced by the greatly increased numbers of older people in the country, we need to know more of the processes and the consequences of aging. (U.S. Public Health Service, 1943, p. 1)

The Assistant Surgeon General, Lawrence Kolb, in his address on the psychiatric significance of aging as a public health problem, said, "Extensive research is needed into all types of mental disease," (U.S. Public Health Service, 1943, p. 17). Anticipating what much later studies would show, he remarked that, "A change in social and cultural patterns that would cause people to live less intensely probably would have some effect on cerebral arteriosclerosis and mental disease" (p. 17).

Winfred Overholser presented the orientation to the conference. He pointed out that the U.S. Bureau of the Census reported a growth in the older population, and added, "These facts have directed the attention not only of sociologists, insurance executives, and public welfare officials, but that of physicians and psychologists as well, toward a closer and more serious study of the various problems incident to later life" (U.S. Public Health Service, 1943, p. 3). He also gave his perspective that would be widely accepted today:

> Aging is a process which begins at birth, and progresses with varying rates of rapidity both as regards the individual and his several parts. Some persons are old at 45, others young at 70. Furthermore, one organ or organ system may age prematurely (as the heart, arteries, or kidneys), whereas others maintain excellent function into much later years. Too much stress has been laid upon chronological age, whereas physiologic and psychological age are far more important. (p. 4)

The 1941 Mental Health Conference prompted research on the psychological and social aspects of aging, along with the medical and biological. The conference gives further evidence of the impact of a changing demography on the thinking about aging leading to the emergence of gerontology as a field of study. Unfortunately, World War II erupted about 6 months after the conference was held and before the conference proceedings were published. This led to a protracted gap in follow-up of the ideas expressed at the conference, and they were not published until 1943 (U.S. Public Health Service, 1943).

One common public and professional view of the 20th century was that ill older persons should rest. This was derived from the experience that people with acute infectious diseases benefited from bed rest. Unfortunately, the "use it and lose it" principle was applied to chronic diseases as well. Persons with heart attacks were put to bed and told to take it easy. In recent years, the principle of "use it and lose it" has been replaced by "use it or lose it." Physical activity has come to be regarded as a desirable component of staying well and treating many chronic illnesses (Schroots et al., 1988).

After World War II, the focus of medicine and public health shifted to chronic diseases away from infectious diseases, whose mortality rates were being dramatically reduced by the introduction of penicillin and other antibiotics. The Gerontological Society of America and the American Geriatrics Society were founded, followed by the Western Gerontological Society, which later became the American Society on Aging.

The emergence of studies of aging is apparent in the volume of research articles published. For example, in the field of the psychology of aging, there were more published research articles in the 1950s than in the previous 100 years (Riegel, 1977). Since the 1950s the number of psychologists specialized in the study of aging has increased at a faster rate than did the number in psychology as a whole.

The publication of books in gerontology was slower than the growth of research articles, the latter being encouraged by the creation of new journals. Apparently book publishers did not recognize the emergence of the need for books about aging, in contrast with the longer established area of child development. The *Handbook of Aging and the Individual* (Birren, 1959) was published in 1959 only after protracted discussions with numerous publishers who shied away from publishing in the field of aging. The first printing by The University of Chicago Press was sold out in 6 months. Now there are publishers that specialize in books and journals about aging. Publishers, businesses, professionals, and institutions have difficulty in estimating the significance of emerging themes and issues, such as those of aging, resulting in lag effects in public and professional knowledge.

An example of one of the ideas that restricted somewhat the growth of research on the behavioral aspects of aging was psychoanalysis. Its founder, Sigmund Freud, held that the basic character of the individual was laid down in the first few years of life. At the National Institute of Mental Health in the 1950s, there was resistance to expanding research on aging. This was a mind-set of reasonable, well-educated leadership, that is, that the study of aging was considerably less important than the study of early life development. This mind-set also delayed the introduction of treatments of mental illnesses with medications because the view was held that the most appropriate treatment was with psychotherapy with an emphasis on psychoanalysis. Was the increase in emphasis on the study of aging due to discovery, insight, or the influence of major changes in the nation's demography? A major influence was the demographic change toward an increasingly older population, but also an emergence of the view of multifactorial causes of the conditions of human life. The paradigms of yesterday are slow to yield to emerging evidence, in the sciences, professions, institutions, and culture (Kenyon, Birren,

& Schroots, 1991). This is relevant to the idea of the impending "agequake" and the extent to which it can be anticipated.

Before the start of the development of the program in gerontology at the University of Southern California in 1965, there was not a single university in California that had courses on aging or had graduate students doing research. Professional schools such as social work, law, education, and public health had no teaching related to aging, nor did any of the disciplines such as biology, sociology, and psychology have specialized teaching and research. In 1965 there wasn't a single medical school with a program of teaching and research on geriatrics and problems of aging.

The activities of the Josiah Macy Jr. Foundation and those of the U.S. Public Health Service were providing leadership before the academic institutions. It would appear that the academic paradigms of the era did not include questions about aging and the life span. Despite the general academic lack of interest in studies of aging, several areas of interest were forming by the 1960s. The literature of this era of research on the biological, behavior, and social aspects of aging has been well reviewed (Binstock & Shanas, 1977; Birren & Schaie, 1977; Finch & Hayflick, 1977), and these efforts seeded gerontology as we know it today.

GERONTOLOGY IN THE PRESENT

In the latter part of the 20th century, public pressures were developing from the rise in the number of older persons. Questions were beginning to be raised in Congress and other public arenas about meeting the needs of an aging population. In 1975 Congress approved the creation of the National Institute on Aging. The body was responding to the rising social pressures of an older society. More funds became available for research on aging. Also, fellowships and training grants became part of the national educational scene.

In recent years the growth of the private sector's interest in aging has interacted with universities. As retirement communities, assisted living facilities, and nursing homes have grown, many positions have been created for staff members educated in background knowledge and skills relevant to serving older persons. Currently California has about 3.5 million persons over the age of 65 and this is expected to double to 7 millon. This will increase to 7 million in approximately 25 years. The demand for qualified staff in the business sector, with training based on solid research, will put increasing pressure on universities to provide such relevant training.

There will also be a parallel increase in the need for research that offers pathways to reducing late-life disabilities and illness (Redfoot & Pandya,

2002). The other side of this is an increased need for providing educational and personal growth for retirees. As the population has been growing older, it has also been growing healthier and more active. A community survey I was involved with in 1992 found that there were more elderly persons who wanted to add new experiences to their lives than required personal services. This clashed with the contemporary view that older persons were essentially dependent. The study contrasted the group of "needers" who required services with those we called the "growers," those persons interested in new learning, such as computer use, taking general university courses, and getting involved in the Elderhostel program. Obviously, the older population is diverse, with many clusters of individuals with quite different needs and wants.

The growth of the older population has been referred to as an "agequake" because it will shake up nations and institutions whose cultures and practices are based on out-of-date models and stereotypes. We are growing older in a changing society that in many ways appears to be increasingly impersonal. It might be said that we are living in an impersonal age in which economic efficiency has nudged out personal contact. Both the development of online banking to handle all deposits and debits and supermarket automated checkout lines are cogent examples. Business has become increasingly efficient by eliminating personal contacts, but it has also contributed to a contemporary impersonal society that may especially impact on older persons who matured in a more personal, "small shop" society.

One of the needs of retired persons today is the establishment and maintenance of personal networks. Social networks help to maintain quality of life and mental health. Health, economic security, and adequate housing are necessary elements in living well, but social contacts are also important. Perhaps the present time will see a growth of interest in research and instruction of individuals who will be specialized in improving the personal lives of the elderly in contrast to increasing daily efficiency of living in the impersonal era.

One of the great scientific advances of recent decades has been the mapping of the human genome. Now we are learning that neighboring genes in the organism can influence the expression of a gene. Genetics are much more complex than previously realized. Furthermore, the expression of a gene is influenced by its environment. This leads us into a new era of biological ecology, not only with respect to the evolution of species but also in the development and aging of an individual.

Clearly, the rapid expansion of life expectancy in the 20th century has been the result of the influences of an improved environment, with reduction of transient nutritional deficiencies and clean water, as well as medical advances and the introduction of antibiotics. But in this picture there is now the need to encourage personal behavior that maximizes the potentials of the human species. What kind of future does such thought portend?

THE FUTURE OF GERONTOLOGY

The agequake that faces America when the longer living boomers retire will be a major factor influencing evolving social policies related to major aspects of life: health care, work, retirement, pensions, housing, and terminal care. The future will likely bring an increasing appreciation of the diversity of America's growing older population. The author served as the outside examiner for a five-student master's degree research project of the Anderson Graduate School at UCLA. A total of 33 national surveys were analyzed with respect to the characteristics of the population with age. About six subgroups of the mature population were identified. At one end were the "explorers," who had enough money and health and wanted to add new things to their lives. Next were the "conservers," who had the same general characteristics of the explorers but wanted to hold on to what they had, and not add. At the other end of the distribution were the "martyrs," who had relatively poor lives but were ready to tell you about how bad life had treated them. A subgroup of these has been described in other contexts as "toxic agers." These individuals are so bitter about their lives that they drive away those who would assist them. Because the aged population is growing, all of these groups will increase, challenging the institutions and professional groups that would serve them to minimize negative influences and maximize the positive. We can expect both late-life bloomers and early-life faders in our changing population, but gerontology is expected to contribute to increasing the numbers of late-life bloomers, increasing the quality of life, and decreasing the number of disabled and unproductive elderly who are unable to maintain independent lives.

Yet in comparison with issues of aging in developing countries, those of America appear to be less demanding. Demographic changes are coming more quickly in developing countries. Asian countries, for example, are rapidly adding years to the lives of their inhabitants, but their cultures are based on ancient customs that don't match well with current needs (Kumar, 2003; Liebig & Rajan, 2003; Ramamurti & Jamuna, 2004). The less-developed regions of the world have over 80% of the world's inhabitants. India and China each have more that a billion people in their populations. The United States has the third-largest population, with about 295 million. However, because of its earlier increase in life expectancy and ethnic and cultural diversity, rapid societal change has been a characteristic of America. Thus the country has been adapting to an older population for a longer time, in contrast to China and India (Liebig & Rajan, 2003).

An example of aging in a developing country is India. India has shown a rapid increase in the number of older persons. Those over 60 years have risen from 12 million in 1901, to 20 million in 1951, and to 75 million in 2001 (Liebig & Rajan, 2003). It is expected to be 179 million in 2031. The explosive growth in India's older population is interacting with changes in urbanization and modernization, resulting in a condition that invites the use of the metaphor that India is facing a major "agequake". Although India is still an agricultural country, large social changes will leave many older persons facing health, housing, and economic problems, placing a strain on family traditions of the daughter-in-laws being the primary caregivers. Very few of the older persons live in institutions for the elderly, perhaps 0.1%. As the educated young move to the cities, older persons are left behind in the agricultural areas. They will need housing and health care in the future that is not currently widely provided by the government. In brief, public policies will have to develop quickly in India to deal with the emerging "agequake".

The rapid need for developing national programs for the elderly is likely to lead India to seek education on the issues of societal aging for some of its university students. Graduate students may seek university placements in countries that have longer traditions of government programs for older persons. In this sense, selected American universities may be targets for the placement of Indian and other Asian students in both research and professional fields. This would seem to contradict the notion that Asian countries have over the centuries developed cultural traditions to care for the elderly. Though this is true, the impending "agequake" threatens many aspects of traditional care, including the roles that women have played in the past.

One forecast for the future is that there will be an increased demand for higher education on the many aspects of aging, including that of effective social policies in dealing with aging populations. This requires exposure to an integrated picture of the needs of an aging population. In the American university tradition, the specialized departments and disciplines each breaks off a piece of the large "jigsaw puzzle" without much concern with the relationship of their knowledge to that of others.

A second view of gerontology of the future is that there will be pressure for integrating knowledge across academic specialties. The big picture is needed to avoid such problems as are being faced with Social Security deficits and the Medicare crisis. A critical factor in the development of social policy is the maintenance of flexibility. Age 65 was adopted as the age of retirement for Social Security in the 1930s, when life expectancy was much lower that it is today.

A more detailed example of the need for maintaining flexibility in formulating age-related policies and regulations is seen in the establishment of age 60 as the age of retirement for commercial airline pilots. Age 60 was adopted by the Federal Aviation Administration (FAA) in 1959 with the recommendation that the retirement age be moved higher or lower depending on evidence from subsequent research. When the age 60 retirement rule was adopted, health screening was in an early stage of development, and it was not highly reliable. In 1 year there were 17 deaths in the cockpits of commercial planes. The FAA wanted to protect the public from casualties in airline crashes that might be attributed to pilot age.

At the time the age 60 regulation was adopted, the Airline Pilots Association attempted in the courts to have the rule overturned. The association was formed by flight captains who were older than the rest of the cockpit crews. The cost of the legal actions required a rise in budget that led the association to increase its membership. It broadened its membership to include copilots, who generally were younger than the captains. A result was that the association reversed its position on the age 60 rule and favored it. Also, the airlines favored keeping the age 60 rule because the retirement costs of older pilots rose with their years of employment. So the age 60 rule has remained in effect for reasons remote from those of its original adoption, protecting the public.

How could flexibility in the age 60 rule be modified in relation to new data? For one thing, in 1959, health assessment was weak. Among other things there were no treadmill tests that would reveal cardiac weaknesses and the probability of heart attacks. In brief, an examining physician might tell a patient that he was healthy, only to have the patient die soon after leaving the doctor's office.

A second factor at the time of the rule adoption was the lack of in-flight performance records that are now maintained. A third factor was the flight simulator that permits evaluation of pilot performance under different simulated conditions. These sources of information permit evaluations of pilot health and performance that are much superior to that of chronological age. Chronological age is merely a convenient index to many unrelated factors that should be evaluated separately.

Today younger pilots who pose flight risks can be distinguished from older pilots who are safer from performance and health points of view. Why isn't the pilot retirement age raised in relation to the evidence gathered by improved technology? An assumption is that the complexities of related economic reasons dominate the decision process and its political context. There are the economics of the employers, the economics of society, and the economics of the individual pilots. These are a long way from issues of protecting the public from accidents and pilot competence. There is rumor of evidence that young pilots commit the most flight errors. If this is so, it should be entered into consideration of evidence-based policy decisions. It also leads to the view that what are often viewed as policy matters of age or aging have other complex economic bases.

In the future gerontology may be expected to provide a broad perspective on evolving public policies that are related to aging. In India today the retirement age for professors is age 60, while retirement age has been uncapped in the United States. Pension policies in developed and developing countries will no doubt be revised as people live longer, are healthier, and are more active. From the perspective of the individual, early pension vesting and portability are important. As the trends toward later retirement and multiple careers become increasingly common, the opportunity of carrying forward one's pension fund to a new employer is important.

There are many other issues besides the complex economic ones facing our aging population. The increasing value of longitudinal data will help detect trends in the population that will in turn determine the directions in public policies regarding aged persons. One contribution of the longitudinal studies is the evidence that there is great diversity in the older population. Not only are there the early needy and dependent, there are also the late-life bloomers and those whose experience can be put to good use. The best use of the productivity of older persons is a present and future challenge to gerontology.

One prospect is the development of senior councils to use the experience of those who have lived through wars, depressions, and natural disasters. Judges, elected officials, and professionals are not commonly recalled to offer judgments on current problems. Emeriti centers that are being developed in universities may help to make experience available to current administrations. Experience may be tapped for advice about such problems as handling student unrest over rising tuition costs, or faculty unease about health care costs and policies about retirement and hiring of new faculty. One may expect that there will be the emergence of senior counselors or "gero coaches."

Given the complexity of the issues of aging facing gerontology, the need for greater communication across disciplines and professions may be a productive topic to discuss with academic retirees. Encouraging cross-disciplinary research and teaching about aging may be facilitated by advice from an emeriti center's members or a council of retired faculty.

A new feature of changing contacts of the elderly with younger generations is the focus of OneGeneration, a California organization to bring toddlers and the elderly into contact. OneGeneration offers daily care for infants and young children in a setting co-located with adult day care for the elderly. Mixing of the young and old in daily activities may be a sign of the future, and more programs will emerge that will reduce the impersonal style of lives of both the young and the old.

There are many other potential issues that will rise to challenge the knowledge base of gerontology in the future. One of the social issues arousing tension is the wishes of dying persons in relation to the values of families and culture. To what extent is the end-of-life care to be decided by the dying person, relatives, professionals, and the courts? The customs of dying, death, and bereavement will likely change as the number of very aged persons exiting life increases (Kuhl, 2002). Traditions of death rituals will undoubtedly change as we shift from the early times when children frequently died and adults died in the prime of their work lives before the children left home. Early in the 20th century, care of orphans was a major social concern, whereas currently many children are sought for adoption. More attention is being given today to the celebration of life as it was lived, with photographs of the deceased and personal eulogies by friends and community members, in contrast to earlier burial rituals.

As the number of older age deaths increases with the demographic changes, there may be new rituals evolving in memorial services. Cemeteries have become huge, and perhaps there will be more emphasis on where to archive our life stories and share them with family and friends than on where to store our bones. At the moment there are relatively few archives for personal histories to be accessed by others after our passing. The rising interest in organizing our autobiographies suggests a growing need for archives of personal histories. One feature of an autobiography archive that is different from a body cemetery is the maintenance of computer accessibility in pace with software updating. It would be a constructive step forward for relatives and friends to access national autobiography archives by e-mail. There are many things about the lives of my parents and my grandparents, for instance, that I would like to know. Knowing the cemetery where they are buried doesn't tell me much about them.

The foregoing examples illustrate the interaction of the many variables involved with aging. There are many more topics than can lead to questions about the impact of the "agequake" upon our culture, institutions, professions, and personal ways of life that gerontology may be called upon to address. The role of religion in later life is receiving more attention, and there is more exchange between theologians and empirical scientists (Kimble & McFadden, 2003). It hardly seems necessary to add that we are in for a profound expansion of databases that provide a basis for developing public policy for the elderly. Maintaining that there will be an expansion of a need for basic research, applied research, and services to the growing older population seems to be an unavoidable conclusion. One way of helping to ensure high quality of planning and oversight is to gather data that will provide evidence for flexible decisions, in contrast to the rigid opinion-based decisions of the past that told us that age 65 was the beginning of old age for all of us.

A SUMMARY PERSPECTIVE ON GERONTOLOGY

Gerontology is one of the most complex subjects facing science in the 21st century. Although it has roots in ancient speculations about length of life, research on aging did not emerge as a major area of academic focus until about 1950. Pressures from the demographic changes in an older population and associated health concerns provided a context in which Congress created the National Institute on Aging in 1975 with funding for research and training.

The diversity of issues about aging and the tendencies for disciplines to specialize have resulted in a great need for integration of information from across subfields of study. The interaction between causal variables further adds to the complexity of phenomena of aging. Although the human genome provides diversity in disease proneness and longevity, the interaction of genes modifies specific expression. Also, the interaction of genetics with physical and social environments leads to the view that human aging is an expression of ecological relationships. It may be expected that more will be learned about the ecology of aging from current and future longitudinal studies, and clues will be gained about prospects for interventions to improve health and the quality of life with advancing age.

The practical issues associated with an aging population are increasingly creating specialties in providing services to the aged. These specialties in turn need a flow of new information from basic and applied research. There seems little reason to doubt that the field of gerontology in terms of research, teaching, and practice will grow dramatically in the coming decades. The "agequake" will continue to challenge our personal and institutional models of aging. Lag effects will become apparent in institutions, cultures, and individuals. Lag effects in our scientific paradigms will also become apparent as we learn more about the complexity of the aging of the human organism in relation to the environment. Increasingly, it is being realized that age itself doesn't cause anything; it is merely a convenient index for initial grouping of data. In the growth of our understanding and explanations of phenomena of aging through research, we will have to continue to replace age with causal variables.

REFERENCES

Achenbaum, W. A. (1979). *Old age in the new land: The American experience since 1790.* Baltimore: Johns Hopkins Press.

Achenbaum, W. A., & Levin, J. S. (1989). What does gerontology mean? *The Gerontologist, 29,* 393–400.

Binstock, R. H., & Shanas, E. (Eds.). (1977). *Handbook of aging and the social sciences.* New York: Van Nostrand Reinhold.

Birren, J. E. (Ed.). (1959). *Handbook of aging and the individual.* Chicago: The University of Chicago Press.

Birren, J. E., & Schaie, K. W. (Eds.). (1977). *Handbook of the psychology of aging.* New York: Van Nostrand Reinhold.

Cole, T. R., & Meyer, D. L. 1991. Aging, metaphor, and meaning: A view from cultural history. In G. M. Kenyon, J. E. Birren, & J. J. F. Schroots, (Eds.), *Metaphors of aging in science and the humanities* (pp. 57–82). New York: Springer.

Cowdry, E. V. (Ed.). (1933). *Arteriosclerosis: A survey of the problem.* New York: Macmillan.

Cowdry, E. V. (Ed.). (1939). *Problems of ageing.* Baltimore: Williams & Wilkins.

Finch, C. E., & Hayflick, L. (Eds.). (1977). *Handbook of the biology of aging.* New York: Van Nostrand Reinhold.

Gruman, G. J. (2003). History of ideas about the prolongation of life: The evolution of prolongevity hypotheses to 1800. Springer.

Kenyon, G. M., Birren, J. E., & Schroots, J. J. F. (1991). *Metaphors of aging in science and the humanities.* New York: Springer.

Kimble, M. A., & McFadden, S. H. (Eds.). (2003). *Aging, spirituality, and religion.* Minneapolis, MN: Fortress Press.

Kuhl, D. (2002). *What dying people want.* New York: Public Affairs.

Kumar, V. (2003). Health status and health care services among older persons in India. In P. S. Liebig & S. I. Rajan (Eds.), *An aging India: Perspectives, prospects, and policies* (pp. 67–83). New York: Haworth Press.

Lee, R. Miller T., and Edwards R. (2003). Special Report: The Growth and Aging of California's Population: Demographic and Fiscal Projections, Characteristics and Service Needs. *Center for the Economics and Demography of Aging. CEDA Papers:* Paper 2003-0002CL. http://repositories.cdlib.org/iber/ceda/papers/2003-0002CL.

Liebig, P. S., & Rajan, S. I. (Eds.). (2003). *An aging India: Perspectives, prospects, and policies.* New York: Haworth Press.

Metchnikoff, E. (1903). *The nature of man.* New York: G. P. Putnam.

Ramamurti, P. V., & Jamuna, D. (2004). *Handbook of Indian gerontology.* New Delhi, India: Serials Publications.

Redfoot, D. L., and S. M. Pandya. (2002). Before the Boom: Trends in Long-Term Supportive Services for Older Americans with Disabilities, AARP Public Policy Institute.

Riegel, K. F. (1977). History of psychological gerontology. In J. E. Birren & K. W. Schaie (Eds.), *Handbook of the psychology of aging* (pp.70–102). New York: Van Nostrand Reinhold.

Schroots, J. J. F., Birren, J. E., & Svanborg, A. (Eds.). (1988). *Health and aging.* New York: Springer.

U.S. Public Health Service. (1938a). *The national health survey: 1935–1936. Illness among employed and unemployed workers* (Sickness and Medical Care Series, Bulletin No. 7). Washington, DC: National Institute of Health.

U.S. Public Health Service. (1938b). *Pneumonia in urban United States: Frequency, severity, and medical care* (Sickness and Medical Care Series, Bulletin No. 11). Washington, DC: National Institute of Health.

U.S. Public Health Service. (1943). *Mental health in later maturity* (Suppl. 168 to the Public Health Reports). Washington, DC: U.S. Government Printing Office.

Index

DATE DUE			
Rec	June	10	